Multidisciplinary Management of Common Bile Duct Stones

Jeffrey W. Hazey
Darwin L. Conwell • Gregory E. Guy
Editors

Multidisciplinary Management of Common Bile Duct Stones

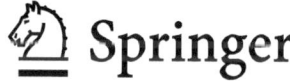

Springer

Editors
Jeffrey W. Hazey, MD, FACS
Chief, Division of General
   and Gastrointestinal Surgery
Department of Surgery
The Ohio State University Wexner
   Medical Center
Columbus, OH, USA

Gregory E. Guy, MD
Division of Vascular and
   Interventional Radiology
Department of Radiology
The Ohio State University Wexner
   Medical Center
Columbus, OH, USA

Darwin L. Conwell, MD
Director, Division of Gastroenterology,
   Hepatology, and Nutrition
Professor of Medicine
Department of Internal Medicine
The Ohio State University Wexner
   Medical Center
Columbus, OH, USA

ISBN 978-3-319-22764-1   ISBN 978-3-319-22765-8   (eBook)
DOI 10.1007/978-3-319-22765-8

Library of Congress Control Number: 2015953227

Springer Cham Heidelberg New York Dordrecht London

Printed on acid-free paper

Springer International Publishing AG Switzerland is part of Springer Science+Business Media
(www.springer.com)

I would like to dedicate this textbook to all physicians (surgeons, gastroenterologists, and radiologists) who tirelessly care for patients, often at personal expense, as well as those who have participated in my training throughout the years and have given me the skills and knowledge to effectively treat patients. I would be remiss if I did not thank my colleagues in surgery who teach me something new every day, often commiserating with me after a long or difficult day. All the patients who allow me to operate on them or try novel techniques (sometimes unproven) are the ones who truly deserve thanks. Finally, I wish to thank my wife, Jeannie, and my daughters, Jessica and Jordan, who tolerate my long hours and fatigue in an effort to make a difference. Without their unwavering support, I would not be able to do anything discussed in the text.

Jeffrey W. Hazey

Foreword

Bile duct stones are not a new problem for surgeons. For decades, a direct open surgical approach to the bile duct was the only definitive therapy for this malady. With the advent of advanced endoscopic, radiologic, and minimally invasive surgical techniques, the treating physician is presented with a myriad of choices and decisions regarding the timing and approach to the stones. Furthermore, the introduction of new surgical procedures for the treatment of gastric disease and morbid obesity often has made access to the biliary tree challenging. In this book, the authors have endeavored to outline each of the techniques for imaging and treating common bile duct stones and to equitably assess the timing and value of each method. It is imperative for practicing surgeons and gastroenterologists to be familiar with the material presented herein in order to provide their patients with the safest and most effective care.

Cleveland, OH, USA   Jeffrey L. Ponsky

Preface

In some large academic medical centers, tradition and culture reign. These "traditions" often lead us to "silos" that exist between specialties, with little cross-fertilization. Often these "turf wars" create a lack of information transfer that ultimately results in inefficient care for patients, and some may argue, less quality care. I truly hope that by outlining a multidisciplinary approach to the management of common bile duct stones, I can educate readers on alternative methods to expand the options available to patients. Collective intelligence will always improve patient care along with increased professionalism between specialties. After all, if all you possess is a hammer, everything begins to look like a nail.

It is with tremendous gratitude I extend to my colleagues and patients who are deserving of the praise that ultimately led to the development of this textbook. As is often the case, this textbook is the work of several professional colleagues who tirelessly care for patients and "fight the good fight" every day, night, and weekend, with little regard for their personal lives. In a similar light, patients consent to sometimes invasive procedures that may put their lives and health at risk in an effort to ameliorate their suffering. It is the patients who allow us to perform sometimes less proven techniques in an effort to advance medical science and improve the quality of health care.

Columbus, OH, USA   Jeffrey W. Hazey

Contents

Contributors

Brandon D. Andrew, M.D. Department of Surgery, The Guthrie Robert Packer Hospital Residency Program in Surgery, Sayre, PA, USA

Eliza W. Beal, M.D. Department of General Surgery, The Ohio State University Wexner Medical Center, Columbus, OH, USA

Sylvester M. Black, M.D., Ph.D. Department of General Surgery, The Ohio State University Wexner Medical Center, Columbus, OH, USA

Suresh Chamarthi, M.B.B.S. Department of Radiology, The Ohio State University Wexner Medical Center, Columbus, OH, USA

Darwin L. Conwell, M.D. Director, Division of Gastroenterology, Hepatology, and Nutrition, Professor of Medicine, Department of Internal Medicine, The Ohio State University Wexner Medical Center, Columbus, OH, USA

Joshua D. Dowell, M.D., Ph.D. Division of Vascular and Interventional Radiology, Department of Radiology, Wexner Medical Center, The Ohio State University, Columbus, OH, USA

Samer El-Dika, M.D., M.Sc. Division of Gastroenterology, Hepatology, and Nutrition, Department of Internal Medicine, The Ohio State University Wexner Medical Center, Columbus, OH, USA

Section of Advanced Therapeutic Endoscopy, Division of Gastroenterology, The Ohio State University Wexner Medical Center, Columbus, OH, USA

Robert D. Fanelli, M.D., M.H.A., F.A.C.S. Department of Surgery, The Guthrie Clinic, Sayre, PA, USA

Clinical Professor of Surgery, The Commonwealth Medical College, Scranton, PA, USA

Clinical Professor of Surgery, SUNY Upstate Medical University, Binghamton, NY, USA

Professor of Surgery, Albany Medical College, Albany, NY, USA

J. Royce Groce, M.D. Division of Gastroenterology, Hepatology, and Nutrition, Department of Internal Medicine, The Ohio State University Wexner Medical Clinic, Columbus, OH, USA

Gregory E. Guy, M.D. Division of Vascular and Interventional Radiology, Department of Radiology, The Ohio State University Wexner Medical Center, Columbus, OH, USA

Jeffrey W. Hazey, M.D., F.A.C.S. Chief, Division of General and Gastrointestinal Surgery, Department of Surgery, The Ohio State University Wexner Medical Center, Columbus, OH, USA

Terence Jackson, M.D. Department of Surgery, University Hospitals Case Medical Center, Cleveland, OH, USA

Sunny Jaiswal, M.D., M.B.A. Department of Radiology, The Ohio State University Wexner Medical Center, Columbus, OH, USA

Edward L. Jones, M.D. Department of Surgery, Denver VA Medical Center and the University of Colorado, Denver, CO, USA

Teresa S. Jones, M.D. Department of Surgery, The Ohio State University Wexner Medical Center, Columbus, OH, USA

Reshi C. Kanuru, M.D. Division of Gastroenterology, Hepatology, and Nutrition, Department of Internal Medicine, The Ohio State University Wexner Medical Center, Columbus, OH, USA

Helmi Khadra, M.D. Department of Surgery, University Hospitals Case Medical Center, Cleveland, OH, USA

Somashekar G. Krishna, M.D., M.P.H. Division of Gastroenterology, Hepatology and Nutrition, Department of Internal Medicine, The Ohio State University Wexner Medical Center, Columbus, OH, USA

Ashwini Kumar, M.B.B.S., M.D. Department of Laparoendoscopic Surgery, University of Miami, Miami, FL, USA

Jourdanton, TX, USA

Nicholas Latchana, M.D., M.S. Department of General Surgery, The Ohio State University Wexner Medical Center, Columbus, OH, USA

Edward Levine, M.D. Department of Internal Medicine, The Ohio State University Wexner Medical Center, Columbus, OH, USA

Annie Lim, D.O. Division of Vascular and Interventional Radiology, Department of Radiology, Wexner Medical Center, The Ohio State University, Columbus, OH, USA

Bill S. Majdalany, M.D. Department of Radiology, University of Michigan, Ann Arbor, MI, USA

Jeffrey Marks, M.D. Department of Surgery, University Hospitals Case Medical Center, Cleveland, OH, USA

Jose M. Martinez, M.D. Department of Surgery, Miller School of Medicine, University of Miami, Miami, FL, USA

Michael Paul Meara, M.D., M.B.A. Division of General and Gastrointestinal Surgery, The Ohio State University Wexner Medical Center, University Hospital East, Columbus, OH, USA

Marty M. Meyer, M.D. Division of Gastroenterology, Hepatology and Nutrition, The Ohio State University Wexner Medical Center, Columbus, OH, USA

Vimal K. Narula, M.D. Department of Surgery, The Ohio State University Wexner Medical Center, Columbus, OH, USA

Veeral M. Oza, M.D. Division of Gastroenterology, Hepatology and Nutrition, Department of Internal Medicine, The Ohio State University Wexner Medical Center, Columbus, OH, USA

Eric M. Pauli, M.D. Division of Minimally Invasive and Bariatric Surgery, Department of Surgery, Penn State Hershey Medical Center, Hershey, PA, USA

Joshua R. Peck, M.D. Division of Gastroenterology, Hepatology and Nutrition, Department of Internal Medicine, The Ohio State University Wexner Medical Center, Columbus, OH, USA

Victorio Pidlaoan, M.D. Division of Gastroenterology, Hepatology and Nutrition, Department of Internal Medicine, The Ohio State University Wexner Medical Center, Columbus, OH, USA

Mohammad H. Shakhatreh, M.D., M.P.H. Division of Gastroenterology, Hepatology, and Nutrition, Department of Internal Medicine, The Ohio State University Wexner Medical Clinic, Columbus, OH, USA

Sheetal Sharma, M.D. Section of Advanced Therapeutic Endoscopy, Division of Gastroenterology, The Ohio State University Wexner Medical Center, Columbus, OH, USA

James Spain, M.D. Department of Radiology, The Ohio State University Wexner Medical Center, Columbus, OH, USA

Jeffrey Weinstein, M.D. Division of Vascular and Interventional Radiology, Department of Radiology, Einstein Medical Center, Philadelphia, PA, USA

Joshua S. Winder, M.D. Division of Minimally Invasive and Bariatric Surgery, Department of Surgery, Penn State Hershey Medical Center, Hershey, PA, USA

Historical Perspective and Treatments for Common Bile Duct Stones

Jeffrey W. Hazey

Introduction

Gallstones have formed in humankind for thousands of years having been found in mummified remains more than 3000 years ago. The first documented account of gallstones in man was made by a pathologist, Antonio Benivieni in 1420. The significance of gallstone disease may not have been known at that time but quickly became apparent at the turn of the twentieth century. On July 15, 1882, Dr. Carl Johann August Langenbuch performed the world's first cholecystectomy [1]. Early manuscripts published by A. W. Mayo Robson in The Lancet, April 12, 1902 highlighted the importance of the link between the surgeon and "concretions" [2]. This was followed in 1909 identifying the role of the surgeon in the treatment of certain forms of jaundice [3]. It was not until 1929 that a more comprehensive discussion of surgical techniques for the gallbladder and bile ducts was published [4]. Fast forward to the twenty-first century with widespread use and acceptance of endoscopic and laparoscopic techniques that have revolutionized the approach to choledocholithiasis. Morbidity and mortality have continued to improve to the point that common bile duct stones are often treated in the outpatient setting. The introduction of Natural Orifice Translumenal Endoscopic Surgery (NOTES) in the last 10 years may be the next step in minimally invasive approaches. Looking back, endoscopic retrograde cholangiopancreatography (ERCP) with its associated techniques (endoscopic sphincterotomy (ES)) was a prelude to NOTES techniques for the therapeutic treatment of common bile duct stones.

Historical Perspective and Treatments

Before the world's first published cholecystectomy, treatment of gallbladder and gallstone disease was relegated to removal of stones, abscess drainage or creation of a cholecystic fistulae. Early reports describe the removal of gallstones and "sewing" the gallbladder wall to the skin or colon effectively creating a cholecytocutaneous fistula or cholecystoenterostomy. Dr. Carl Johann August Langenbuch performed the world's first cholecystectomy at the Lazarus Krankenhaus in Berlin Germany in 1882 [1]. This case was first reported in the Berliner Klinische Wochenschrift in November 1882. Bela Halpert celebrated this achievement with an article published in the Archives of Surgery in 1932, "Fiftieth Anniversary

J.W. Hazey, M.D., F.A.C.S. (✉)
Chief, Division of General and Gastrointestinal Surgery, Department of Surgery, The Ohio State University Wexner Medical Center, N729 Doan Hall, 410 W 10th Ave, Columbus, OH 43210, USA
e-mail: jeffrey.hazey@osumc.edu

© Springer International Publishing Switzerland 2016
J.W. Hazey et al. (eds.), *Multidisciplinary Management of Common Bile Duct Stones*,
DOI 10.1007/978-3-319-22765-8_1

of the Removal of the Gallbladder. Carl Langenbuch—Master Surgeon of the Biliary System" [5, 6]. In April 1883, Langenbuch remarked, "the gallbladder should be removed not because it contains gallstones but because it forms them" (Fig. 1.1). By 1889, Langenbuch had performed 24 cholecystectomies culminating in 1896 with a historical sketch of the development of surgery of the biliary system. He died in 1901 of peritonitis following appendicitis.

It was in 1890, Courvoisier first removed a gallstone from the common bile duct by direct incision (Fig. 1.2). The first attempts to describe the relationship between gallstones and their significance when located in the biliary tree/common bile duct was made by A. W. Mayo Robson in 1902 when he published a paper read before the Royal Medical and Chirurgical Society March 25th 1902. The paper titled, "The Surgical Treatment of Obstruction in the Common Bile Duct by Concretions" specifically referenced the operation of choledochotomy. In this publication, Robson referenced 60 patients who underwent extraction of common bile duct stones. It was here that some of the first principles of surgery for common bile duct stones were established. He is quoted as stating, "no operation should, as a rule, be concluded until it is clearly made out that the ducts, including the hepatic and common ducts, are quite free from concretions, otherwise disappointment and dissatisfaction are certain to follow." He goes on to note that the common bile duct has to be "attacked" in 1 of every 5–6 cases. He noted that cholecystoenterostomy leaves the cause untouched and never be performed. His mortality in the first 60 cases is quoted at 16.6 % but was able to show significant improvement over time with a reported mortality of 5 % or less at the end of the trial (Fig. 1.3) [2].

In an address on "Certain Forms of Jaundice Capable of Relief or Cure by Surgical Treatment" in 1909, Robson described choledocholithiasis as a frequent cause of jaundice and reiterated his stance on surgery of the common bile duct. He states, "with very few exceptions common duct cholelithiasis is not a condition in which short-circuiting the obstruction should be

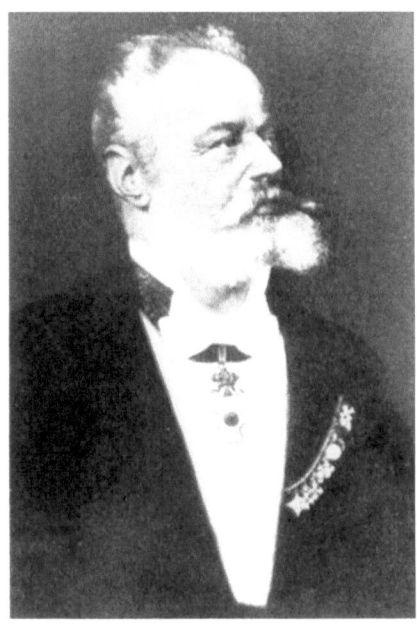

Fig. 1.1 Carl Langenbuch. (© 2013 J.H.M.B. Stoot, R.J.S. Coelen, J.L.A. van Vugt, and C.H.C. Dejong. Originally published in General Introduction: Advances in Hepatic Surgery, In: *Hepatic Surgery*, Prof. Hesham Abdeldayem (Ed.), under Creative Commons Attribution license CC BY 3.0. Available from: DOI: 10.5772/54710.)

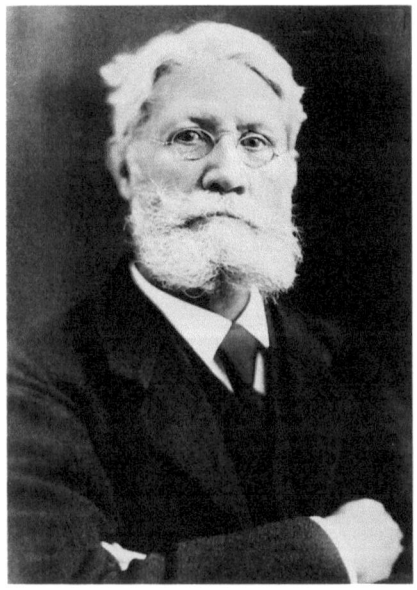

Fig. 1.2 Ludwig Courvoisier. (From Wellcome Library, London; reproduced under Creative Commons Attribution license CC BY 4.0.)

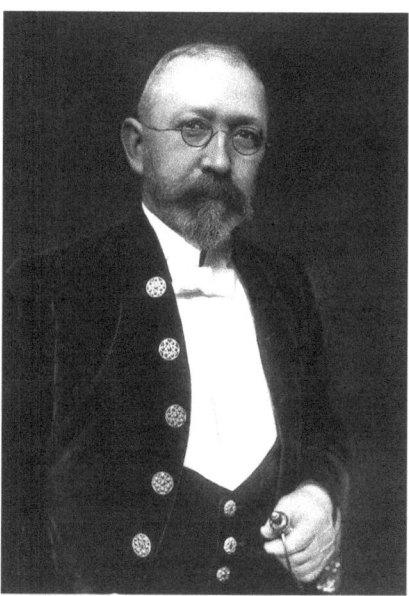

Fig. 1.3 A. W. Mayo Robson. (From Wellcome Library, London; reproduced under Creative Commons Attribution license CC BY 4.0.)

history from Langenbuch to modern day NOTES procedures for cholecystectomy [8]. Both publications are concise and well worth review for the reader interested in our surgical history.

Modern-Day Multidisciplinary Management

As one can imagine, with technological evolution the management of common bile duct stones has increasingly become less invasive and less morbid for patients. Medical management of common bile duct stones shows limited success and is mostly relegated to prophylaxis in an attempt to prevent stone formation primarily or after a procedure to remove common bile duct stones and their source. Nonoperative or noninvasive methods like extra-corporal shockwave lithotripsy (ESWL) have been used with some success in large part due to the heterogeneity of common bile duct stones and implications of retained fragments within the biliary tree.

employed, as the cause is capable of radical cure by means of a direct operation with under improved technique is most successful, as I can testify by an experience of about 200 operations, which in the last 150 have resulted in the recovery of 97 %" [3].

Almost 20 years passed before the Bradshaw Lecture was published in The Lancet in 1929 when R. P. Rowlands gave a comprehensive lecture on surgery of the gallbladder and bile ducts. Rowlands outlined the slow progress that had been made to date and commented on surgeons' trepidation with surgery in the upper abdomen. He presented a series of 9531 autopsies and noted a 8.4 % rate of cholelithiasis. Radiography initially was used to detect calcified gallstones or a calcified gallbladder wall but the advent of cholecystography by Graham in 1923 was hailed as a great advance [4].

The surgical heritage of cholecystectomy is well outlined by L. William Traverso in his article published in The American Journal of Surgery in 1976 in a brief culminating in Langenbuch first cholecystectomy in 1882 [7]. Nat Soper's manuscript in the World Journal of Surgery outlines our

The majority of patients with common bile duct stones are managed by gastroenterologists using endoscopic techniques, surgeons using operative techniques (both open and minimally invasive) or interventional radiologists utilizing percutaneous approaches. Training today tends to "specialize" the ability to do various techniques both between specialties and within each specialty. As an example, few surgeons are trained to perform ERCP necessitating a referral to gastroenterology in the event a patient requires nonoperative common bile duct stone removal. Similarly, when the common bile duct is inaccessible endoscopically and/or the patient is not a candidate for surgery (or refuses surgical intervention) percutaneous techniques may be employed by an interventional radiologist. Within the specialty of surgery, surgeons may not be trained or comfortable performing a laparoscopic or open common bile duct exploration. The level of comfort and training may dictate the technique offered to patients or result in a referral or transfer to a surgeon comfortable with these techniques. In this same spirit, not all gastroenterologists are trained in ERCP. In addition, invasive ERCP trained gastroenterologists through credentialing are differentiated to perform only diagnostic or both diagnostic and therapeutic ERCP. The relative shortage of gastroenterology coverage in the USA can result in limited endoscopic availability when managing common bile duct stones. Smaller rural hospitals may have limited gastroenterologic "coverage" and those that are available may not perform ERCP or only diagnostic ERCP. In situations such as these, surgical treatment of common bile duct stones is necessary (if the surgeon(s) are comfortable with the technique) or referral to an institution with expertise is undertaken. Occasionally, gastroenterologists credentialed to perform diagnostic ERCP may place a 7 french stent (does not require an endoscopic sphincterotomy) in an effort to temporize the obstruction until a patient can be referred for definitive care.

The chapters to follow are an attempt by the authors to summarize and stress the notion that often, but not always, management of patients with common bile duct stones are a multidisciplinary effort. Knowledge and skill of surgeons, gastroenterologists, and radiologists are meant to be complementary. The overarching goal is to provide timely definitive care for patients with common bile duct stones using the least invasive and least morbid techniques to maximize the "value" of care for patients. As is most often the case, skills acquired by one of these specialists may not be mastered or in the armamentarium of one of the other specialists. It is imperative physicians are knowledgeable of the various techniques offered to patients with common bile duct stones. Different healthcare environments may offer different capabilities in large part due to the fact that surgeon, gastroenterology or interventional radiology "coverage" may not be available. Knowledge of the "options" available to patients will empower physicians and patients to receive timely, appropriate care. In some circumstances, referral or transfer to a facility that can provide less invasive or more definitive techniques in the management of common bile duct stones is appropriate.

We hope the reader can reference the techniques outlined in this textbook to help treat and guide care for patients with common bile duct stones. Similarly, physicians may now reference a single text that addresses management across specialties and will no longer need to read multiple texts (i.e., surgical text, gastroenterology text or radiology text) in order to get an overview of treatment options. I want to thank the authors for their contributions as this text is a true reflection of collegiality and professionalism across disciplines.

References

1. Langenbuch C. Ein Fall von Exstirpation der Gallenblase wegen chronischer Cholelithiasis: Heilung. Berliner Klin Wochenschr. 1882;19:725–7.
2. Mayo Robson AW. The surgical treatment of obstruction in the common bile-duct by concretions, with especial reference to the operation of choledochotomy as modified by the author, illustrated by 60 cases. Lancet. 1902;159(4102):1023–7.
3. Mayo Robson AW. An address on certain forms of jaundice capable of relief or cure by surgical treatment with a consideration of the operation of cholecystenterostomy based on an experience of 64 cases. Lancet. 1909;173(4458):371–4.
4. Rowlands RP. Surgery of the gall-bladder and bile-ducts. Lancet. 1929;214(5543):1075–81.
5. Sprakman R. 100th anniversary of the first cholecystectomy. A reprinting of the 50th anniversary article from the archives of surgery, July 1932. Arch Surg. 1982;117(12):1525.
6. Halpert B. Carl Langenbuch. Master surgeon of the biliary system. Arch Surg. 1932;25:178–82.
7. Traverso LW. Carl Langenbuch and the first cholecystectomy. Am J Surg. 1976;132(1):81–2.
8. Soper NJ. Cholecystectomy: from Langenbuch to natural orifice transluminal endoscopic surgery. World J Surg. 2011;35(7):1422–7.

Joshua S. Winder and Eric M. Pauli

Introduction

Choledocholithiasis, or the presence of formed stones within the common bile duct (CBD), represents a common and challenging problem in modern health care (Fig. 2.1). The diagnosis and treatment of CBD stones is not always straightforward and has been the source of ongoing debate [1, 2]. In Westernized societies, patients who present with symptomatic cholelithiasis have concomitant CBD stones in 3–15 % of cases [3–5]. Secondary stones, or those formed within the gallbladder and then migrate into the CBD, represent the majority of CBD stones in the USA [6]. The clinical spectrum from CBD stones can vary widely ranging from silent, or asymptomatic, to biliary obstruction, jaundice, cholangitis, and gallstone pancreatitis. As such, the incidence of CBD stones is underestimated in the literature, as most cases of CBD stones are diagnosed incidentally at time of cholecystectomy or present as complications of CBD stones. In this chapter we explore the spectrum of CBD disease and its prevalence in at-risk populations.

J.S. Winder, M.D. • E.M. Pauli, M.D. (✉)
Division of Minimally Invasive and Bariatric Surgery,
Department of Surgery, Penn State Hershey Medical
Center, 500 University Drive, MC H149, Hershey,
PA 17033, USA
e-mail: jwinder@hmc.psu.edu; epauli@hmc.psu.edu

The Burden of Gallstone Disease

Overall Gallstone Disease Burden

To better understand CBD stones in the USA, one must appreciate the extent of gallstone disease as this is the major contributor to CBD stones in this population [6, 7]. Gallstones are extremely prevalent in Western societies and represent a significant health problem. In the USA it is reported that 15 % of the adult population have gallstones, which equates to 20–25 million adults. The burden of gallstone disease in Europe is similar with median prevalence of 5.9–21.9 % [8]. In the USA, an estimated 700,000 cholecystectomies are performed annually [9]. For those patients with asymptomatic stones, 1–3 % will develop complications annually including cholecystitis, obstructive jaundice, cholangitis, and pancreatitis [10]. Because of this, the direct and indirect cost of gallstone disease in the USA totals ~$6.2 billion which has increased over the past 30 years [11–13]. Gallstone disease is also one of the leading causes of hospital admissions, with an estimated 1.8 million ambulatory care visits annually [14]. The overall mortality due to gallstone-related disease is relatively low at 0.6 % with an estimated 1092 deaths in 2004 in the USA. These numbers have been steadily decreasing which is largely attributed to the more effective treatment modalities available for ascending cholangitis. Additionally, the mortality rate was highest

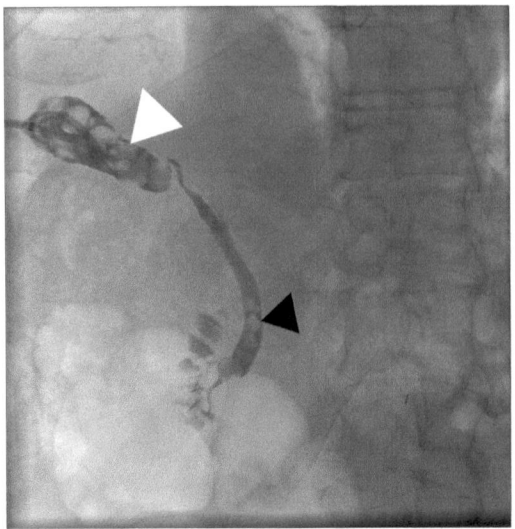

Fig. 2.1 Cholecystogram demonstrating cholelithiasis (*white arrowhead*) and concomitant choledocholithiasis (*black arrowhead*)

in older individuals with 85 % of all deaths occurring in patients >65 years old [12]. Globally, the estimated mortality of biliary disease is estimated at 2.5 deaths per 100,000 population in 2010 which is a decrease from 3.1 deaths per 100,000 population in 1990 [15].

Pancreatitis Disease Burden

Gallstones play a key role in the etiology of acute pancreatitis. Between 40 and 70 % of all cases of acute pancreatitis can be attributed to gallstones [6, 7]. In 2003, acute pancreatitis was the most common discharge diagnosis for patients admitted to gastroenterology with hospitalization rates of 0.52 per 1000 US population for Caucasians and 0.76 per 1000 for African Americans [16]. The total direct and indirect cost of pancreatitis in the USA in 2004 was ~$3.7 billion. Rates of both ambulatory care visits and hospitalizations for pancreatitis have risen over the past 30 years, which may be a reflection of the increased obesity rates over the same time period. In 2004, pancreatitis was the 11th most common underlying cause of death from digestive diseases and the 5th most common nonmalignant cause, just after peptic ulcer disease. Pancreatitis was listed as underlying

cause of death among 49 % of the 7142 death certificates on which it was found [17]. Fifty-six percent of deaths due to pancreatitis occurred among persons age >65 years old [12, 17].

Cholangitis Disease Burden

The most common causes of ascending cholangitis in the USA are biliary obstruction due to gallstones (60 %), followed by malignant obstruction of the CBD, fibrotic strictures, and lastly parasitic infection [18]. Unfortunately, reported rates of cholangitis do not differentiate the underlying causes when reported in the literature, though the majority of cases in the USA are due to CBD stones. The age adjusted hospitalization rate for cholangitis for males and females in the USA in 2006 was 1.76 per 100,000. This represented a 24 % decrease from 30 years prior. Hospitalization rates were highest in patients >70 years old and highest in Asian/Pacific islanders followed by Native American populations. African Americans had the lowest hospitalization rates [19]. The age-adjusted in hospital mortality for patients with cholangitis was 48.9 per 100,000 in 2006. This represented a 73 % decline from 30 years prior [19]. Additionally, the mortality has also steadily dropped over the same time period. Mortality from acute cholangitis was >50 % prior to 1980, 10–30 % from 1981 to 1990, and 2–10 % after 2000 [20–23]. This decline likely represents a move from open surgical biliary drainage to endoscopic biliary decompression and duct clearance during that same time period [24, 25].

Cost of Choledocholithiasis

A significant amount of resources and effort is spent on the diagnosis and treatment of CBD stones. Laparoscopic intraoperative cholangiogram (IOC) at the time of cholecystectomy incurs a cost of US$706–739 per case [26]. Howard et al. performed a cost-effectiveness analysis comparing magnetic resonance cholangiopancreatography (MRCP) as the diagnostic imaging modality vs. endoscopic retrograde cholangio-pancreatography (ERCP) and found that in postcholecystectomy patients, the strategy of using MRCP first, followed by ERCP if MRCP is positive, has an average total health system cost of $6305, compared with the strategy of using ERCP first with an average total health system cost of $7004 [27]. Arguedas et al., reported the average Medicare reimbursement rates obtained on a retrospective sampling of 35 patients admitted for acute biliary pancreatitis and found the cost for therapeutic ERCP, IOC, MRCP, and endoscopic ultrasound were $1006, $699, $700, and $525 respectively [28]. The cost of admission for mild biliary pancreatitis is further increased when the recommendation for cholecystectomy during the same admission is followed [29].

Populations with the Highest Incidence of Biliary Stones

There is very little data on the incidence of primary CBD stones. However, we can infer from the high proportion of CBD stone complications that are due to secondary stones that those patients at higher risk of developing gallstones will also carry a higher risk of developing choledocholithiasis (and one of its potential complications). It is with this in mind that we review the following populations and disease states with the highest incidence of gallstones.

Ethnicity

Ethnicity plays a key role in the formation of biliary stones. Cholesterol stones predominate in Western societies while brown pigmented stones are more common in Asia [30]. Cholesterol stones are primarily made up of cholesterol monohydrate crystals and comprise 80 % of the gallstones present in the US population [31]. Prevalence rates vary widely between different ethnic groups and geographic regions (Fig. 2.2). The highest rates of cholelithiasis are in Native Americans with reported rates as high as 64 % of women and 29 % of men [32]. Mexican-Americans seem to also be at higher risk for stone formation, though this seems to be directly related to the inherited risk from their native Central American ancestry [33–35]. Native populations of South America seem to be similarly affected by stone disease with 49.4 % of women and 12.6 % of men who are native Mapuche Indians of Chile affected [36]. The rate of stones in white Americans is approximately 16.6 % in women and 8.6 % in men, while the rates in black Americans are approximately 13.9 % of women and 5.3 % of men [9, 11]. In Europe, Norway and East Germany have the highest rates of cholelithiasis at 21.9 % and 19.7 % respectively [8]. Prevalence rates were somewhat lower in Italy at 11 % [37], with the lowest rates in sub-Saharan African populations (<5 %) [11].

In Japan the incidence of gallstones is fairly low at 3.2 % [38]. Although secondary CBD stones predominate in the USA and Westernized cultures, primary CBD stones are most common in Asian cultures. In Taiwan the overall prevalence of gallstones was 4.6 % in men and 5.4 % in women [39]. Southeast Asian including Taiwan, Hong Kong, and Singapore experience a higher number of primary bile duct stones than Western populations [40]. The incidence of intrahepatic bile duct stones in all patients with gallstones in Taiwan is >50 %, with concomitant extra hepatic bile duct stones in 70 % of cases [40]. In these populations, intrahepatic stones can be present concomitantly with extrahepatic (CBD) stones. However, the composition of these stones seems to differ in that intrahepatic stones have a higher cholesterol component, while extrahepatic stones are made primarily of bilirubin.

Age

The prevalence of gallstones increases with age in all racial and ethnic groups regardless of sex [41]. For example, in Italy 5–8 % of young women have gallstones compared to 25–30 % of women over the age of 50 [37]. The type of stones seems to change with age as well with pigmented stones becoming more common than cholesterol stones in older populations [42]. Men have increasing rates of cholelithiasis much later in life than women with total prevalence approaching 8 % in all ages compared to 25.3 % in men >60 years of age [9].

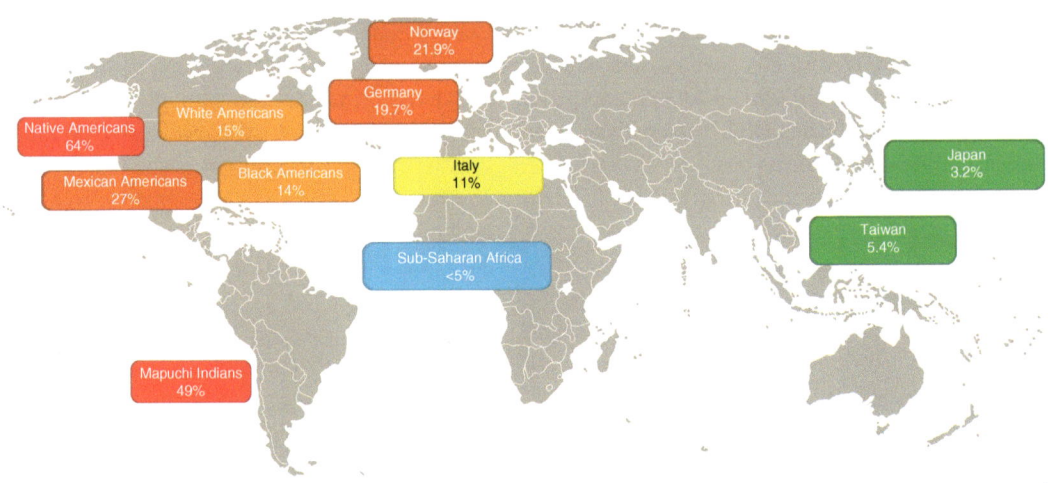

Fig. 2.2 Prevalence of gallstones throughout the world. Rates are highest among Native American populations and lowest among sub-Saharan African tribes

Gender, Pregnancy and Estrogen

In the vast majority of studies the prevalence of gallstones is higher in women than men of the same age in all ethnic and racial groups. However, this difference seems to narrow with increasing age as mentioned earlier [43]. Parity has been found to play a role in the prevalence of gallstones with women having a history of previous pregnancy at higher risk of stone formation [44]. During pregnancy biliary sludge, which may be a precursor to stone formation, develops in up to 30 % of women [45]. Gallstones have been found to form in 1–3 % of pregnant women [46]. These findings seem to be related to estrogen as parity, oral contraceptive use, and estrogen replacement therapy are all established risk factors for cholesterol stone formation [47–49]. It is felt that female sex hormones adversely affect bile secretion and gallbladder function. Estrogen increases the amount of cholesterol secreted into the bile while decreasing the amount of bile salts secreted. Progestins further diminish bile salt secretion while also impairing gallbladder emptying, leading to bile stasis and a relative lithogenic state compared to nonpregnant females.

Obesity

Obesity has been shown to increase the development of gallstones [50, 51]. The mechanisms by which this occurs include increased levels of cholesterol synthesis and higher cholesterol to bile salt concentration within the bile. Increased synthesis of bile is due to the increased activity of the rate-limiting step in cholesterol synthesis, the hepatic enzyme 3-hydroxyl-3-methyl-glutaryl co-enzyme A (HMG-CoA) reductase. This allows for more rapid precipitation of cholesterol crystals and stone formation. Both women and men who are obese synthesize higher amounts of cholesterol and secrete higher levels of cholesterol into the bile [52]. Based on Body Mass Index (BMI) currently in the USA approximately 35.5 % of adult males and 35.8 % of adult females are obese based on a BMI >30 kg/m^2 and 6.3 % of all adults were morbidly obese with a BMI >40 kg/m^2 [53]. This number had been increasing over the past few decades though it seems to have leveled off based on epidemiologic data collected in 2010. At least 25 % of morbidly obese individuals have evidence of gallstones [54]. Women have an even higher risk of stones when coupled with obesity. In one series, women with a BMI >32 kg/m^2 had an age-adjusted relative risk of having gallstones of 6.0 compared with nonobese controls [55].

Diet and TPN

Diet and lifestyle changes in the past century have been linked to stone formation. This is evident in Westernized societies and those with developing economies. A clear example is that of postwar Japan. Following World War II, Japan underwent extensive Westernization. As a result, the presence of gallstones doubled in the late 1940s. This was also associated with a transition in composition of those stones from pigmented subtypes to more cholesterol stones. The change also resulted in a higher ratio of women with gallstones than men [56].

Diets high in cholesterol, fatty acids, carbohydrates, and legumes have higher rates of cholelithiasis [57–61]. Alternatively, unsaturated fat, coffee, fiber, vitamin C, calcium, and moderate ingestion of alcohol reduce the risk [62–65]. Total parenteral nutrition (TPN) is a well-know risk factor for developing microlithiasis (biliary sludge) in critically ill patients [66]. In one series after 4 weeks of TPN, half of patients had sludge on ultrasonography and after 6 weeks, all patients displayed evidence of sludge [67].

Bariatric Surgery and Rapid Weight Loss

Another risk factor for the formation of stones occurs in patients who undergo weight-loss surgery and experience a large amount of rapid weight loss. Gallstone disease is prevalent in patients who undergo bariatric surgery with the incidence as high as 30–52 % [68, 69]. Predisposing factors in the setting of bariatric surgery include increased cholesterol concentrations in bile, increased secretion of calcium and mucin into bile that occurs during rapid weight loss, and increased concentration of arachidonic acid derivatives [70–72]. The dietary changes adopted by bariatric patients including fasting and restriction also promote bile stasis [73]. This risk seems to be the greatest immediately after the surgery when the rate of weight loss is the highest [74]. With an obesity epidemic in Western countries, bariatric patients and surgical weight loss patients represent an enlarging percentage of patients with CBD stones. As will be discussed in later chapters, choledocholithiasis management following certain types of bariatric surgical procedures (Rou-en-Y gastric bypass and duodenal switch) can be quite challenging as direct peroral access to the biliary tree is often not feasible.

Chronic Disease

Cirrhosis is a well-established risk factor for stone formation with prevalence rates as high as 30 % [75, 76]. Stones in these patients tend to be of the pigmented subtype as opposed to cholesterol stones [77]. One study found a higher prevalence of stones in patients with Child class 2 or 3 cirrhosis compared with patients with a high BMI [75].

Patients with ileal Crohn's disease have a two to threefold increased risk of developing stones [78]. One of the proposed mechanisms for this occurrence is the failure of the terminal ileum to absorb bile acids which are then transported to the colon where biological detergents solubilize unconjugated bilirubin which is then transported back to the liver and concentrated in the bile where it precipitates and forms pigmented stones [79].

Cystic fibrosis is associated with bile acid malabsorption. The prevalence of stones in patients with cystic fibrosis is increased 10–30 % [80]. Sickle cell disease results in chronic hemolysis and excess bilirubin secretion. This leads to the formation of black pigmented stones (Fig. 2.3). Spinal cord injury is associated with a nearly three times higher risk of gallstones [81]. The etiology of cholelithiasis in patients with spinal cord injury is not fully understood but is thought to be due to abnormal gallbladder motility and stasis, abnormal enterohepatic circulation, and abnormal biliary lipid secretion [82].

Incidence of Stones Based on Location of Origin: Primary vs. Secondary

Primary Choledocholithiasis

CBD stones can be divided into two general categories: primary and secondary. Primary stones are those that form within the intra or extra-hepatic bile ducts, excluding the gallbladder (Fig. 2.4). Secondary stones are those that form within the gallbladder and then migrate through the cystic

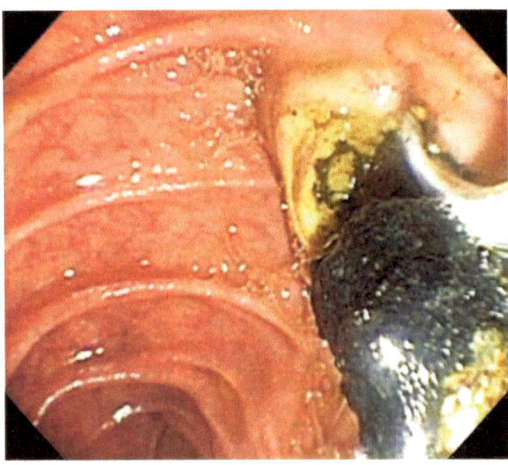

Fig. 2.3 Endoscopic view during ERCP of black-pigmented stone impacted at the sphincter of Odi

duct into the intra or extra-hepatic bile ducts. Primary stones are uncommon in Western populations. Historically there have been reported cases of primary CBD stones in patients with congenital gallbladder agenesis though this is rare [83]. Primary CBD stones occur more commonly in Asian populations as discussed earlier. The reason for this difference is not fully understood, but likely relies on a combination of bile stasis, bile infection, malnutrition, and parasitic infection [84].

Secondary Choledocholithiasis

As mentioned earlier, secondary stones represent the vast majority of CBD stones in the USA and Westernized populations [6, 7]. The total number of patients with secondary CBD stones is likely underestimated as many of these patients are asymptomatic. It is likely that many small stones are passed without incident. Furthermore, it is unknown whether small stones that are passed into the CBD then increase in size until they become symptomatic. Not all gallstones have the ability to pass through the cystic duct into the CBD due to their size and the spiral mucosal folds within the cystic duct known as the valves of Heister [85]. Gallstones larger than the cystic duct are more likely to result in cholecystitis and chronic pain than in choledocholithiasis (Fig. 2.5).

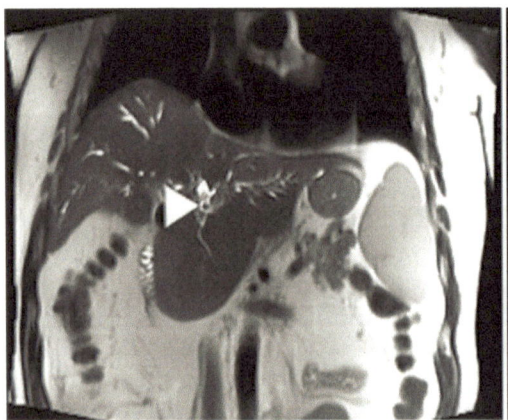
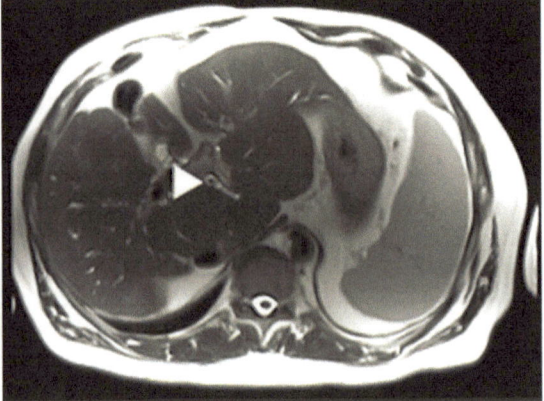

Fig. 2.4 Axial and coronal T2 weighted magnetic resonance imaging (MRI) views of primary intrahepatic stones (marked by *arrowhead*) formed in the setting of strictured biliary tree in a patient with primary sclerosing cholangitis

Fig. 2.5 Opened specimen following cholecystectomy and CBD exploration showing larger stone retained within the gallbladder and smaller stone retrieved from CBD

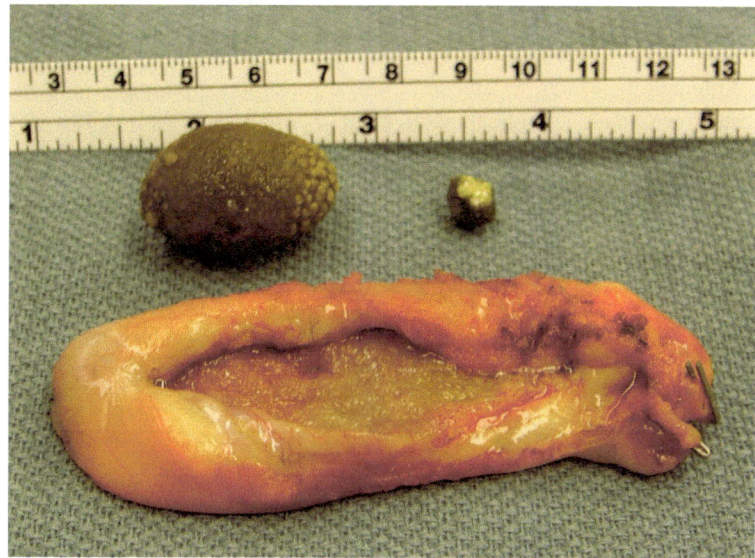

Retained Choledocholithiasis

Retained stones are a subset of secondary stones and represent gallstones that were present during the time of cholecystectomy that were either unrecognized and within the CBD or migrated through the cystic duct at the time of operation. Uncommonly, a long cystic duct stump may be left in situ at the time of cholecystectomy that still contains gallstones that pose a risk for migration (Fig. 2.6). In one study to better understand the natural history of retained stones, researchers examined 997 patients who underwent laparoscopic cholecystectomy and found that 3.4 % demonstrated evidence of choledocholithiasis. In one-third of those patients with CBD stones, the stone spontaneously passed within 6 weeks of the operation. All of the patients remained asymptomatic over that period, and in the patients where the stone did not spontaneously pass, the stone was removed with ERCP [86]. When examining patients who had previously undergone cholecystectomy who presented later with signs and symptoms consistent with CBD stones, one study showed that the median time to presentation from their operation was 4 years. In this study, 31 % of those patients presented with clinical complica-

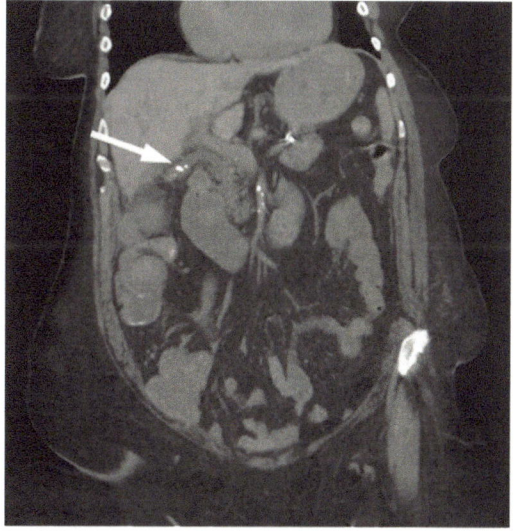

Fig. 2.6 Coronal CT image of patient with retained stones (*white arrow*) in a long cystic duct after laparoscopic cholecystectomy

tions from their CBD stones including obstructive jaundice, cholangitis, and gallstone pancreatitis [87]. These studies suggest that the majority of retained stones are either passed spontaneously, or remain asymptomatic for prolonged periods following surgery.

Conclusions

Although the exact prevalence of CBD stones is unknown, their complications remain a highly morbid, and costly problem for health care today. It is reasonable to infer that patients with a higher propensity for forming gallstones will suffer from a higher rate of stone migration and CBD stone complications. Knowing which populations are more commonly affected by CBD stones will assist the clinician in the proper assessment and treatment of those affected by this relatively common disease process.

References

1. Clayton ES, Connor S, Alexakis N, Leandros E. Meta-analysis of endoscopy and surgery versus surgery alone for common bile duct stones with the gallbladder in situ. Br J Surg. 2006;93(10):1185–91. doi:10.1002/bjs.5568.
2. Iranmanesh P, Frossard JL, Mugnier-Konrad B, Morel P, Majno P, Nguyen-Tang T, et al. Initial cholecystectomy vs sequential common duct endoscopic assessment and subsequent cholecystectomy for suspected gallstone migration: a randomized clinical trial. JAMA. 2014;312(2):137–44. doi:10.1001/jama.2014.7587.
3. Metcalfe MS, Ong T, Bruening MH, Iswariah H, Wemyss-Holden SA, Maddern GJ. Is laparoscopic intraoperative cholangiogram a matter of routine? Am J Surg. 2004;187(4):475–81. doi:10.1016/j.amjsurg.2003.12.047.
4. Riciardi R, Islam S, Canete JJ, Arcand PL, Stoker ME. Effectiveness and long-term results of laparoscopic common bile duct exploration. Surg Endosc. 2003;17(1):19–22. doi:10.1007/s00464-002-8925-4.
5. Schirmer BD, Winters KL, Edlich RF. Cholelithiasis and cholecystitis. J Long-Term Eff Med Implants. 2005;15(3):329–38.
6. Lowenfels AB, Maisonneuve P, Sullivan T. The changing character of acute pancreatitis: epidemiology, etiology, and prognosis. Curr Gastroenterol Rep. 2009;11(2):97–103.
7. Gullo L, Migliori M, Olah A, Farkas G, Levy P, Arvanitakis C, et al. Acute pancreatitis in five European countries: etiology and mortality. Pancreas. 2002;24(3):223–7.
8. Aerts R, Penninckx F. The burden of gallstone disease in Europe. Aliment Pharmacol Ther. 2003;18 Suppl 3:49–53.
9. Everhart JE, Khare M, Hill M, Maurer KR. Prevalence and ethnic differences in gallbladder disease in the United States. Gastroenterology. 1999;117(3):632–9.
10. Friedman GD. Natural history of asymptomatic and symptomatic gallstones. Am J Surg. 1993;165(4):399–404.
11. Shaffer EA. Epidemiology and risk factors for gallstone disease: has the paradigm changed in the 21st century? Curr Gastroenterol Rep. 2005;7(2):132–40.
12. Everhart JE, Ruhl CE. Burden of digestive diseases in the United States part I: overall and upper gastrointestinal diseases. Gastroenterology. 2009;136(2):376–86. doi:10.1053/j.gastro.2008.12.015.
13. Sandler RS, Everhart JE, Donowitz M, Adams E, Cronin K, Goodman C, et al. The burden of selected digestive diseases in the United States. Gastroenterology. 2002;122(5):1500–11.
14. Shaheen NJ, Hansen RA, Morgan DR, Gangarosa LM, Ringel Y, Thiny MT, et al. The burden of gastrointestinal and liver diseases, 2006. Am J Gastroenterol. 2006;101(9):2128–38. doi:10.1111/j.1572-0241.2006.00723.x.
15. Stewart B, Khanduri P, McCord C, Ohene-Yeboah M, Uranues S, Vega Rivera F, et al. Global disease burden of conditions requiring emergency surgery. Br J Surg. 2014;101(1):e9–22. doi:10.1002/bjs.9329.
16. Fagenholz PJ, Fernandez-del Castillo C, Harris NS, Pelletier AJ, Camargo Jr CA. Direct medical costs of acute pancreatitis hospitalizations in the United States. Pancreas. 2007;35(4):302–7. doi:10.1097/MPA.0b013e3180cac24b.
17. Everhart JE, Ruhl CE. Burden of digestive diseases in the United States Part III: liver, biliary tract, and pancreas. Gastroenterology. 2009;136(4):1134–44. doi:10.1053/j.gastro.2009.02.038.
18. Qureshi WA. Approach to the patient who has suspected acute bacterial cholangitis. Gastroenterol Clin N Am. 2006;35(2):409–23. doi:10.1016/j.gtc.2006.05.005.
19. Jamal MM, Yamini D, Singson Z, Samarasena J, Hashemzadeh M, Vega KJ. Decreasing hospitalization and in-hospital mortality related to cholangitis in the United States. J Clin Gastroenterol. 2011;45(10):e92–6. doi:10.1097/MCG.0b013e31822f364c.
20. Andrew DJ, Johnson SE. Acute suppurative cholangitis, a medical and surgical emergency. A review of ten years experience emphasizing early recognition. Am J Gastroenterol. 1970;54(2):141–54.
21. Tai DI, Shen FH, Liaw YF. Abnormal pre-drainage serum creatinine as a prognostic indicator in acute cholangitis. Hepato-Gastroenterology. 1992;39(1):47–50.
22. Thompson J, Bennion RS, Pitt HA. An analysis of infectious failures in acute cholangitis. HPB Surg. 1994;8(2):139–44. discussion 45.
23. Lee CC, Chang IJ, Lai YC, Chen SY, Chen SC. Epidemiology and prognostic determinants of patients with bacteremic cholecystitis or cholangitis. AmJGastroenterol.2007;102(3):563–9.doi:10.1111/j.1572-0241.2007.01095.x.
24. Lai EC, Mok FP, Tan ES, Lo CM, Fan ST, You KT, et al. Endoscopic biliary drainage for severe acute cholangitis. N Engl J Med. 1992;326(24):1582–6. doi:10.1056/NEJM199206113262401.
25. McNabb-Baltar J, Trinh QD, Barkun AN. Biliary drainage method and temporal trends in patients admitted with cholangitis: a national audit. Can J Gastroenterol. 2013;27(9):513–8.

26. Livingston EH, Miller JA, Coan B, Rege RV. Costs and utilization of intraoperative cholangiography. J Gastrointest Surg. 2007;11(9):1162–7. doi:10.1007/s11605-007-0209-9.
27. Howard K, Lord SJ, Speer A, Gibson RN, Padbury R, Kearney B. Value of magnetic resonance cholangiopancreatography in the diagnosis of biliary abnormalities in postcholecystectomy patients: a probabilistic cost-effectiveness analysis of diagnostic strategies. Int J Technol Assess Health Care. 2006;22(1):109–18.
28. Arguedas MR, Dupont AW, Wilcox CM. Where do ERCP, endoscopic ultrasound, magnetic resonance cholangiopancreatography, and intraoperative cholangiography fit in the management of acute biliary pancreatitis? A decision analysis model. Am JGastroenterol.2001;96(10):2892–9.doi:10.1111/j.1572-0241.2001.04244.x.
29. Tenner S, Baillie J, DeWitt J, Vege SS. American College of G. American College of Gastroenterology guideline: management of acute pancreatitis. Am J Gastroenterol. 2013;108(9):1400–15. doi:10.1038/ajg.2013.218. 16.
30. Shaffer EA. Gallstone disease: Epidemiology of gallbladder stone disease. Best Pract Res Clin Gastroenterol. 2006;20(6):981–96. doi:10.1016/j.bpg.2006.05.004.
31. Wittenburg H. Hereditary liver disease: gallstones. Best Pract Res Clin Gastroenterol. 2010;24(5):747–56. doi:10.1016/j.bpg.2010.07.004.
32. Everhart JE, Yeh F, Lee ET, Hill MC, Fabsitz R, Howard BV, et al. Prevalence of gallbladder disease in American Indian populations: findings from the Strong Heart Study. Hepatology. 2002;35(6):1507–12. doi:10.1053/jhep.2002.33336.
33. Everhart JE. Gallstones and ethnicity in the Americas. J Assoc Acad Minor Phys. 2001;12(3):137–43.
34. Diehl AK, Stern MP. Special health problems of Mexican-Americans: obesity, gallbladder disease, diabetes mellitus, and cardiovascular disease. Adv Intern Med. 1989;34:73–96.
35. Maurer KR, Everhart JE, Ezzati TM, Johannes RS, Knowler WC, Larson DL, et al. Prevalence of gallstone disease in Hispanic populations in the United States. Gastroenterology. 1989;96(2 Pt 1):487–92.
36. Miquel JF, Covarrubias C, Villaroel L, Mingrone G, Greco AV, Puglielli L, et al. Genetic epidemiology of cholesterol cholelithiasis among Chilean Hispanics, Amerindians, and Maoris. Gastroenterology. 1998;115(4):937–46.
37. Barbara L, Sama C, Morselli Labate AM, Taroni F, Rusticali AG, Festi D, et al. A population study on the prevalence of gallstone disease: the Sirmione Study. Hepatology. 1987;7(5):913–7.
38. Nomura H, Kashiwagi S, Hayashi J, Kajiyama W, Ikematsu H, Noguchi A, et al. Prevalence of gallstone disease in a general population of Okinawa, Japan. Am J Epidemiol. 1988;128(3):598–605.
39. Chen CH, Huang MH, Yang JC, Nien CK, Etheredge GD, Yang CC, et al. Prevalence and risk factors of gallstone disease in an adult population of Taiwan: an epidemiological survey. J Gastroenterol Hepatol. 2006;21(11):1737–43.doi:10.1111/j.1440-1746.2006. 04381.x.
40. Kim MH, Sekijima J, Lee SP. Primary intrahepatic stones. Am J Gastroenterol. 1995;90(4):540–8.
41. Chen CY, Lu CL, Huang YS, Tam TN, Chao Y, Chang FY, et al. Age is one of the risk factors in developing gallstone disease in Taiwan. Age Ageing. 1998;27(4):437–41.
42. Einarsson K, Nilsell K, Leijd B, Angelin B. Influence of age on secretion of cholesterol and synthesis of bile acids by the liver. N Engl J Med. 1985;313(5):277–82. doi:10.1056/NEJM198508013130501.
43. The epidemiology of gallstone disease in Rome, Italy. Part I. Prevalence data in men. The Rome Group for Epidemiology and Prevention of Cholelithiasis (GREPCO). Hepatology. 1988;8(4):904–6
44. Attili AF, Capocaccia R, Carulli N, Festi D, Roda E, Barbara L, et al. Factors associated with gallstone disease in the MICOL experience. Multicenter Italian Study on Epidemiology of Cholelithiasis. Hepatology. 1997;26(4):809–18. doi:10.1002/hep.510260401.
45. Maringhini A, Ciambra M, Baccelliere P, Raimondo M, Orlando A, Tine F, et al. Biliary sludge and gallstones in pregnancy: incidence, risk factors, and natural history. Ann Intern Med. 1993;119(2):116–20.
46. Valdivieso V, Covarrubias C, Siegel F, Cruz F. Pregnancy and cholelithiasis: pathogenesis and natural course of gallstones diagnosed in early puerperium. Hepatology. 1993;17(1):1–4.
47. Thijs C, Knipschild P. Oral contraceptives and the risk of gallbladder disease: a meta-analysis. Am J Public Health. 1993;83(8):1113–20.
48. Hulley S, Grady D, Bush T, Furberg C, Herrington D, Riggs B, et al. Randomized trial of estrogen plus progestin for secondary prevention of coronary heart disease in postmenopausal women. Heart and Estrogen/progestin Replacement Study (HERS) Research Group. JAMA. 1998;280(7):605–13.
49. Cirillo DJ, Wallace RB, Rodabough RJ, Greenland P, LaCroix AZ, Limacher MC, et al. Effect of estrogen therapy on gallbladder disease. JAMA. 2005;293(3):330–9. doi:10.1001/jama.293.3.330.
50. Grundy SM, Duane WC, Adler RD, Aron JM, Metzger AL. Biliary lipid outputs in young women with cholesterol gallstones. Metab Clin Exp. 1974;23(1):67–73.
51. Grundy SM, Metzger AL, Adler RD. Mechanisms of lithogenic bile formation in American Indian women with cholesterol gallstones. J Clin Invest. 1972;51(12):3026–43. doi:10.1172/JCI107130.
52. Bennion LJ, Grundy SM. Effects of obesity and caloric intake on biliary lipid metabolism in man. J Clin Invest. 1975;56(4):996–1011. doi:10.1172/JCI108180.
53. Flegal KM, Carroll MD, Kit BK, Ogden CL. Prevalence of obesity and trends in the distribution of body mass index among US adults, 1999-2010. JAMA. 2012;307(5):491–7. doi:10.1001/jama.2012.39.

54. Li VK, Pulido N, Fajnwaks P, Szomstein S, Rosenthal R, Martinez-Duartez P. Predictors of gallstone formation after bariatric surgery: a multivariate analysis of risk factors comparing gastric bypass, gastric banding, and sleeve gastrectomy. Surg Endosc. 2009;23(7):1640–4. doi:10.1007/s00464-008-0204-6.

55. Maclure KM, Hayes KC, Colditz GA, Stampfer MJ, Speizer FE, Willett WC. Weight, diet, and the risk of symptomatic gallstones in middle-aged women. N Engl J Med. 1989;321(9):563–9. doi:10.1056/NEJM198908313210902.

56. Kameda H, Ishihara F, Shibata K, Tsukie E. Clinical and nutritional study on gallstone disease in Japan. Jpn J Med. 1984;23(2):109–13.

57. Lee DW, Gilmore CJ, Bonorris G, Cohen H, Marks JW, Cho-Sue M, et al. Effect of dietary cholesterol on biliary lipids in patients with gallstones and normal subjects. Am J Clin Nutr. 1985;42(3):414–20.

58. Tsai CJ, Leitzmann MF, Willett WC, Giovannucci EL. Long-chain saturated fatty acids consumption and risk of gallstone disease among men. Ann Surg. 2008;247(1):95–103. doi:10.1097/SLA.0b013e31815792c2.

59. Scragg RK, McMichael AJ, Baghurst PA. Diet, alcohol, and relative weight in gall stone disease: a case-control study. Br Med J. 1984;288(6424):1113–9.

60. Tsai CJ, Leitzmann MF, Willett WC, Giovannucci EL. Dietary carbohydrates and glycaemic load and the incidence of symptomatic gall stone disease in men. Gut. 2005;54(6):823–8. doi:10.1136/gut.2003.031435.

61. Nervi F, Covarrubias C, Bravo P, Velasco N, Ulloa N, Cruz F, et al. Influence of legume intake on biliary lipids and cholesterol saturation in young Chilean men. Identification of a dietary risk factor for cholesterol gallstone formation in a highly prevalent area. Gastroenterology. 1989;96(3):825–30.

62. Tsai CJ, Leitzmann MF, Willett WC, Giovannucci EL. The effect of long-term intake of cis unsaturated fats on the risk for gallstone disease in men: a prospective cohort study. Ann Intern Med. 2004;141(7):514–22.

63. Leitzmann MF, Willett WC, Rimm EB, Stampfer MJ, Spiegelman D, Colditz GA, et al. A prospective study of coffee consumption and the risk of symptomatic gallstone disease in men. JAMA. 1999;281(22):2106–12.

64. Leitzmann MF, Tsai CJ, Stampfer MJ, Rimm EB, Colditz GA, Willett WC, et al. Alcohol consumption in relation to risk of cholecystectomy in women. Am J Clin Nutr. 2003;78(2):339–47.

65. Simon JA, Hudes ES. Serum ascorbic acid and gallbladder disease prevalence among US adults: the Third National Health and Nutrition Examination Survey (NHANES III). Arch Intern Med. 2000;160(7):931–6.

66. Guglielmi FW, Boggio-Bertinet D, Federico A, Forte GB, Guglielmi A, Loguercio C, et al. Total parenteral nutrition-related gastroenterological complications. Dig Liver Dis. 2006;38(9):623–42. doi:10.1016/j.dld.2006.04.002.

67. Messing B, Bories C, Kunstlinger F, Bernier JJ. Does total parenteral nutrition induce gallbladder sludge formation and lithiasis? Gastroenterology. 1983;84(5 Pt 1):1012–9.

68. D'Hondt M, Sergeant G, Deylgat B, Devriendt D, Van Rooy F, Vansteenkiste F. Prophylactic cholecystectomy, a mandatory step in morbidly obese patients undergoing laparoscopic Roux-en-Y gastric bypass? J Gastrointest Surg. 2011;15(9):1532–6. doi:10.1007/s11605-011-1617-4.

69. Tucker ON, Fajnwaks P, Szomstein S, Rosenthal RJ. Is concomitant cholecystectomy necessary in obese patients undergoing laparoscopic gastric bypass surgery? Surg Endosc. 2008;22(11):2450–4. doi:10.1007/s00464-008-9769-3.

70. Shiffman ML, Shamburek RD, Schwartz CC, Sugerman HJ, Kellum JM, Moore EW. Gallbladder mucin, arachidonic acid, and bile lipids in patients who develop gallstones during weight reduction. Gastroenterology. 1993;105(4):1200–8.

71. Shiffman ML, Sugerman HJ, Kellum JM, Moore EW. Calcium in human gallbladder bile. J Lab Clin Med. 1992;120(6):875–84.

72. Shiffman ML, Sugerman HJ, Kellum JM, Moore EW. Changes in gallbladder bile composition following gallstone formation and weight reduction. Gastroenterology. 1992;103(1):214–21.

73. Marzio L, Capone F, Neri M, Mezzetti A, De Angelis C, Cuccurullo F. Gallbladder kinetics in obese patients. Effect of a regular meal and low-calorie meal. Dig Dis Sci. 1988;33(1):4–9.

74. Al-Jiffry BO, Shaffer EA, Saccone GT, Downey P, Kow L, Toouli J. Changes in gallbladder motility and gallstone formation following laparoscopic gastric banding for morbid obesity. Can J Gastroenterol. 2003;17(3):169–74.

75. Conte D, Fraquelli M, Fornari F, Lodi L, Bodini P, Buscarini L. Close relation between cirrhosis and gallstones: cross-sectional and longitudinal survey. Arch Intern Med. 1999;159(1):49–52.

76. Acalovschi M, Badea R, Dumitrascu D, Varga C. Prevalence of gallstones in liver cirrhosis: a sonographic survey. Am J Gastroenterol. 1988;83(9):954–6.

77. Alvaro D, Angelico M, Gandin C, Ginanni Corradini S, Capocaccia L. Physico-chemical factors predisposing to pigment gallstone formation in liver cirrhosis. J Hepatol. 1990;10(2):228–34.

78. Whorwell PJ, Hawkins R, Dewbury K, Wright R. Ultrasound survey of gallstones and other hepatobiliary disorders in patients with Crohn's disease. Dig Dis Sci. 1984;29(10):930–3.

79. Brink MA, Slors JF, Keulemans YC, Mok KS, De Waart DR, Carey MC, et al. Enterohepatic cycling of bilirubin: a putative mechanism for pigment gallstone formation in ileal Crohn's disease. Gastroenterology. 1999;116(6):1420–7.

80. Vitek L, Carey MC. Enterohepatic cycling of bilirubin as a cause of 'black' pigment gallstones in adult life. Eur J Clin Investig. 2003;33(9):799–810.

81. Xia CS, Han YQ, Yang XY, Hong GX. Spinal cord injury and cholelithiasis. Hepatobiliary Pancreat Dis Int. 2004;3(4):595–8.

82. Apstein MD, Dalecki-Chipperfield K. Spinal cord injury is a risk factor for gallstone disease. Gastroenterology. 1987;92(4):966–8.

83. Gerwig Jr WH, Countryman LK, Gomez AC. Congenital absence of the gallbladder and cystic duct: report of six cases. Ann Surg. 1961;153:113–25.

84. Chen HH, Zhang WH, Wang SS, Caruana JA. Twenty-two year experience with the diagnosis and treatment of intrahepatic calculi. Surg Gynecol Obstet. 1984;159(6):519–24.

85. Turner MA, Fulcher AS. The cystic duct: normal anatomy and disease processes. Radiographics. 2001;21(1):3–22. doi:10.1148/radiographics.21.1.g01ja093. questionnaire 288–94.

86. Collins C, Maguire D, Ireland A, Fitzgerald E, O'Sullivan GC. A prospective study of common bile duct calculi in patients undergoing laparoscopic cholecystectomy: natural history of choledocholithiasis revisited. Ann Surg. 2004;239(1):28–33. doi:10.1097/01.sla.0000103069.00170.9c.

87. Cox MR, Budge JP, Eslick GD. Timing and nature of presentation of unsuspected retained common bile duct stones after laparoscopic cholecystectomy: a retrospective study. Surg Endosc. 2014. doi:10.1007/s00464-014-3907-x.

Sunny Jaiswal and Suresh Chamarthi

Biliary Anatomy

The biliary system consists of intrahepaticand extrahepatic ducts, and the intrahepatic portion of the biliary tree is further subdivided into right and left sides. The branches of the left and right intrahepatic biliary tree run parallel to the corresponding portal venous system branches. The right hepatic duct (RHD) drains the segments of the right hepatic lobe and consists of two major branches. The right posterior duct (RPD) drains the posterior segments (VI and VII), and the right anterior duct (RAD) drains the anterior segments (V and VIII). The left hepatic duct drains segments II–IV. The common hepatic duct (CHD) is formed when the RHD and LHD converge. The cystic duct most commonly joins the CHD below the confluence of the LHD and RHD to form the common bile duct (CBD). The CBD then unites with the duct of Wirsung, which originates in the pancreas, to enter the duodenum. The sphincter of Oddi, which consists of smooth muscle, surrounds the common channel of these two ducts.

S. Jaiswal, M.D., M.B.A. (✉)
S. Chamarthi, M.B.B.S.
Department of Radiology, The Ohio State University Wexner Medical Center, Columbus, OH, USA
e-mail: Sunny.Jaiswal@osumc.edu;
Suresh.Chamarthi@osumc.edu

This is considered the standard anatomy and occurs in approximately 58 % of people as shown on Fig. 3.1 [1].

Some variation of the standard biliary anatomy occurs in approximately 40 % of the population. The most common variation in the intrahepatic biliary tree is drainage of the RPD into the LHD. This variant occurs in approximately 13–19 % of the population [1–3]. The RPD may also empty into the rightward aspect of the RAD, instead of coursing posterior to the RAD, in about 12 % of the population [3]. Another common variant of the main hepatic biliary branches is the simultaneous confluence of the RPD, RAD, and LHD to form the CHD. This so-called "triple confluence" occurs in 11 % of the population [1, 2]. Other less common variants include drainage of the RPD directly into the CHD (aberrant hepatic duct) and accessory hepatic ducts [4].

The cystic duct joins the CHD to form the CBD. The site of cystic duct insertion into CHD is approximately halfway between the porta hepatis and the ampulla of Vater. However, the site of insertion can be variable and can occur anywhere between the porta hepatis and the ampulla of Vater [5]. The cystic duct usually enters the CHD from the right lateral aspect in 49.9 % of cases [5]. It can also enter from the medial aspect in approximately 18.4 % or from anterior or posterior aspect in approximately 31.7 % [5]. The cystic duct usually runs parallel to the CHD for a short distance.

© Springer International Publishing Switzerland 2016
J.W. Hazey et al. (eds.), *Multidisciplinary Management of Common Bile Duct Stones*,
DOI 10.1007/978-3-319-22765-8_3

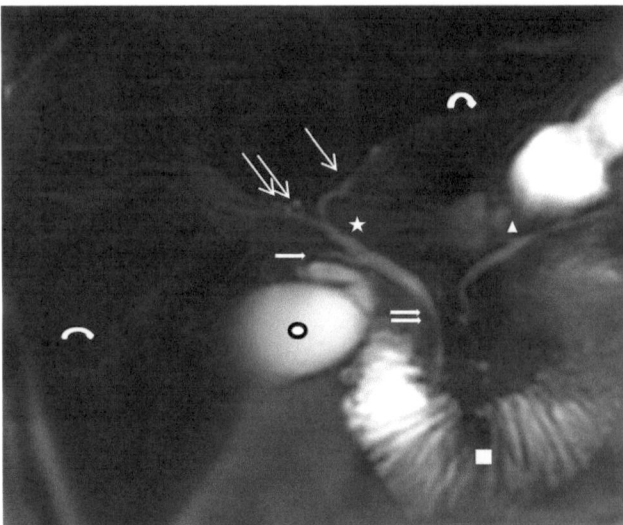

Fig. 3.1 Normal biliary anatomy. Magnetic resonance cholangiopancreatography (MRCP) of a normal biliary tree. The intrahepatic ducts can be seen centrally and demonstrate smooth tapering as they extend to the periphery of the liver (*curved arrow*). They are only faintly seen in the periphery of the liver. The right hepatic duct (*double long arrows*) and left hepatic duct (*single long arrow*) join to form the common hepatic duct (*star*). The gallbladder (*oval*) is partially seen with the cystic duct (*single thick arrow*) joining common hepatic duct to form the common bile duct (*double thick arrows*). The common bile duct (CBD) tapers smoothly as it reaches the duodenum (*square*). Pancreatic duct (*triangle*) is partially seen extending to the CBD

The cystic duct has a variably longer parallel course relative to the CHD in 10.6 % of patients and varies in length from 1.5 to 9.5 cm [5].

Imaging of the Biliary Tree

The biliary tree can be imaged by a number of different modalities including fluoroscopy, ultrasound (US), computed tomography (CT) and magnetic resonance imaging (MRI). Each modality has its relative advantages and disadvantages with respects to imaging the biliary tree. US is readily available and does not expose the patient to ionizing radiation. Unfortunately, US is operator dependent and is prone to artifact, which may result in limited visualization of the biliary tree. CT is also readily available and can provide good information on the biliary tree. However, not all stones are visible by CT, and there are associated radiation risks. MRI/MRCP avoids the risk of radiation and allows for detailed anatomical delineation of the biliary tree but is less readily available than US or CT and can be limited by artifact. Fluoroscopic detection of CBD stones involves direct contrast injection into the common bile duct and is done mainly through an adjunctive procedure—either t-tube cholangiography in the postoperative setting or endoscopic retrograde cholangiopancreatography (ERCP) or percutaneous transhepatic cholangiography (PTC). As these methods use iodinated contrast to outline the stone in the bile duct, the collective sensitivity and specificity of these procedures is high. On the other hand, these procedures (t-tube cholangiography aside) have a defined risk profile, are done under moderate or deep sedation or general anesthesia and confer the risk of exposure to ionizing radiation. Thus, the patient assumes procedural and anesthetic risks with ERCP and PTC that are not present with US, CT, or MRI. ERCP and PTC are covered in detail elsewhere in this text.

Detection of Choledocholithiasis

Choledocholithiasis refers specifically to stones in the common bile duct. The detection of CBD stones varies with the various imaging modalities and depends upon many factors. The factors

Fig. 3.2 MRI of dilated ducts. MRCP demonstrating dilatation of the right and left intrahepatic biliary tree and of the common bile duct (*star*). The bile ducts can easily be seen extending to the periphery of the liver. A distal common bile duct stone is depicted as a rounded low signal structure (*arrow*) outlined by the bright signal from the fluid in the surrounding biliary tree

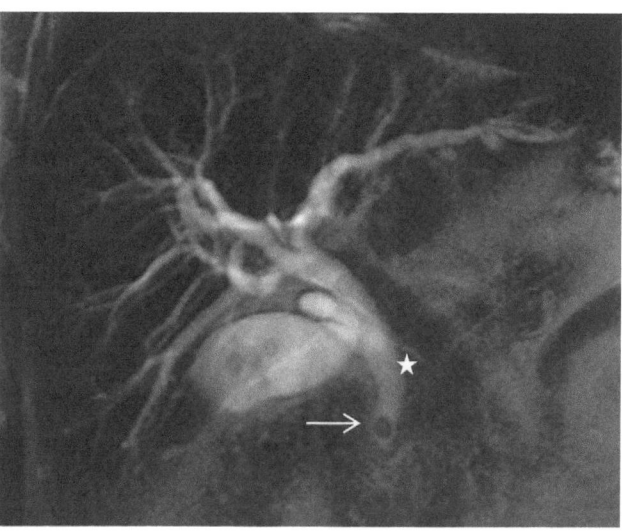

which may influence the diagnosis of CBD stones are the contents of the stone, the presence or absence of direct and indirect findings of choledocholithiasis, the technological factors of a given imaging modality and the diligence of the interpreting physician.

Cholesterol is the main component of approximately 80 % of gallstones, with 10 % being pure cholesterol [6]. Pigmented stones have less than 25 % cholesterol, and the major component is calcium bilirubinate [6]. Calcium carbonate is a less common constituent of all gallstones. Approximately 15–20 % of gallstones contain enough calcium to be visible on plain radiographs [7]. Therefore plain radiographs cannot detect bile duct stones in most cases. Similarly, because of the variable calcium content, not all bile duct stones may be seen with CT.

The radiological diagnosis of choledocholithiasis is inextricably tied to the presence or absence of direct and indirect imaging findings. The unassailable direct finding is the detection of an object (US or CT) or filling defect (MRCP) in the common bile duct. Although other objects (tumor, thrombus, fungal debris as examples) or filling defects (air) may mimic stones, there are other characteristics which may help differentiate stones from other potential diagnoses. Stones are often seen in the dependent posterior location of the biliary tree and may be outlined by fluid.

Stones are also often geometric and angulated and may have a lamellated appearance. It should be noted that the direct visualization of a common bile duct stone may be limited by the imaging technique, the inherent shortcomings of the modality in use and the size of the stone.

The most frequent indirect sign of choledocholithiasis is biliary duct dilatation (Fig. 3.2). Under physiological conditions, the CBD measures 6–7 mm in diameter. There is controversy whether or not the duct caliber increases with age or after cholecystectomy. The intrahepatic bile ducts (IBDs) are smaller in caliber, smoothly taper as they extend to the periphery of the liver and are not easily visible in the peripheral third of the liver. They are often faintly seen with intravenous contrast enhanced CT or contrast enhanced gradient echo T1-weighted MR imaging, but can be seen better with MRCP. The normal nondilated small intrahepatic bile ducts are difficult to visualize on ultrasound. The larger main right and left bile ducts can be identified as tubular structures running anterior to and in parallel with the right and left branches of the portal vein and measure up to 2 mm in diameter in the nondilated system. Therefore, when dilated bile ducts are found, a search for the cause of obstruction should ensue. Other indirect findings of CBD stones are generally the result of inflammation caused by the stones. These indirect findings

Fig. 3.3 Ultrasound demonstrating a common duct stone. Grayscale ultrasound image in the longitudinal plane demonstrates a round echogenic structure (*arrow*), representing a stone, with posterior acoustic shadowing (*double arrow*) in the dilated common bile duct (*star*)

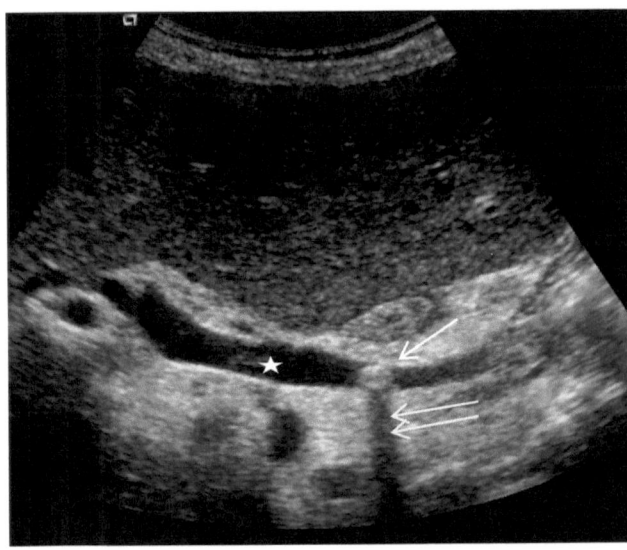

include periductal edema, biliary epithelial thickening and duct mural enhancement.

Finally, the diligence of the interpreting physician commonly comes into play. Because of the content of the stones and because of the inherent technical factors of the various imaging modalities, common bile duct stones are frequently not seen on initial imaging. The proper clinical scenario and/or the presence of indirect imaging findings of CBD stones should prompt the interpreting physician to recommend further evaluation.

Diagnosis by Ultrasound Imaging

The sensitivity of ultrasound in the detection of common duct stones ranges from 72 to 84 % [8–10]. Meticulous scanning technique permits identification of small stones in minimally dilated ducts or non-dilated ducts. The common duct should be scanned in both longitudinal and transverse planes. The patient should be scanned in different positions including decubitus, upright, and semi-upright positions. Liver and water-filled stomach and duodenum can be used as acoustic windows for better visualization of the common bile duct. Tissue harmonic imaging improves both contrast resolution and the detection of acoustic shadow and is therefore recommended for routine assessment of the biliary tree [11].

The stones are typically echogenic, appearing bright on ultrasound, with posterior acoustic shadowing (Fig. 3.3). Up to 10 % of stones may not cause posterior acoustic shadowing [12, 13], especially in the distal duct. Factors that may lower the sensitivity of detecting stones on ultrasound include gas in the duodenum, lack of dilatation of biliary tree, and absence of bile pool around stones. Gas in the ducts can mimic stones due to high reflectivity and shadowing. Gas can also obscure underlying stones.

Endoscopic ultrasound (EUS) has been shown to have a higher sensitivity of approximately 94 % for the detection of common duct stones [14]. EUS is covered more thoroughly in another section of this text.

Diagnosis by CT

The reported sensitivity of standard CT for choledocholithiasis is between 72 and 88 % [15–17]. CT with intravenous contrast allows for better visualization of the biliary tree (Fig. 3.4) although often non-contrast CT is adequate. When choledocholithiasis is diagnosed by standard CT, it is often depicted as a calcified object in the common bile duct. It should, however, be noted that the CT appearances of stones may vary, as on

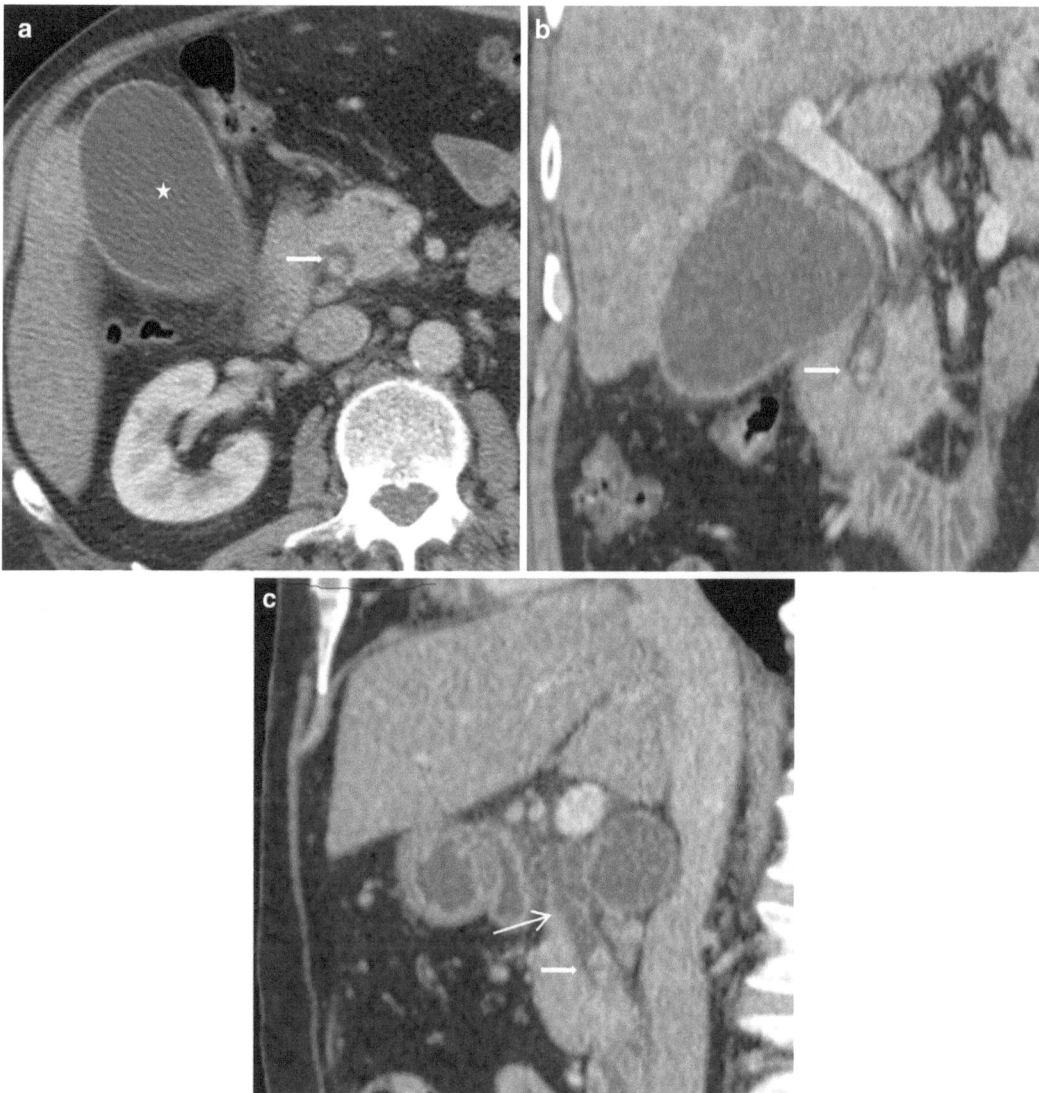

Fig. 3.4 CT Demonstrating stones in the distal common bile duct. Axial (**a**), Coronal (**b**), and Sagittal (**c**) images at the level of the common bile duct (*thin arrow*, **c**) showed a distended gallbladder (*star*, **a**) with mild wall thicken-ing. The common bile duct is mildly dilated and in the distal duct there are two hyperdense rounded structures representing stones (*thick arrows*, **a–c**)

radiographs, ranging from being heavily calcified to being slightly less radiopaque than bile to having gas attenuation as the result of foci of nitrogen gas contained within the stone [18]. The common bile duct can be traced to the pancreatic head on most contrast and non-contrast enhanced CT's. Coronal reconstructions also help visualize the common bile duct.

CT cholangiography can also be performed by giving iopodic acid intravenously. The patient is imaged after several hours when contrast is excreted, thus opacifying the biliary tree. This technique has a sensitivity reported to be about 92 % [19]. CT cholangiography is not readily available at all institutions, takes planning and time for excretion to occur, and carries the risk of renal tubular deposition of uric acid from the iopodic acid. However, it can be considered for patients who are not candidates for MRI.

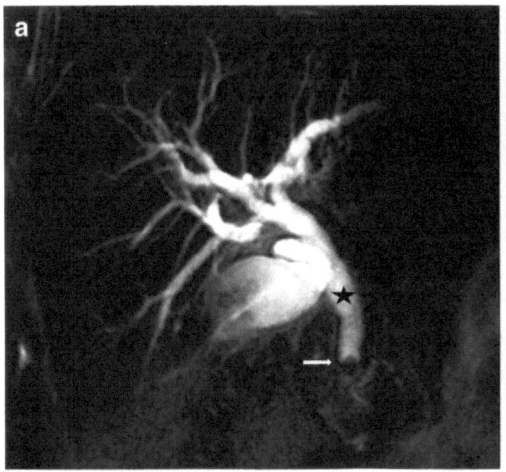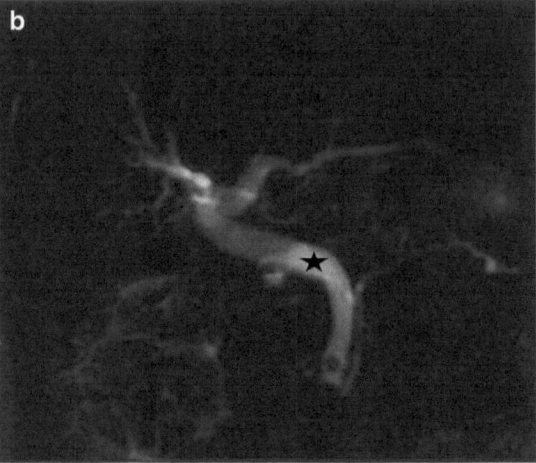

Fig. 3.5 MRCP demonstrating a common bile duct stone. MRCP images from two separate patients demonstrate a dilated biliary tree and a dilated common bile duct (*star*, **a** and **b**) in each patient. In the distal CBD of each patient, there is a rounded low signal structure (*arrow*, **a** and **b**) which represents a stone and which is causing upstream dilatation of the biliary tree

Diagnosis by MRI

MRI is often requested in the setting of the clinical suspicion of CBD stones based on a patient's symptoms, suggestive laboratory data or when US or CT findings are not definitive. Unlike CT, no radiation risk is present. MR cholangiopancreatography (MRCP) has a reported sensitivity and specificity of 89–100 % and 83–100 %, respectively [20, 21]. MRCP uses a T2 weighted sequence. The biliary tree stands out as high (bright) signal on T2 weighted imaging. As with CT, detection rates improve when slice thickness of 3 mm or less is acquired. This allows one to trace the biliary tree to the duodenum. High sensitivity and specificity for the detection of biliary filling defects and of stones is likely because all stones manifest as relatively low-signal-intensity (dark) foci with T2 weighting (Fig. 3.5). Because of its very high contrast resolution, MR cholangiography can demonstrate calculi as small as 2 mm despite its limited spatial resolution compared with ERCP [22]. However, it should be noted that although tiny stones have been detected, MRI can easily miss stones smaller than 3 mm [23].

It is important to note that air can mimic the appearance of a CBD stone as depicted on MR. Since calcium and air both demonstrate low signal on T2 weighted images they both appear as filling defects in the CBD. Some clues for distinction would be that air, unlike stones, is often in the nondependent portion of the duct.

Differential Diagnosis

Although biliary obstruction is often caused by stones, there are several other benign and malignant conditions that can result in biliary obstruction. Malignancies to consider include cholangiocarcinoma, ampulla of Vater carcinoma, and pancreatic adenocarcinoma. Benign processes that may cause biliary obstruction include parasite infections, other inflammatory conditions, strictures, iatrogenic causes and dilated periductal veins.

Cholangiocarcinoma

Cholangiocarcinoma is a primary malignant tumor of the bile ducts and may develop at any level within the biliary tree. When the tumor involves the confluence of the left and right hepatic ducts at the

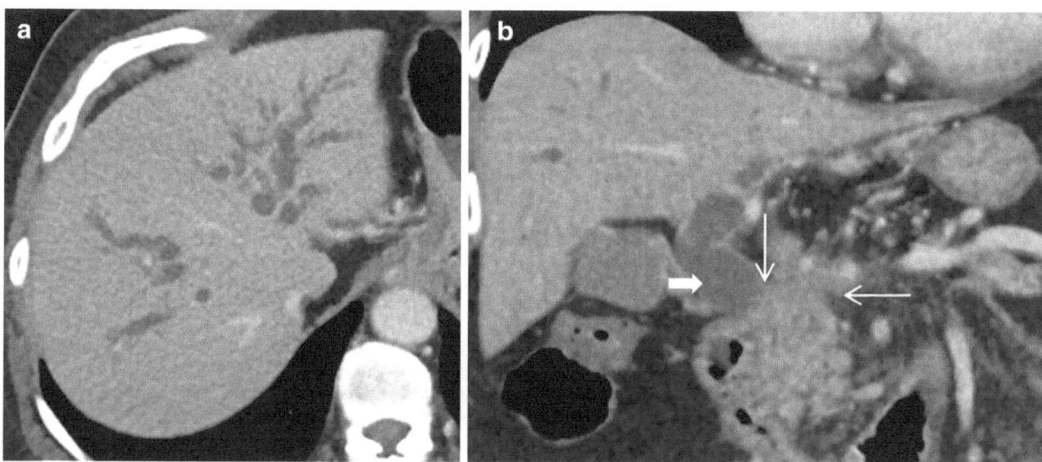

Fig. 3.6 Biliary ductal dilatation caused by pancreatic mass. Axial (**a**) and Coronal (**b**) CT images demonstrate dilated intrahepatic ducts (*star*, **a**). The common bile duct (*thick arrow*, **b**) is also dilated to the pancreatic head where there is an infiltrative mass (*thin arrows*, **b**) involving the head of the pancreas

porta hepatis, it is referred to as a Klatskin tumor. Dilatation of the biliary tree can be followed to the point of obstruction where it may be possible to detect a solid poorly defined mass.

Ampulla of Vater Carcinoma

Carcinoma of the ampulla of Vater is a relatively uncommon tumor accounting for about 1 % of all adenocarcinomas and for approximately 5 % of gastrointestinal tract carcinomas [24]. Imaging studies demonstrate the obstructive effects of the tumor on the biliary or pancreatic ducts. However, although the double-duct sign (dilatation of both common bile duct and pancreatic duct) may be obvious, the tumor itself is often not apparent with imaging [25, 26].

Pancreatic Adenocarcinoma

Tumors in the head of the pancreas can result in early biliary obstruction and often result in the clinical presentation of jaundice. Ultrasound is usually performed to rule out choledocholithiasis and look for biliary dilatation in patients who present with jaundice and abdominal pain.

Multidetector computed tomography is the preferred initial imaging modality in patients with clinical suspicion for pancreatic cancer (Fig. 3.6). MRI has assumed an increasingly prominent role in the diagnosis of pancreatic cancer and is currently used interchangeably with MDCT.

Parasites

Parasitic involvement of the liver and/or biliary tree is an important differential diagnosis in patients with jaundice. Parasites such as *Ascaris lumbricoides* (round worm), *Clonorchis sinensis*, and *Fasciola hepatica* can infest biliary tree. Parasitic infestations can result in biliary obstruction, cholangitis, and even cholangiocarcinoma. Worms can be visualized in dilated biliary tree on imaging.

Mirizzi's syndrome

Mirizzi's syndrome refers to obstruction of the common hepatic duct due to extrinsic compression from an impacted stone in the cystic duct or in Hartmann's pouch of the gallbladder. Several studies demonstrated that this condition has been estimated to occur in 0.7–1.8 % of all cholecystectomies [27–30]. Predisposing factors in the development of Mirizzi's syndrome include a long cystic duct coursing parallel to the common hepatic duct and low insertion of the cystic duct into the CBD [31, 32].

Features that suggest Mirizzi's syndrome on ultrasound include the following [33]: dilatation of the biliary tree above the level of the gallbladder neck, the presence of a stone impacted in the gallbladder neck and an abrupt change in bile duct caliber from dilated common hepatic duct above the level of the stone to non-dilated common bile duct below the level of the stone.

The main role of CT in patients with suspected Mirizzi's syndrome is to exclude a malignancy in the area of porta hepatis or in the liver. MRI and MRCP are playing an increasingly important role and have the additional advantage of showing the extent of inflammation around the gallbladder that may help differentiate Mirizzi's syndrome from other gallbladder pathologies such as gallbladder malignancy. Typical MRCP features of Mirizzi's syndrome include cholelithiasis, a stone in the cystic duct, focal stricture of the CHD, dilatation of the intrahepatic bile ducts and proximal CHD, and a normal-caliber distal CBD [31, 34, 35].

References

1. Puente SG, Bannura GC. Radiological anatomy of the biliary tract: variations and congenital abnormalities. World J Surg. 1983;7:271–6.
2. Mortele KJ, Ros PR. Anatomic variants of the biliary tree: MR cholangiographic findings and clinical applications. AJR Am J Roentgenol. 2001;177:389–94.
3. Gazelle GS, Lee MJ, Mueller PR. Cholangiographic segmental anatomy of the liver. RadioGraphics. 1994;14:1005–13.
4. Mortelé KJ, Rocha TC, Streeter JL, et al. Multimodality imaging of pancreatic and biliary congenital anomalies. RadioGraphics. 2006;26(3):715–31.
5. Turner MA, Fulcher AS. The cystic duct: normal anatomy and disease processes. RadioGraphics. 2001;21:13–22.
6. Bortoff GA, Chen MY, Ott DJ, Wolfman NT, Routh WD. Gallbladder stones: imaging and intervention. RadioGraphics. 2000;20:751–66.
7. Zeman RK. Cholelithiasis and cholecystitis. In: Gore RM, Levine MS, Laufer I, editors. Textbook of gastrointestinal radiology. Philadelphia, PA: Saunders; 1994. p. 1636–74.
8. Laing FC, Jeffrey RB, Wing VW. Improved visualisation of choledocholithiasis by sonography. AJR Am J Roentgenol. 1984;143:949–52.
9. Dong B, Chen M. Improved sonographic visualisation of choledocholithiasis. J Clin Ultrasound. 1987; 15:185–90.
10. Rickes S, Treiber G, Mönkemüller K, et al. Impact of the operator's experience on value of high-resolution transabdominal ultrasound in the diagnosis of choledocholithiasis: a prospective comparison using endoscopic retrograde cholangiography as the gold standard. Scand J Gastroenterol. 2006;41:838–43.
11. Ortega D, Burns PN, Hope Simpson D, et al. Tissue harmonic imaging: is it a benefit for bile duct sonography? AJR Am J Roentgenol. 2001;176(3):653–9.
12. Kane RA. The biliary system. In: Goldberg BB, Kurtz AB, editors. Gastrointestinal ultrasonography. Edinburgh: Churchill Livingstone; 1988. p. 75–137.
13. Dewbury KC, Smith CL. The misdiagnosis of common bile duct stones with ultrasound. Br J Radiol. 1983;56:625–30.
14. Tse F, Liu L, Barkun AN, Armstrong D, Moayyedi P. EUS: a meta-analysis of test performance in suspected choledocholithiasis. Gastrointest Endosc. 2008;67(2):235–44.
15. Anderson SW, Lucey BC, Varghese JC, Soto JA. Accuracy of MDCT in the diagnosis of choledocholithiasis. AJR Am J Roentgenol. 2006;187:174–80.
16. Neitlich JD, Topazian M, Smith RC, Gupta A, Burrell MI, Rosenfield AT. Detection of choledocholithiasis: comparison of unenhanced helical CT and endoscopic retrograde cholangiopancreatography. Radiology. 1997;203:753–7.
17. Anderson SW, Rho E, Soto JA. Detection of biliary duct narrowing and choledocholithiasis: accuracy of portal venous phase multidetector CT. Radiology. 2008;247:418–27.
18. Chan WC, Joe BN, Coakley FV, et al. Gallstone detection at CT in vitro: effect of peak voltage setting. Radiology. 2006;241:546–53.
19. Soto JA, Alvarez O, Munera F, Velez SM, Valencia J, Ramirez N. Diagnosing bile duct stones: comparison of unenhanced helical CT, oral contrast-enhanced CT cholangiography and MR cholangiography. AJR Am J Roentgenol. 2000;175:1127–34.
20. Hekimoglu K, Ustundag Y, Dusak A, et al. MRCP vs. ERCP in the evaluation of biliary pathologies: review of current literature. J Dig Dis. 2008;9:162–9.
21. Romagnuolo J, Bardou M, Rahme E, Joseph L, Reinhold C, Barkun AN. Magnetic resonance cholangiopancreatography: a meta-analysis of test performance in suspected biliary disease. Ann Intern Med. 2003;139:547–57.
22. Fulcher AS, Turner MA, Capps GW, Zfass AM, Baker KM. Half-Fourier RARE MR cholangiopancreatography: experience in 300 subjects. Radiology. 1998;207:21–32.

23. Yeh BM, Liu PS, Soto JA, Corvera CA, Hussain HK. MR imaging and CT of the biliary tract. RadioGraphics. 2009;29:1669–88.
24. Karayiannakis AJ, Kakolyris S, Kouklakis G, et al. Synchronous carcinoma of the ampulla of Vater and colon cancer. Case Rep Gastroenterol. 2011;5(2):301–7.
25. Zeman RK, Burrell MI. Gallbladder and bile duct imaging: a clinical radiologic approach. New York: Churchill Livingstone; 1987. p. 575.
26. Pandolfo I, Scribano E, Blandino A, et al. Tumors of the ampulla diagnosed by CT hypotonic duodenography. J Comput Assist Tomogr. 1990;14:199–200.
27. Mishra MC, Vashishtha S, Tandon R. Biliobiliary fistula: preoperative diagnosis and management implications. Surgery. 1990;108:835.
28. Corlette MB, Bismuth H. Biliobiliary fistula. A trap in the surgery of cholelithiasis. Arch Surg. 1975; 110:377.
29. Redaelli CA, Büchler MW, Schilling MK, et al. High coincidence of Mirizzi syndrome and gallbladder carcinoma. Surgery. 1997;121:58.
30. Beltran MA, Csendes A, Cruces KS. The relationship of Mirizzi syndrome and cholecystoenteric fistula: validation of a modified classification. World J Surg. 2008;32:2237–44.
31. Menias CO, Surabhi VR, Prasad SR, Wang HL, Narra VR, Chintapalli KN. Mimics of cholangiocarcinoma: spectrum of disease. RadioGraphics. 2008;28(4): 1115–29.
32. Ahlawat SK, Singhania R, Al-Kawas FH. Mirizzi syndrome. Curr Treat Options Gastroenterol. 2007; 10(2):102–10.
33. Becker CD, Hassler H, Terrier F. Preoperative diagnosis of the Mirizzi syndrome: limitations of sonography and computed tomography. AJR Am J Roentgenol. 1984;143(3):591–6.
34. Choi BW, Kim MJ, Chung JJ, Chung JB, Yoo HS, Lee JT. Radiologic findings of Mirizzi syndrome with emphasis on MRI. Yonsei Med J. 2000;41(1):144–6.
35. Kim PN, Outwater EK, Mitchell DG. Mirizzi syndrome: evaluation by MRI imaging. Am J Gastroenterol. 1999;94(9):2546–50.

Making the Diagnosis: Gastroenterology

Joshua R. Peck, Nicholas Latchana, Samer El-Dika, and Sheetal Sharma

Introduction

Choledocholithiasis describes the presence of a stone impacted in the common bile duct (CBD). Though usually found in the gallbladder, 10–15 % of patients with gallstones will have stone migration into the bile duct (secondary choledocholithiasis) [1]. A further complicating matter is that stones can form spontaneously in the CBD, known as primary choledocholithiasis. Certain medical and anatomical conditions, such as cystic fibrosis, and periampullary diverticulum predispose individuals to forming stones in the CBD [2]. Recognizing that stones can form even after a cholecystectomy is crucial for physicians to not miss potentially treatable causes of disease.

There are multiple well-established risk factors for CBD stones. Non-black race (particularly Native Americans), female gender, and pregnancy have been shown to have increased risk [3]. Individuals with obesity as well as those who undergo rapid weight loss (as seen in bariatric surgery) are also at increased risk [4, 5]. Certain medical comorbidities, such as those with Crohn's disease, hemolytic anemias, primary sclerosing cholangitis, and cirrhosis are more likely to have stones [6–9]. Lastly, patients on certain medications, such as oral contraceptive therapies as well as total parenteral nutrition (TPN) have been shown to increase risk of stone formation [9, 10].

J.R. Peck, M.D. (✉)
Division of Gastroenterology, Hepatology, and Nutrition, Department of Internal Medicine, The Ohio State University Wexner Medical Center, Columbus, OH, USA
e-mail: Joshua.Peck@osumc.edu

N. Latchana, M.D., M.S.
Department of General Surgery, The Ohio State University Wexner Medical Center, Columbus, OH, USA

S. El-Dika, M.D., M.Sc.
Division of Gastroenterology, Hepatology, and Nutrition, Department of Internal Medicine, The Ohio State University Wexner Medical Center, Columbus, OH, USA

Section of Advanced Therapeutic Endoscopy, Division of Gastroenterology, The Ohio State University Wexner Medical Center, Columbus, OH, USA

S. Sharma, M.D.
Section of Advanced Therapeutic Endoscopy, Division of Gastroenterology, The Ohio State University Wexner Medical Center, Columbus, OH, USA
e-mail: Sheetal.Sharma@osumc.edu

Physical Examination

Choledocholithiasis can range in presentation from asymptomatic to overt presentation with decompensated cholangitis [11]. It can be detected incidentally during workup in up to 7–20 % of patients with gallbladder stones awaiting cholecystectomy. CBD stones can otherwise vary in symptom presentation, ranging from biliary colic, obstructive jaundice, cholangitis, or acute pancreatitis. The right upper quadrant pain of choledocholithiasis may mirror classic biliary colic; however, symptoms tend to last longer (greater than 6 h, where classical biliary colic tends to last less than an hour). Less common presentations include biliary fibrosis and choledochoduodenal fistulas.

Cholangitis is perhaps the most feared complication of choledocholithiasis, with retrospective studies indicating CBD stones were present in 28–70 % of affected individuals [12]. The classically taught physical exam findings are Charot's triad of right upper quadrant pain, jaundice, and fevers but recent series have found all three present in only 15–20 % of patients [13]. Reynald's pentad, which adds hypotension and altered mental status to the triad, is even less common. It is imperative to recognize and treat acute cholangitis, as the mortality ranges from 11 to 30 % [14–16].

Laboratory Findings

As would be expected with an obstructive CBD stone, laboratory values tend to show a cholestatic pattern. Multiple studies have shown the most utility is the negative predictive value of liver biochemical tests [17, 18]. Whereas the negative predictive value of completely normal liver biochemical test is estimated to be more than 97 %, the positive predictive value of abnormal liver tests is estimated at only 15 %. As abnormal lab values increase, so does the likelihood of CBD stones [19].

In patients with cholangitis, labs typically show a cholestatic and inflammatory pattern. Labs demonstrating cholestasis may include an elevated alkaline phosphatase (ALP) and γ-glutamyl transpeptidase (GGT), which are elevated in approximately 90 % of individuals with cholangitis. Other cholestatic labs include elevated total and direct bilirubin, as well as elevated serum transaminases, with aspartate alanine aminotransferase (ALT) tending to be higher than aspartate transaminase.

Inflammatory labs may include an elevated white blood cell count, c-reactive protein, and erythrocyte sedimentation rate [20].

As with other causes of acute pancreatitis, patients who present with gallstone pancreatitis typically have elevations in serum amylase and lipase greater than three times the upper limit of normal. The diagnosis of gallstone pancreatitis is supported with concurrent elevation in serum ALT ≥ 150 IU/L [21], and carries a 95 % positive predictive value in diagnosing acute gallstone pancreatitis in patients with acute pancreatitis. AST levels are also frequently elevated.

Imaging

Because laboratory data can be normal in patients with choledocholithiasis, imaging of the CBD serves as an adjunct in establishing the presence of a CBD stone. Transabdominal ultrasonography (US) is the preferred initial imaging modality in patients with symptoms concerning for cholecystitis or symptomatic cholelithiasis. Though the sensitivity is poor for detecting actual impacted stones in the CBD, sensitivity approaches 77–87 % for detecting the common finding of a dilated CBD [17]. Ductal dilation of 6 mm or greater has been shown to correlate with high likelihood of choledocholithiasis, even when a stone is not visualized. US offers numerous other benefits as the initial imaging test of choice, including the relatively low cost, lack of radiation, and availability at most locations (including the emergency room). A significant limitation of ultrasonography is that it is highly operator dependent.

In multiple healthcare settings, computed tomography (CT) scans of the abdomen are frequently obtained in patients presenting with abdominal pain, who then go one to be diagnosed with choledocholithiasis. Abdominal CT has an increased sensitivity and specificity as compared to US (65–88 % and 73–97 %, respectively). Due to the associated radiation, the need for iodinated contrast agents and the associated nephrotoxicity, and relatively higher cost of CT, US is still the preferred initial method to evaluate for CBD stones.

Abdominal X-ray (AXR) without adjunct fluoroscopic endoscopy (i.e., ERCP) has a very limited role in the diagnosis or management of choledocholithiasis. It lacks significant sensitivity and only picks up on large, calcified stones. Only an estimated 10 % of gallstones are radiolucent [22]. AXR is of most use in excluding nonbiliary intraabdominal pathology which may mimic biliary symptoms (i.e., severe constipation, ileus, small bowel obstruction).

ERCP is the only endoscopic procedure which can both identify and treat CBD stones. It has a sensitivity of 89 % and a specificity of nearly 100 % in identifying CBD stones [23]. ERCP is an invasive procedure which carries a relatively high morbidity of 5 % and mortality of <1 % which is greatly influenced by the experience of the performing endoscopist [24]. Adverse events include pancreatitis, bleeding, and perforations, among many others. ERCP for suspected or confirmed CBD stones is advocated to primarily prevent cholangitis and cholecystitis. Those with ERCP and stone clearance should have a laparoscopic cholecystectomy within several weeks, as delays have shown in increase recurrent biliary events [25]. Because of the high risk of procedural complications, the role of first-line ERCP in choledocholithiasis is generally reserved for patients at high-risk for having a CBD stone, or in patients presenting with cholangitis [26].

Magnetic Resonance Cholangiopancreatography (MRCP) is the most sensitive (85–92 %) and specific (93–97 %) noninvasive method to evaluate for CBD stones [17]. It is considered by many practitioners as the gold standard for the detection of choledocholithiasis given the overall safety profile and lack of ionizing radiation. An important limitation is that the sensitivity is decreased for smaller stones (under 6 mm) in the distal duct as well as stones in a dilated distal duct. Endoscopic ultrasonography (EUS) has equal sensitivity and specificity to MRCP in the detection of most CBD stones [17]. It does offer advantages to MRCP which make it a very useful modality in a variety of situations. First, it is superior to MRCP in detecting small stones (<5 mm) as well as evaluating for biliary sludge, particularly those near the ampulla [27]. Second, in many situations it can be immedi-

ately followed by an ERCP. This is often advantageous because it eliminates delay in treatment that patients often experience in having an MRCP performed, waiting for interpretation of images, and then needing to schedule a procedure potentially on a separate day Recent studies have demonstrated that EUS prior to ERCP allows for a significant reduction in unnecessary ERCP in those with suspected CBD obstruction The ability to perform both exams simultaneously, also prevents delays and decreases risk of interval cholangitis [28, 29]. Additionally, EUS can be performed on certain populations who are unable to undergo magnetic resonance imagining, such as those with defibrillators, pacemakers, and other metal hardware in the body. Lastly, it is possible to perform the procedure bedside in critically ill patients who may not be able to safely travel for an MRCP.

EUS does have limitations, especially when compared with MRCP. The most obvious and significant difference is that EUS is an invasive procedure which requires sedation. Though complications are rare (0.1–0.3 %) [17], they do still harbor significant morbidity and mortality not seen with MRCP. In addition, EUS may have limited accessibility based on both the training of the endoscopist as well as equipment availability at smaller centers. Lastly, EUS may be extremely difficult or even impossible in patients who have abnormal anatomy (i.e., after Roux-en-Y bypass, Billroth II surgery, or in severe pyloric stenosis) [30].

How to Approach Patient with Suspected or Confirmed Stones

Most individuals with confirmed choledocholithiasis will need a cholecystectomy. The rationale behind removing the gallbladder is to reduce the risk of recurrent CBD stones both from stones concurrently contained within the gallbladder as well as from de novo formation. Studies have shown increased risk of recurrent biliary disease without cholecystectomy, such as recurrent cholecystitis, biliary colic, choledocholithiasis, and gallstone pancreatitis. For example, the risk of recurrent gallstone pancreatitis ranges from 75 to 90 % of persons with an intact gallbladder; the risk decreases to <10 % in individuals after cholecystectomy [31, 32].

High Risk of Choledocholithiasis

Approaching the patient with suspected choledocholithiasis can be a daunting task, as decisions need to be made which are associated with significant medical costs and possibly morbidities. As demonstrated above, there is neither a clear cut laboratory, nor transabdominal ultrasonographic marker that is 100 % sensitive or specific for the presence of a CBD stone. Missing a CBD stone in a patient can be a serious event, as there is an associated increased risk in developing recurrent cholecystitis, cholangitis, or pancreatitis.

Given the diagnostic challenge, guidelines have been made to assist the practitioner in categorizing patients presenting with biliary symptoms by risk of having a CBD stone, as well as the subsequent therapeutic approach [17]. Very strong predictors include a visualized CBD stone on ultrasonography, clinical ascending cholangitis, or a serum total bilirubin of >4 mg/dL. If either of the aforementioned symptoms are present, the patient has a >50 % chance of having choledocholithiasis and it places the patient in the "high risk" category [25].

Strong predictors of choledocholithiasis include ultrasonographic findings of a dilated CBD >6 mm in individuals with an intact gallbladder, as well as a serum total bilirubin level of 1.8–4 mg/dL. Individuals with both of these findings are also stratified in the "high risk" category.

Individuals in the "high risk" category should proceed to either ERCP or cholecystectomy with IOC. Deciding between the two depends on multiple factors including institutional resources available and the individual's severity of illness [33]. For example, in the unstable patient it is generally preferred to first go to ERCP to decompress the duct. After stability is achieved it is up to the discretion of the surgeon when to progress with cholecystectomy. An important situation to

consider is that of the patient presenting with overt cholangitis, whether or not a stone is visualized on imaging. In these patients, the endoscopist should proceed first with an ERCP to decompress the CBD. Other populations of note include those with an unacceptable operative risk, such as those with decompensated cirrhosis. In these patients, performing an ERCP should be the first procedure undertaken. Afterwards, a multidisciplinary discussion weighing risks versus benefits of cholecystectomy can be undertaken and specific patient factors accounted for

Intermediate Risk of Choledocholithiasis

Moderate predictors of a CBD stone include age >55 years old, clinical gallstone pancreatitis, or the presence of abnormal liver biochemical tests other than bilirubin (i.e., AST/ALT, GGT, or ALP). The presence of one or more of these predictors, or if one but not both of the strong predictors are found, this places individuals in the "intermediate risk" category and portends a 10–50 % risk of choledocholithiasis. Patients with an intermediate risk of CBD stones can be approached in a variety of different ways, and the specific approach will vary by institutional resources and experience.

Broadly, the approach can be categorized as preoperative versus intraoperative. The preoperative approach is designed to initially evaluate for a CBD stone with the minimally invasive method, and use that information to determine whether an ERCP prior to cholecystectomy or an intraoperative cholangiogram (IOC) with stone retrieval at the time of surgery. As discussed in a separate chapter, the decision to proceed with ERCP vs IOC varies based on a multitude of factors. To evaluate for a stone, one can chose EUS or MRCP. As previously mentioned, there are distinct advantages to each procedure and the decision on which to use is individualized. If a stone is noted on either of those modalities, an ERCP should be the next step to clear the duct prior to cholecystectomy. At institutions where EUS and MRCP are not available, one can proceed to either preoperative ERCP or directly to surgery with either IOC or laparoscopic ultrasonography, as discussed in a separate chapter.

An alternative approach is to evaluate for the presence of a CBD stone during the time of cholecystectomy. This can be either with an IOC or laparoscopic US. If no stone is found, the surgeon can proceed directly with a cholecystectomy. If a stone is found at that time, either an intraductal or transductal approach can be done to remove it. In the event that the surgeon is unable to perform stone removal, either because of technical limitations or lack of proper equipment, a postoperative ERCP can be performed [34–36].

Low Risk of Choledocholithiasis

Individuals with symptomatic cholelithiasis who lack any of the previously mentioned criteria have a less than 10 % chance of harboring a CBD stone [17, 18]. In this group, it is not cost efficient to perform any further evaluation for choledocholithiasis. It is therefore recommended that these patients can directly proceed to cholecystectomy without preoperative CBD stone evaluation. Whether patients in the "low risk" group should have routine IOC during cholecystectomy is an area of debate, and is outside the realm of this chapter.

Gallstone Pancreatitis

Gallstone pancreatitis may be triggered by the transient migration of a gallstone, but can present with a coexisting CBD stone as well. Gallstone pancreatitis can also present simultaneously with cholangitis. The role of ERCP is well established in patients with gallstone pancreatitis who demonstrate disease in the CBD. There is however no evidence to support its role in gallstone pancreatitis without either cholangitis, a CBD stone or dilated CBD seen on imaging, or increasing liver tests. In patients with persistent elevated liver tests or a dilated CBD, EUS or MRCP should be considered to evaluate for a stone prior to proceeding with ERCP [37].

What If ERCP Is Unsuccessful?

Uncommonly, ERCP may be unsuccessful at removing a CBD stone. This is typically from difficult anatomy, either as a result of surgery (i.e., Roux-en-Y, Billroth II), duodenal diverticulum, biliary strictures, or technical difficulty cannulating the sphincter of Oddi [38]. Options including repeating ERCP on a subsequent day or transfer to a tertiary center with more experience in ERCP have been shown to carry a high success rate of 88–96 % when the initial ERCP failed [25, 39]; however, the decision should be on a case-by-case basis depending on the etiology of failed procedure. Another option is a rendezvous procedure, where an interventional radiologist (IR) performs percutaneous transhepatic cholangiography (PTC) and places a transpapillary guidewire. The endoscopist can then use the guidewire during the ERCP to assist with cannulation. A newer method of biliary access is EUS guided wire placement, with subsequent ERCP using the wire once again as a guide. This depends greatly on local expertise, but can be superior to IR placement in specific clinical scenarios when done in a tertiary care center. Lastly, it may be appropriate to proceed directly to surgery for IOC and either open or laparoscopic exploration of the CBD can be undertaken. Regardless of the method chosen, all patients with a high suspicion for a CBD stone or with an identified CBD stone ultimately need exploration of the CBD.

Timing

Cholangitis

Because individuals with choledocholithiasis can exhibit a wide spectrum of severity, the urgency of stone removal and ultimately cholecystectomy is dependent on the initial presentation. In persons who present with cholangitis, the decision on when to proceed with ERCP is based upon stability and initial response to antibiotics. In individuals with persistent signs of end-organ damage despite aggressive fluid resuscitation and appropriate antibiotic use, emergent ERCP is indicated for source control of sepsis.

Current recommendations are for stable individuals with cholangitis who respond to fluid and antibiotics to have an ERCP within 24–48 h of presentation [12], and ideally before 72 h [25]. Furthermore, newer evidence shows that delay of more than 72 h has been shown to carry an increase in morbidity and mortality, as well as increased hospital length-of-stay and overall cost [40]. If a patient has hemodynamic or clinical deterioration during this time, they should be brought more urgently for ERCP.

Gallstone Pancreatitis

Patients who present with gallstone pancreatitis and concurrent cholangitis should have an ERCP within 24 h of presentation, with the urgency depending on clinical stability and response to fluids and antibiotics. In patients with gallstone pancreatitis and labs or imaging showing biliary obstruction who do not have cholangitis, the optimal timing of ERCP has not been established. Worsening jaundice or ductal dilation indicates the need for more acute intervention [41].

Choledocholithiasis

For patients at high risk for choledocholithiasis or imaging confirming its presence who do not have cholecystitis, cholangitis, or gallstone pancreatitis, the optimal timing for ERCP is not fully established. The decision on when to perform ERCP is dependent on the patient's clinical stability, physician/endoscopy availability, and the severity of symptoms. The rationale for clearance of the duct in these patients who may have minimal to no symptoms is based upon studies showing a 21–34 % risk of CBD stones spontaneously migrating [25, 42, 43]. Migrated stones can cause both pancreatitis and cholangitis, which each carry increased morbidity and mortality.

Cholecystectomy

The timing of cholecystectomy for all patients with CBD disease depends upon the presentation. For individuals who present with isolated choledocholithiasis who undergo preoperative ERCP, cholecystectomy should be performed within 2 weeks [25]. Postponing surgery after 2 weeks has been shown to carry an increased risk of interval development of cholecystitis, recurrent choledocholithiasis, biliary colic, and gallstone pancreatitis [44]. Furthermore, delay is associated with higher rates of conversion to open cholecystectomy which carries increased morbidity and length of stay [45].

Without a cholecystectomy, patients with gallstone pancreatitis have up to a 30 % chance of developing recurrent pancreatitis, cholecystitis, or cholangitis within 6–18 weeks [32]. Patients presenting with mild or moderate gallstone pancreatitis (as categorized by the absence of organ failure $\geq$48 h) should have a cholecystectomy during the same hospitalization and within 1 week of presentation [46, 47]. In patients with severe pancreatitis (organ failure $\geq$ 48 h) or in those with necrotizing pancreatitis, cholecystectomy should be delayed at least 3 weeks due to increased infectious complications [46].

Cholecystectomy is indicated in surgically fit patients with cholangitis found to have concurrent gallstones or choledocholithiasis [48]. Due to concerns for infection and technical challenges in early operation, data is limited on the optimal timing of surgery. A study has shown reduced complications and recurrent disease when performed within 6 weeks of initial presentation [49].

Pre-procedural Labs

Current guidelines do not recommend routine testing of coagulation studies and hemoglobin/hematocrit prior to endoscopic intervention, unless patients have known bleeding disorders, anticoagulant use, or other conditions associated with acquired coagulopathies [50]. Many patients presenting with biliary illness requiring endoscopic or surgical treatment will be hospitalized and frequently have a variety of lab results available. Prior to either ERCP or surgical intervention, it is commonplace to ensure an INR ≤ 1.5 and a platelet count of ≥50 K/UL to reduce the risk of procedural bleeding. In patients with known bleeding or anemia, ensuring a hgb ≥ 7 g/dL (≥8 g/dL if known cardiac disease) is also prudent.

Pre-procedural Medications

Patients may be on medications which can increase risk of procedural bleeding, such as antiplatelet drugs and anticoagulants. A thorough discussion of the different medications and their pre-procedural management is outside the realm of this chapter. It is important to consider all the medications an individual is on, and discuss with the patient and other physicians assisting in management the risks, benefits, and alternatives to stopping drugs which may increase the risk of bleeding.

There is a limited role for routine antimicrobial use prior to endoscopy. Current guidelines support antibiotic prophylaxis before ERCP when obstructive biliary tract disease is known or suspected and there may be incomplete biliary drainage [51]. They also recommend antibiotic prophylaxis prior to ERCP in patients who have had liver transplantation. Antimicrobial selection should include drugs with enteric gram-negative and enterococci coverage. As of 2007, the American Heart Association no longer recommends prophylactic antibiotics against infective endocarditis in patients undergoing endoscopic procedures [52].

References

1. Tazuma S. Epidemiology, pathogenesis, and classification of biliary stones (common bile duct and intrahepatic). Best Pract Res Clin Gastroenterol. 2006;20(6):1075–83.
2. Oak JH, Paik CN, Chung WC, Lee K-M, Yang JM. Risk factors for recurrence of symptomatic common bile duct stones after cholecystectomy. Gastroenterol Res Pract. 2012;2012:6pages.
3. Sampliner RE, Bennett PH, Comess LJ, Rose FA, Burch TA. Gallbladder disease in Pima Indians. Demonstration of high prevalence and early onset by cholecystography. N Engl J Med. 1970;283(25):1358–64.
4. The epidemiology of gallstone disease in Rome, Italy. Part I. Prevalence data in men. The Rome Group for Epidemiology and Prevention of Cholelithiasis (GREPCO). Hepatology. 1988;8(4):904–6.
5. Liddle RA, Goldstein RB, Saxton J. Gallstone formation during weight-reduction dieting. Arch Intern Med. 1989;149(8):1750–3.
6. Lapidus A, Bangstad M, Astrom M, Muhrbeck O. The prevalence of gallstone disease in a defined cohort of patients with Crohn's disease. Am J Gastroenterol. 1999;94(5):1261–6.
7. Murakami J, Shimizu Y. Hepatic manifestations in hematological disorders. Int J Hepatol. 2013;2013:484903.
8. Conte D, Fraquelli M, Dieci MG, Lodi L, Dottorini F, Aimo GP, et al. Close relation between cirrhosis and gallstones. Cross sectional and longitudinal survey. Arch Intern Med. 1999;159(1):49–52.
9. Racine A, Bijon A, Fournier A, Mesrine S, Clavel-Chapelon F, Carbonnel F, et al. Menopausal hormone therapy and risk of cholecystectomy: a prospective study based on the French E3N cohort. Can Med Assoc J. 2013;185(7):555–61.
10. Dawes LG, Muldoon JP, Greiner MA, Bertolotti M. Cholecystokinin increases bile acid synthesis with total parenteral nutrition but does not prevent stone formation. J Surg Res. 1997;67(1):84–9.
11. Desai R, Shokouhi BN. Common bile duct stones - their presentation, diagnosis and management. Indian J Surg. 2009;71(5):229–37.
12. Kimura Y, Takada T, Kawarada Y, Nimura Y, Hirata K, Sekimoto M, Yoshida M, Mayumi T, Wada K, Miura F, Yasuda H, Yamashita Y, Nagino M, Hirota M, Tanaka A. Definitions, pathophysiology, and epidemiology of acute cholangitis and cholecystitis: Tokyo Guidelines. J Hepato-Biliary-Pancreat Surg. 2007;14(1):15–26.
13. Kinney TP. Management of ascending cholangitis. Gastrointest Endosc Clin N Am. 2007;17(2):289–306.
14. Chijiiwa K, Kozaki N, Naito T, Kameoka N, Tanaka M. Treatment of choice for choledocholithiasis in patients with acute obstructive suppurative cholangitis and liver cirrhosis. Am J Surg. 1995;170(4):356–60.
15. Csendes A, Diaz JC, Burdiles P, Maluenda F, Morales E. Risk factors and classification of acute suppurative cholangitis. Br J Surg. 1992;79(7):655–8.
16. Thompson J, Bennion RS, Pitt HA. An analysis of infectious failures in acute cholangitis. HPB Surg. 1994;8(2):139–45.
17. Maple JT, Ben-Menachem T, Anderson MA, Appalaneni V, Banerjee S, Cash BD, et al. The role of endoscopy in the evaluation of suspected choledocholithiasis. Gastrointest Endosc. 2010;71(1):1–9.

18. Yang MH, Chen TH, Wang SE, Tsai YF, Su CH, Wu CW, et al. Biochemical predictors for absence of common bile duct stones in patients undergoing laparoscopic cholecystectomy. Surg Endosc. 2008;22(7):1620–4.

19. Onken JE, Brazer SR, Eisen GM, Williams DM, Bouras EP, DeLong ER, et al. Predicting the presence of choledocholithiasis in patients with symptomatic cholelithiasis. Am J Gastroenterol. 1996;91(4):762–7.

20. Mosler P. Diagnosis and management of acute cholangitis. Curr Gastroenterol Rep. 2011;13(2):166–72.

21. Tenner S, Dubner H, Steinberg W. Predicting gallstone pancreatitis with laboratory parameters - a meta-analysis. Am J Gastroenterol. 1994;89(10):1863–6.

22. Cheifetz AS. Oxford American handbook of gastroenterology and hepatology. Oxford: Oxford University Press; 2011. p. 246–7.

23. Prat F, Amouyal G, Amouyal P, Pelletier G, Fritsch J, Choury AD, et al. Prospective controlled study of endoscopic ultrasonography and endoscopic retrograde cholangiography in patients with suspected commonbileduct lithiasis. Lancet. 1996;347(8994):75–9.

24. Adler DG, Baron TH, Davila RE, Egan J, Hirota WK, Leighton JA, et al. ASGE guideline: the role of ERCP in diseases of the biliary tract and the pancreas. Gastrointest Endosc. 2005;62(1):1–8.

25. Maple JT, Ikenberry SO, Anderson MA, Appalaneni V, Decker GA, Early D, et al. The role of endoscopy in the management of choledocholithiasis. Gastrointest Endosc. 2011;74(4):731–44.

26. Surlin V, Săftoiu A, Dumitrescu D. Imaging tests for accurate diagnosis of acute biliary pancreatitis. World J Gastroenterol. 2014;20(44):16544–94.

27. Tham TCK. Approach to jaundice. Gastrointestinal emergencies. Hoboken, NJ: Wiley-Blackwell; 2009. p. 25–33.

28. Benjaminov F, Stein A, Lichtman G, Pomeranz I, Konikoff FM. Consecutive versus separate sessions of endoscopic ultrasound (EUS) and endoscopic retrograde cholangiopancreatography (ERCP) for symptomatic choledocholithiasis. Surg Endosc. 2013;27(6):2117–21.

29. Zaheer A, Anwar M, Donohoe C, O'Keeffe S, Mushtaq H, Kelleher B, Clarke E, Kirca M, McKiernan S, Mahmud N, Keeling N, MacMathuna P, O'Toole D. The diagnostic accuracy of endoscopic ultrasound in suspected biliary obstruction and its impact on endoscopic retrograde cholangiopancreatography burden in real clinical practice: a consecutive analysis. Eur J Gastroenterol Hepatol. 2013;25(7):850–7.

30. Adams MA, Hosmer A, Wamsteker EJ, Anderson MA, Elta GH, Kubiliun NM, Kwon RS, Piraka CR, Scheiman JM, Waljee AK, Hussain HK, Elmunzer BJ. Predicting the likelihood of a persistent bile duct stone in patients with suspected choledocholithiasis: accuracy of existing guidelines and the impact of laboratory trends. Gastrointest Endosc. 2015;82(1):88–93.

31. Gurusamy KS, Farouk M, Tweedie JH. UK guidelines for management of acute pancreatitis: is it time to change? Gut. 2005;54(9):1344–5.

32. Hernandez V, Pascual I, Almela P, Anon R, Herreros B, Sanchiz V, et al. Recurrence of acute gallstone pancreatitis and relationship with cholecystectomy or endoscopic sphincterotomy. Am J Gastroenterol. 2004;99(12):2417–23.

33. Ng T, Amaral JF. Timing of endoscopic retrograde cholangiopancreatography and laparoscopic cholecystectomy in the treatment of choledocholithiasis. J Laparoendosc Adv Surg Tech A. 1999;9(1):31–7.

34. Kharbutli B, Velanovich V. Management of preoperatively suspected choledocholithiasis: a decision analysis. J Gastrointest Surg. 2008;12(11):1973–80.

35. Clayton ES, Connor S, Alexakis N, Leandros E. Meta-analysis of endoscopy and surgery versus surgery alone for common bile duct stones with the gallbladder in situ. Br J Surg. 2006;93(10):1185–91.

36. Rhodes M, Sussman L, Cohen L, Lewis MP. Randomised trial of laparoscopic exploration of common bile duct versus postoperative endoscopic retrograde cholangiography for common bile duct stones. Lancet. 1998;351(9097):159–61.

37. Kapetanos DJ. ERCP in acute biliary pancreatitis. World J Gastrointest Endosc. 2010;2(1):25–8.

38. Sanchez A, Rodriguez O, Bellorin O, Sanchez R, Benitez G. Laparoscopic common bile duct exploration in patients with gallstones and choledocholithiasis. JSLS. 2010;14(2):246–50.

39. Swan MP, Bourke MJ, Williams SJ, Alexander S, Moss A, Hope R, et al. Failed biliary cannulation: clinical and technical outcomes after tertiary referral endoscopic retrograde cholangiopancreatography. World J Gastroenterol. 2011;17(45):4993–8.

40. Khashab MA, Tariq A, Tariq U, Kim K, Ponor L, Lennon AM, et al. Delayed and unsuccessful endoscopic retrograde cholangiopancreatography are associated with worse outcomes in patients with acute cholangitis. Clin Gastroenterol Hepatol. 2012;10(10):1157–61.

41. Carroll JK, Herrick B, Gipson T, Lee SP. Acute pancreatitis: diagnosis, prognosis, and treatment. Am Fam Physician. 2007;75(10):1513–20.

42. Oría A, Alvarez J, Chiapetta L, Fontana JJ, Iovaldi M, Paladino A, Bianchi R, Frider B, et al. Risk factors for acute pancreatitis in patients with migrating gallstones. JAMA Surg. 1989;124(11):1295–6.

43. Frossard JL, Hadengue A, Amouyal G, Choury A, Marty O, Giostra E, Sivignon F, Sosa L, Amouyal P. Choledocholithiasis: a prospective study of spontaneous common bile duct stone migration. Gastrointest Endosc. 2000;51(2):175–9.

44. de Vries A, Donkervoort SC, van Geloven AA, Pierik EG. Conversion rate of laparoscopic cholecystectomy after endoscopic retrograde cholangiography in the treatment of choledocholithiasis: does the time interval matter? Surg Endosc. 2005;19(7):996–1001.

45. Schiphorst AH, Besselink MG, Boerma D, Timmer R, Wiezer MJ, van Erpecum KJ, Broeders IA, van Ramshorst B. Timing of cholecystectomy after endoscopic sphincterotomy for common bile duct stones. Surg Endosc. 2008;22(9):2046–50.

46. Uhl W, Müller C, Krähenbühl L, Schmid SW, Schölzel S, Büchler MW. Acute gallstone pancreatitis: timing of laparoscopic cholecystectomy in mild and severe disease. Surg Endosc. 1999;13(11):1070–6.

47. Aboulian A, Chan T, Yaghoubian A, Kaji AH, Putnam B, Neville A, Stabile BE, de Virgilio C. Early chole-cystectomy safely decreases hospital stay in patients with mild gallstone pancreatitis: a randomized pro-spective study. Ann Surg. 2010;251(4):615–9.

48. Nagino M, Takada T, Kawarada Y, Nimura Y, Yamashita Y, Tsuyuguchi T, Wada K, Mayumi T, Yoshida M, Miura F, Strasberg S, Pitt HA, Belghiti J, Fan S-T, Liau K-H, Belli G, Chen X-P, Lai EC-S, Philippi BP, Singh H, Supe A. Methods and timing of biliary drainage for acute cholangitis: Tokyo guidelines. J Hepatobiliary Pancreat Surg. 2007;14(1):68–77.

49. Li VK, Yum JL, Yeung YP. Optimal timing of elective laparoscopic cholecystectomy after acute cholangitis and subsequent clearance of choledocholithiasis. Am J Surg. 2010;200(4):483–8.

50. Levy MJ, Anderson MA, Baron TH, Banerjee S, Dominitz JA, Gan SI, et al. Position statement on rou-tine laboratory testing before endoscopic procedures. Gastrointest Endosc. 2008;68(5):827–32.

51. Khashab MA, Chithadi KV, Acosta RD, Bruining DH, Chandrasekhara V, Eloubeidi MA, et al. Antibiotic prophylaxis for GI endoscopy. Gastrointest Endosc. 2015;81(1):81–9.

52. Wilson W, Taubert KA, Gewitz M, Lockhart PB, Baddour LM, Levison M, et al. Prevention of infec-tive endocarditis: guidelines from the American Heart Association: a guideline from the American Heart Association Rheumatic Fever, Endocarditis and Kawasaki Disease Committee, Council on Cardiovascular Disease in the Young, and the Council on Clinical Cardiology, Council on Cardiovascular Surgery and Anesthesia, and the Quality of Care and Outcomes Research Interdisciplinary Working Group. J Am Dent Assoc. 2008;139(Suppl):3S–24.

Making the Diagnosis: Surgery, a Rational Approach to the Patient with Suspected CBD Stones

Robert D. Fanelli and Brandon D. Andrew

Introduction

Choledocholithiasis is a frequent complication of gallstone disease, occurring in 5–15 % of patients undergoing cholecystectomy. The risk of choledocholithiasis increases with age, with common bile duct stones (CBDS) identified in 30–60 % of patients over age 70 who are undergoing cholecystectomy. CBDS often are occult and asymptomatic, and are not associated with biochemical abnormalities [1–3]. It appears that as many as 30 % of CBDS will be passed spontaneously, but it is not possible to predict reliably which patients will pass stones spontaneously, or if all CBDS will be passed without intervention. CBDS are a significant problem because they may cause pancreatitis, jaundice, and ascending cholangitis, and may lead to significant morbidity, and even mortality.

R.D. Fanelli, M.D., M.H.A., F.A.C.S. (✉)
Department of Surgery, The Guthrie Clinic,
Sayre, PA, USA

Clinical Professor of Surgery, The Commonwealth
Medical College, Scranton, PA, USA

Clinical Professor of Surgery, SUNY Upstate Medical
University, Binghamton, NY, USA

Professor of Surgery, Albany Medical College,
Albany, NY, USA

B.D. Andrew, M.D.
Department of Surgery, The Guthrie Robert Packer
Hospital Residency Program in Surgery, Sayre, PA, USA

CBDS can be classified into primary stones and secondary stones. Primary stones are those which form in the intrahepatic or extrahepatic bile ducts, and largely are composed of calcium bilirubinate and small amounts of cholesterol and calcium salts; these also are referred to as pigment stones. Secondary CBDS are those that form in the gallbladder, largely composed of cholesterol, bile salts, and phospholipids, and then advance into the common bile duct through the cystic duct. In the USA, secondary CBDS are much more common than primary CBDS.

Principles of Management

CBDS can be managed preoperatively, intraoperatively, or postoperatively. The determination as to when CBDS are addressed largely depends on when CBDS are identified. Therefore, in order to pursue the most efficient approach to the management of CBDS, a high degree of suspicion must be maintained when evaluating and treating patients with gallstone disease, especially those considered to be at a higher than average risk for CBDS.

The primary goal in treating patients with gallstone disease in general is to reduce the likelihood of recurring symptoms, and to limit the likelihood of related comorbid conditions like sepsis and pancreatitis. Our goal as surgeons is to ensure the lowest possible rate of untreated

© Springer International Publishing Switzerland 2016
J.W. Hazey et al. (eds.), *Multidisciplinary Management of Common Bile Duct Stones*,
DOI 10.1007/978-3-319-22765-8_5

CBDS across all patients, and to accomplish this goal with cost-efficiency. Our approach involves stratifying patients appropriately with regard to their individual risks for CBDS, and using each patient's determined risk to algorithmically guide clinical management. Proper assessment is important to the efficient utilization of clinical resources as well. Patients with CBDS identified initially in the operating room often require longer blocks of time for treatment, altering the experience of subsequently scheduled patients, staff, and the availability of equipment for colleagues.

Risk Stratification

Risk stratification for CBDS is based on clinical history, physical examination findings, biochemical and imaging data, and the results of invasive investigations. A variety of risk stratification algorithms exist which strive to place the patient in groups of essentially, low, intermediate, or high risk for CBDS. No predictive model has been shown completely accurate in diagnosing CBDS; however, algorithmic approaches can be used to guide further diagnostic interventions [4]. Table 5.1 demonstrates relative risks of CBDS based on commonly utilized evaluation tools [2].

It is generally agreed that patients considered at low risk for CBDS may be taken to surgery directly, without the need for significant further evaluation for CBDS, and that patients at high risk for CBDS will require definitive preoperative evaluation, typically involving an invasive biliary intervention given that most of these patients already exhibit strong direct or indirect evidence of CBDS. It is, however, patients at intermediate risk for CBDS, who will require the most exhaustive preoperative evaluation guided by utility data and, to some extent, by available local expertise.

Preoperative Diagnostic Evaluation

Relevant Clinical Scenarios

CBDS can present as biliary colic, symptomatic or asymptomatic jaundice, bile duct stricture, acute pancreatitis, cholangitis with or without

Table 5.1 Clinical predictors for CBDS

Moderate risk	
• Liver function test other than bilirubin abnormal	
• Age > 55 years	
• Gallstone pancreatitis on presentation	
Strong risk	
• Bilirubin greater than 1.8 but less than 4.0 mg/dL	
• Dilated bile duct on transabdominal ultrasound > 8 mm	
Very strong risk	
• Bilirubin > 4 mg/dL	
• CBDS identified on transabdominal ultrasound	
• Cholangitis on presentation	
Predictors present	Risk for CBDS
None	Low
One, two, or three moderate	Intermediate
One strong with/without moderate	Intermediate
Two strong	High
One or more very strong	High

Adapted from ASGE Standards of Practice Committee [2]

sepsis, or concomitantly with biliopancreatic malignancy, or CBDS may be silent. Certain scenarios, like biliary pancreatitis and cholangitis, can inform the diagnosis of CBDS. Somewhat counterintuitively, there is evidence that biliary pancreatitis may not be a good indicator of persistent CBDS. Since pancreatitis occurs after stones pass through the ampulla, a clinical history of biliary pancreatitis might actually be an indicator that invasive CBD evaluation often will not be necessary. Borie et al. demonstrated that the risk of CBDS declined after the onset of, and recovery from, biliary pancreatitis, presumably due to the fact that CBDS already have passed through the ampulla [5]. A prospective population-based cohort study of 1171 patients showed that the presence of CBDS was not significantly predicted by pancreatitis, or by cholecystitis, and that the greatest agreement between elevated liver chemistries and CBDS was seen in elective patients without a history of pancreatitis or cholecystitis [6]. This and other analyses, suggests that patients who present with biliary pancreatitis are subjected to invasive biliary interventions more often than necessary, given their actual risk of CBDS [5]. Clearly, there is the need for alternative approaches to the evaluation of patients considered high risk for CBDS to avoid unnecessarily invasive methods, and their associated risks and complications. Ascending cholangitis, on the other hand, is associated with a very high risk of persistent CBDS, and there is widespread agreement that patients presenting with biliary sepsis should proceed to ERCP without much further investigation, the focus being placed instead on sepsis rescue [2, 7].

Physical Examination Findings

Jaundice in a patient presenting with right upper quadrant pain may indicate the presence of CBDS. A prospective study showed that jaundice was a significant predictor of common bile duct stones on univariate analysis but not on multiple logistic regression [7]. A patient with jaundice without other signs of acute biliary obstruction should have non-biliary causes of jaundice ruled out as part of the initial evaluation, and certainly, prior to any invasive evaluations of the biliary tree.

Biochemical Tests

Choledocholithiasis is a dynamic disease process. CBDS may cause intermittent obstruction as they migrate through the common bile duct (CBD), or they may become trapped within the CBD in obstructive or nonobstructive patterns. These phenomena may cause variable elevations of the liver chemistries. Additionally, the lag time between obstruction and the rising and falling of liver chemistries impairs their diagnostic utility [8].

There are a number of clinical scenarios associated with elevated liver chemistries, mimicking CBDS: Sphincter of Oddi dysfunction, spontaneous passage of CBDS, extrinsic compression of the CBD by an inflamed gallbladder or pancreas, secretory hepatic dysfunction associated with generalized illness, hepatic hypoperfusion, or Gilbert's syndrome, to name just a few. Falsely negative liver chemistries can be noted in patients with partially obstructing or nonobstructing CBDS, or migration of cholecystolithiasis into the CBD after blood sampling has been performed, for example [6]. False negative liver chemistry results, however, are found infrequently, as suggested by a study involving routine MRCP screening of patients with gallstone disease, which revealed that only 4 % of patients with normal liver chemistries had CBDS, which amounted to a negative predictive value of 96 % [3]. In general, improvement in liver chemistries coinciding with an improvement in clinical symptoms can suggest spontaneous clearance of CBDS, while increasing chemistry levels point toward retained CBDS [9, 10].

Liver chemistries routinely are used in the evaluation of biliary disease. Individual chemistries have at best a moderate predictive value for CBDS; they have greater utility in excluding choledocholithiasis. Bilirubin, alkaline phosphatase, γ-glutamyl transpeptidase (GGT), AST, and ALT each has positive predictive values ranging from 25 to 50 %, while their negative predictive values range from 94 to 99 % [1–3, 6, 7, 11, 12]. Table 5.2 demonstrates sensitivity and specificity ranges for laboratory and imaging tests commonly utilized in evaluating patients for CBDS.

Combined elevations of individual liver chemistries can be more predictive, but these analyses remain most useful in the exclusion of CBDS from consideration. If there are no other risk factors for CBDS, and all liver chemistries are normal, the patient is low risk for CBDS. Any elevation of individual liver chemistries places the patient at intermediate risk, and bilirubin has been demonstrated to be the most predictive chemistry for CBDS, along with alkaline phosphatase as a close second. Please refer to Table 5.1 for complete risk stratification [2].

Al-Jiffry et al. suggest that both abnormal ultrasound (US) and elevated liver chemistries are required to submit a patient for ERCP; bilirubin >4 mg/dL without US findings was not sufficient to warrant an ERCP according to these authors. Those patients instead proceeded to laparoscopic cholecystectomy (LC) with intraoperative cholangiogram (IOC). In our practice, these patients routinely are evaluated using endoscopic ultrasound (EUS), which will be discussed in a subsequent section. The abnormal US require-

Table 5.2 Sensitivity and specificity ranges for laboratory and imaging studies commonly utilized in the evaluation for CBDS

Laboratory studies for detecting CBDS	Sensitivity	Specificity
Total bilirubin (TB)	34–49 %	60–88 %
Alkaline phosphatase (AP)	41–80 %	88–73 %
Gamma glutamyl transpeptidase (GGT)	63–84 %	72–73 %
Aspartate transaminase (AST)	44–64 %	79–86 %
Alanine transaminase (ALT)	50–72 %	68–81 %
At least one component elevated from the panel		
TB–AP–GGT–AST–ALT	52–88 %	53–91 %
Imaging studies for detecting CBDS	Sensitivity	Specificity
Transabdominal ultrasound (US)	20–58 %	68–91 %
Computed tomography (CT)	50–88 %	84–98 %
Magnetic resonance cholangiopancreatography (MRCP)	85–95 %	91–100 %
Endoscopic retrograde cholangiopancreatography (ERCP)	89–93 %	98–100 %
Endoscopic ultrasound (EUS)	89–98 %	94–100 %
Intraoperative cholangiography (IOC)	97–100 %	93–100 %
Laparoscopic ultrasound (LUS)	71–100 %	96–100 %

ment posed by Al-Jiffry et al. is reported to have eliminated unnecessary ERCP in 58.6 % of patients who, at the time of LC with IOC, did not have stones on IOC [13]. Importantly, this study was conducted in a region with a high incidence of hepatitis, sickle cell anemia, and secondary polycythemia, rendering reliance on bilirubin levels alone confusing and insufficient as a significant predictor for CBDS; alkaline phosphatase >300 U/L was associated with an odds ratio of 30 for CBDS [13].

Plaisier et al. suggested that the combination of a more than twofold elevated total bilirubin and alkaline phosphatase was a predictor for CBD stones [14]. Topal et al. found that patients with CBDS or CBD dilatation identified on US, the additional variables of an alkaline phosphatase level greater than 670 U/L, amylase level greater than 95 U/L, age greater than 60 years, and clinically significant fever also were predictive of CBDS. Three or more abnormal values revealed a predictive probability of 75–80 %, while finding that all variables were abnormal was associated with a predictive probability of 90 % [15].

These final two studies discussed, and several others, highlight the unreliable nature of liver chemistries in predicting CBDS, and introduce the notion that positive US findings could be important in stratifying patients at risk for CBDS.

Ultrasound

Limited right upper quadrant abdominal US frequently is used in the evaluation of abdominal pain suspected to be of biliary origin. Transabdominal US is not particularly well suited for direct identification of CBDS, however. Reported sensitivity and specificity for US detection of CBDS range from 20 to 58 %, and 68 to 91 %, respectively [1, 8].

These wide ranges and generally poor sensitivity and specificity can be attributed to the physical limitations related to US. The shape of the CBD wall and lack of a refractive border between stones and the CBD wall compromise the ability of US to identify CBDS. Furthermore, overlying body fat or intestinal gas interferes with US transduction. Detecting CBDS in the intraduodenal and intrapancreatic CBD is limited by these same factors. However, Rickes et al. did show that experienced ultrasonographers have a higher accuracy for diagnosing CBDS (83 % vs 64 %) compared to less experienced operators [16], and that improved training may enhance the utility of ultrasound in the evaluation of patients suspected of having CBDS.

Importantly, US, when used as part a comprehensive diagnostic algorithm, is clinically useful, because US can be used to detect signs which are themselves suggestive of CBDS. A normal sized CBD on US, combined with normal levels of bilirubin and alkaline phosphatase, has a negative predictive value for CBDS of 95 %. A dilated CBD on US alone is enough to raise the risk of CBDS to intermediate [2, 9, 13, 17]. Furthermore, an abnormally dilated CBD on US, reported as 6 mm in some studies and 8 mm in others, in addition to abnormal liver chemistries, is a trigger for ERCP in a less invasive treatment algorithm [13]. Grande et al., devised a formula which used the number of gallstones, the common bile duct diameter, bilirubin and alkaline phosphatase levels to predict choledocholithiasis with a sensitivity and specificity of 92.9 and 99.3 % [18]. Thus, US is a critical diagnostic tool that lends value to ordinary liver chemistry assays and guides further management of the patient suspected of having CBDS.

US measurement of CBD diameter is useful even after intervention for biliary pathology. The CBD diameter decreases after endoscopic sphincterotomy (ES) and extraction of CBDS in patients with dilated CBD due to stones. CBD diameter diminishes on average by 35 % after ES; persistent dilation raises concern for retained or additional CBDS. In a study in which the CBD diameter was measured before and after ES, all patients who did not manifest a decreased CBD diameter were found to have residual CBDS on ERCP [19]. An important caveat is the observation that patients with an intact gallbladder manifest reduced levels of CBD dilation in the presence of CBDS due to the gallbladder serving as a capacitive reservoir which off-loads pressure, thus reducing the likelihood and degree of CBD dilation [17].

Computed Tomography

While computed tomography (CT) has high diagnostic utility for abdominal pathology in general, CT has not contributed much to the success of diagnosing CBDS. Despite advances in CT technology, sensitivity and specificity remains limited. Various reports show sensitivity and specificity ranging from 50 to 88 % and 84 to 98 %, respectively [20, 21]. Sensitivity is

diminished when cholesterol stones are present, the most common composition of secondary CBDS in the USA and Western countries. Patients with CBDS smaller than 5 mm who undergo CT have an inferior diagnostic rate compared with patients with CBDS larger than 5 mm (57 % vs 81 %) [20]. Although CT often is performed in patients with suspected abdominal pathology, in patients suspected of having CBDS, additional imaging may be needed in the event of a negative CT.

Computed Tomography Cholangiography

CT cholangiography, abdominal CT performed after administration of contrast characterized for biliary excretion, rarely is used clinically. Comparatively, magnetic resonance imaging (MRI) and magnetic resonance cholangiopancreatography (MRCP) have better performance characteristics, while avoiding radiation exposure and contrast toxicity associated with CT cholangiography [2, 22]. Furthermore, obstructive cholestasis, often manifested with elevated liver chemistries, impairs biliary excretion of contrast used for CT cholangiography, limiting utility in many patients suspected of CBDS.

Magnetic Resonance Cholangiopancreatography

MRCP is most often utilized in the evaluation of patients at intermediate risk for CBDS; low risk patients typically will not benefit from MRCP imaging, and high risk patients often require direct intervention like ERCP or CBD exploration. MRCP has a sensitivity of 85–95 % and a specificity of 91–100 % for CBDS [1, 2, 15, 23–27]. Sensitivity is poorer for smaller stones, but is dependent on slice thickness used during MRI image acquisition. At a slice thickness of 5 mm, sensitivity for the detection of CBDS smaller than 6 mm, is 33–71 % [1, 24], while a slice thickness of 3 mm was associated with sensitivity of 100 % for CBDS as small as 3 mm in a single study [28]. A negative MRCP accompanying clinical improvement and normalization of biochemical assessment often indicates spontaneous clearance of CBDS [10].

Diagnostic algorithms should endeavor to utilize MRCP over ERCP when possible, and when EUS is unavailable, as MRCP is noninvasive, has virtually no complications compared to a serious adverse event rate of 1–7 % for ERCP [10]. Additionally, in many settings, MRCP is less expensive than ERCP. Using MRCP evaluation for patients suspected of CBDS but who lack high degree risk factors, may help avoid unnecessary ERCP in those approximately 43–80 % of patients who ultimately have a negative MRCP [13, 23, 24, 29].

Endoscopic Retrograde Cholangiopancreatography

ERCP has therapeutic as well as diagnostic capabilities. ERCP can detect CBD stones with a sensitivity of 89–93 % and specificity of 98–100 % [1, 2, 24], in studies where the diagnostic gold standard was ES and duct sweeping with a balloon or basket. Smaller CBDS can be missed with ERCP, although adjacent procedures like cholangioscopy may decrease the miss rate further; it isn't clear if the smallest stones are clinically significant [2, 30]. Despite a CBD clearance rate of 85–92 %, ERCP is saddled with a morbidity rate of 2–7 % with complications including pancreatitis, hemorrhage, and bowel perforation among others. The mortality rate for ERCP is approximately 1 %. ERCP, whether performed preoperatively or postoperatively adds cost to the management of patients suspected of having CBDS, unless it is utilized only for patients in whom the preoperative risk for CBDS exceeded 80 % [31]. If local expertise is available, laparoscopic CBD exploration (LCBDE) is more cost-efficient when CBDS are confirmed intraoperatively using IOC, than is postoperative ERCP. Exceptions to this observation are patients unable to tolerate prolongation of the laparoscopic procedure, or when conversion to open surgery is required by lack of suitable equipment

or surgical expertise. If LCBDE is unavailable, other considerations include intraoperative ERCP, postoperative ERCP, or intraoperative placement of a laparoscopic endobiliary stent to facilitate postoperative ERCP; stenting has not been subjected to a comparative cost analysis but may reduce costs of postoperative ERCP by eliminating the need for inpatient hospitalization after LC while awaiting ERCP [32–34]. Preoperative ERCP is preferred to postoperative ERCP only when a very high risk of CBDS has been identified preoperatively [35].

Less invasive preoperative studies such as MRCP, or using EUS-guided ERCP, can avoid unnecessary ERCP in 30–80 % of patients, and consequently, avoid the complications associated with ERCP [13, 23, 24, 29, 36]. Again, ERCP should be limited, when possible, to patients who will benefit from its therapeutic capabilities; those with high risk for biliary obstruction or CBDS visualized on preoperative imaging studies or during IOC [2, 37].

Endoscopic Ultrasound

EUS has been shown to have excellent accuracy for the diagnoses of CBDS. With a sensitivity of 89–98 % and a specificity of 94–100 % [2, 27, 38], EUS is comparable to ERCP, although less likely to cause complications than ERCP. Despite its lack of therapeutic capability, EUS as a diagnostic bridge to ERCP can prevent unnecessary ERCP in patients who do not have CBDS demonstrated on EUS. This approach, called EUS-guided ERCP, avoided ERCP in 30–75 % of patients, resulted in fewer complications, and was less costly than ERCP [36, 39, 40]. In patients who have known CBDS, or who need biliary decompression for biliary sepsis, ERCP remains more cost-effective [36, 39].

Some institutions have employed wire-guided intraductal ultrasound (IDUS) probes, which can be used to ultrasonographically visualize the CBD and guide therapeutic interventions during ERCP. Accuracy of IDUS was 97 %; higher than the sensitivity of ERCP alone [41, 42]. Authors attributed the improved accuracy to detection of small CBDS, but the clinical significance of these smaller stones is unknown.

It is most desirable to confirm the diagnosis of CBDS prior to surgery. Even when expertise in LCBDE is available, preoperative identification of CBDS allows for more accurate operative scheduling and resource utilization. However, there are times when preoperative analysis is limited, where suspicion for CBDS is low until a distended CBD is recognized intraoperatively, or other factors suggest the need for further evaluation for CBDS.

Intraoperative Diagnostic Evaluation

Intraoperative Cholangiography

IOC has a technical success rate between 75 and 100 %, with sensitivity and specificity of 97–100 % and 93–100 % respectively [43–45]. IOC can be used routinely during laparoscopic cholecystectomy, as we recommend, or employed selectively in those patients with intermediate risk for CBDS as an alternative to another imaging modality such as MRCP [2, 46]. Although some cite uncommon iodinated contrast reactions during IOC and comparable sensitivity and specificity for CBDS as reasons to replace this procedure with more costly preoperative MRCP, we continue to advocate for the routine use of IOC as an important skill for surgeons to master in order to be prepared for laparoscopic endobiliary stenting and LCBDE [1, 47].

Routine versus selective use of IOC is widely debated in literature. Proponents of selective IOC state that a selective policy yields acceptably high positive results, and that asymptomatic common bile duct stones often resolve spontaneously and do not usually pose a problem after laparoscopic cholecystectomy [48]. Arguments in a favor of routine IOC include the fact that the IOC findings can change management in as many as 5–10 % of patients [43], can reduce CBD injuries, identify anatomical variations and is cost-effective [49, 50]. Furthermore, routine use of IOC promotes skill development, improves efficiency of utilization,

and facilitates resident teaching in institutions training surgical residents [46]. IOC was considered an important component in the safe performance of LC by expert surgeons engaged in a recent Delphi consensus organized by the Society of American Gastrointestinal and Endoscopic Surgeons (SAGES) [51].

Laparoscopic Ultrasound

Laparoscopic ultrasound (LUS) can be used in place of IOC for patients with intermediate risk of CBDS, and just as for IOC, some advocate its routine use. Sensitivity and specificity are 71–100 % and 96–100 % respectively [2, 50, 52]. However, evaluation of the intrapancreatic and intraduodenal and ampullary CBD, where many CBDS are found, can be limited, especially in less experienced hands [1]. The learning curve appears to be significant compared to IOC; however, LUS can be completed in just 4–10 min, compared to 10–20 min for IOC in this single study, and with a higher technical completion rate then IOC [43].

Additional Considerations

Anatomic Findings

There are variants in the anatomic relationships of the cystic duct and CBD which might influence the risk for CBDS. Tsitouridis et al. found that 11 % of patients evaluated for CBDS had a low insertion of the cystic duct, defined as an insertion point in the distal third of the bile duct with respect to the distance between the hepatic hilum and the ampulla of Vater (Fig. 5.1), and those patients had a significantly higher rate of CBDS compared with patients without a low cystic duct insertion [53]. Those patients with low cystic duct insertion also had a higher rate of CBD dilatation.

An oblique CBD, a CBD positioned less than 45° from horizontal, also may increase the risk of CBDS (Fig. 5.2). In patients with CBDS undergoing ERCP, oblique CBD was associated with increased risks of chronic pancreatitis, biliary

Fig. 5.1 Low insertion of the cystic duct into the CBD (*red arrow*) is associated with a higher incidence of CBDS

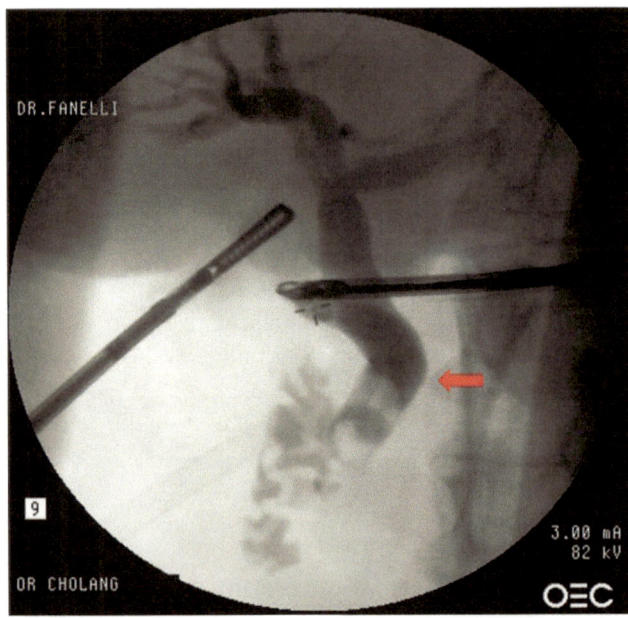

Fig. 5.2 Patients with an oblique CBD have increased risk for chronic pancreatitis, biliary fistula, recurrent CBDS, and are more likely to need multiple ERCP and to be diagnosed with CBDS after surgery

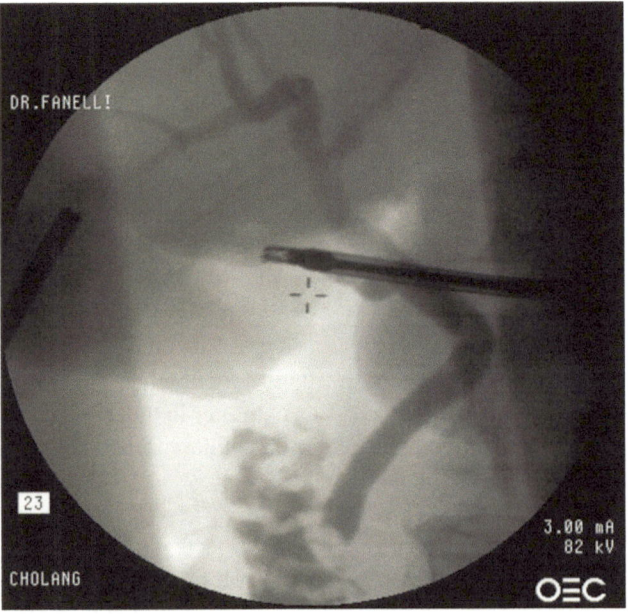

fistulae, recurrent CBDS, the need for multiple ERCP, and more frequent diagnoses of CBDS after surgery. Patients with oblique CBD were older, and more often had undergone prior biliary procedures, which may be confounding factors or themselves causes of oblique CBD [54].

Periampullary diverticulae (PAD) are diverticulae arising along the duodenal wall, such as adjacent to the Ampulla of Vater. The prevalence of PAD increases with age; they rarely are found in patients less than 40 years of age. PAD are associated with an increased risk of recurrent CBDS and are associated with larger CBD diameter [55]. PAD typically are found in patients undergoing evaluation for CBDS; it is unclear whether they increase the risk of CBDS, but they may complicate performance of ERCP and ES when necessary.

Putting It All Together

An Algorithmic Approach to the Patient with Suspected CBDS

In clinical practice, patients suspected of having CBDS undergo risk stratification using noninvasive assessments. Patients are stratified into three groups as demonstrated earlier in Table 5.1; low risk, intermediate risk, and high risk for CBDS. Once stratified, patients are then treated using an algorithmic approach (Fig. 5.3). Low risk patients are scheduled directly for LC with routine IOC; in this patient group, no further preoperative evaluation for CBDS is necessary. IOC is used to improve patient safety, build on nascent resident

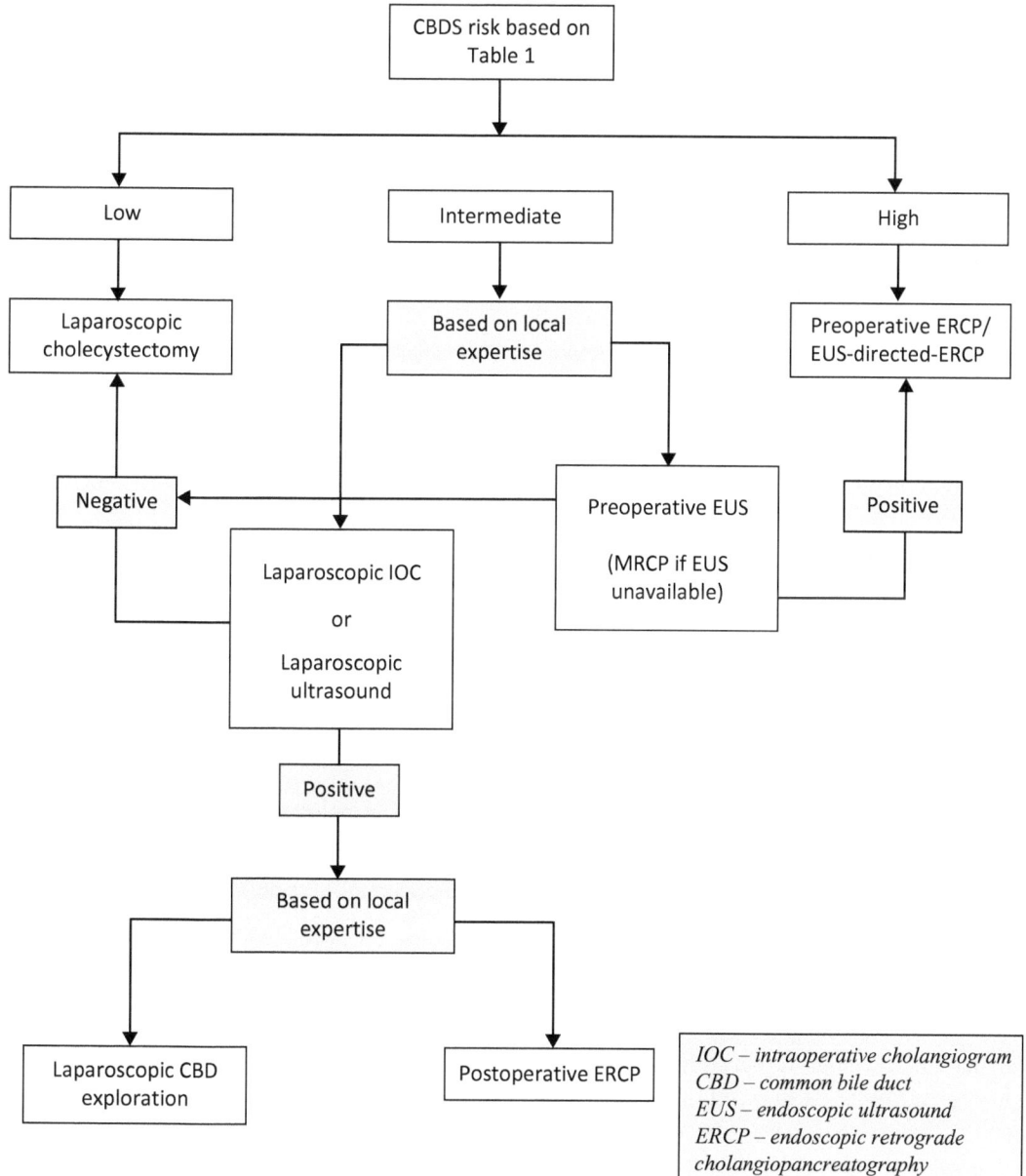

Fig. 5.3 Management of patients with CBDS based on risk stratification (Adapted in part from ASGE Standards of Practice Committee [2].)

skill sets, and to detect smaller and occult CBDS, currently of unknown clinical significance.

Patients at high risk for CBDS most often have an indication to undergo preoperative ERCP alone or EUS-directed-ERCP. It is our practice to offer patients with direct evidence of CBDS, like CBDS visualized on US, CT, or MRCP, an ERCP without additional study unless there are signs that spontaneous clearance of CBDS has occurred. In this setting, we prefer EUS-directed-ERCP. Patients who present with indirect evidence of CBDS like abnormal liver chemistries in concert with a dilated CBD without confirmation of CBDS, a recent history of resolving biliary pancreatitis, or chemistries that are improving, or a CBD diameter that has diminished on serial studies, are offered EUS-directed-ERCP since a good number of these patients will have spontaneously cleared CBDS. We find this approach to lessen the frequency of adverse outcomes associated with ERCP by reserving that intervention for patients proven to have current CBDS. Because one of us performs EUS as well as ERCP (RDF), this approach fits well with the clinical flow of our practice. In settings where EUS is unavailable, MRCP as an additional diagnostic measure and directed ERCP for patients at high risk for CBDS remains a most reasonable option.

The challenge of any algorithmic approach to patients with suspected CBDS is the management of intermediate risk patients. It is important that any algorithm used is consistent with the goal of minimizing morbidity and mortality of treatments, while reducing costs. Sarli et al. found that the use of a risk stratification system for diagnosing of CBDS seemed to reduce the use of intravenous cholangiography, ERCP, and IOC performed [56]. Similarly, Al-Jiffry was able to reduce the use of MRCP as well as ERCP by following a diagnostic algorithm [13].

In our practice, we approach the intermediate risk patient preferentially with EUS, although if timing and scheduling do not permit this approach, we then advocate for direct LC with IOC. When either EUS or IOC are negative, we proceed with standard LC. When preoperative EUS is positive, we provide ERCP immediately following EUS, in the same setting, and schedule the patient for LC

as their clinical condition suggests. When IOC is positive for CBDS, we prefer LCBDE for patients with 1–3 stones, especially those that can be flushed through the ampulla after administration of glucagon or intraductal administration of local anesthetic, or can be removed using transcystic LCBDE techniques. It is our belief that choledochotomy should be avoided unless it represents the only option for removing CBDS, and therefore, patients with larger CBDS or greater numbers of CBDS than three are preferentially treated by laparoscopic endobiliary stent placement and postoperative ERCP. One advantage of this approach is that patients may be discharged home the same day as LC after laparoscopic endobiliary stenting, and then return for elective outpatient ERCP; this eliminates the costly inpatient stay from LC through completion of ERCP that has been reported by some centers.

An algorithmic approach to the evaluation and management of patients suspected of having CBDS represents a rational, coherent, and cost-efficient method. From the surgical perspective, the stratification outlined in Table 5.1 and the algorithm presented in Fig. 5.3 represent an effective approach to patients suspected of harboring CBDS.

References

1. Desai R, Shokouhi BN. Common bile duct stones - their presentation, diagnosis and management. Indian J Surg. 2009;71(5):229–37.
2. ASGE, Committee SoP, Maple JT, Ben-Menachem T, Anderson MA, Appalaneni V, et al. The role of endoscopy in the evaluation of suspected choledocholithiasis. Gastrointest Endosc. 2010;71(1):1–9.
3. Nebiker CA, Baierlein SA, Beck S, von Flue M, Ackermann C, Peterli R. Is routine MR cholangiopancreatography (MRCP) justified prior to cholecystectomy? Langenbeck's Arch Surg. 2009;394(6):1005–10.
4. Topal B, Fieuws S, Tomczyk K, Aerts R, Van Steenbergen W, Verslype C, et al. Clinical models are inaccurate in predicting bile duct stones in situ for patients with gallbladder. Surg Endosc. 2009;23(1):38–44.
5. Borie F, Fingerhut A, Millat B. Acute biliary pancreatitis, endoscopy, and laparoscopy. Surg Endosc. 2003;17(8):1175–80.
6. Videhult P, Sandblom G, Rudberg C, Rasmussen IC. Are liver function tests, pancreatitis and cholecystitis

predictors of common bile duct stones? Results of a prospective, population-based, cohort study of 1171 patients undergoing cholecystectomy. HPB. 2011;13(8):519–27.

7. Sheen AJ, Asthana S, Al-Mukhtar A, Attia M, Toogood GJ. Preoperative determinants of common bile duct stones during laparoscopic cholecystectomy. Int J Clin Pract. 2008;62(11):1715–9.

8. Einstein DM, Lapin SA, Ralls PW, Halls JM. The insensitivity of sonography in the detection of choledocholithiasis. AJR Am J Roentgenol. 1984;142:725-8.

9. Almadi M, Barkun JS, Barkun AN. Management of suspected stones in the common bile duct. CMAJ. 2012;184(8):884–92.

10. Sakai Y, Tsuyuguchi T, Yukisawa S, Tsuchiya S, Sugiyama H, Miyakawa K, et al. Diagnostic value of magnetic resonance cholangiopancreatography for clinically suspicious spontaneous passage of bile duct stones. J Gastroenterol Hepatol. 2008;23(5):736–40.

11. Peng WK, Sheikh Z, Paterson-Brown S, Nixon SJ. Role of liver function tests in predicting common bile duct stones in acute calculous cholecystitis. Br J Surg. 2005;92(10):1241–7.

12. Yang MH, Chen TH, Wang SE, Tsai YF, Su CH, Wu CW, et al. Biochemical predictors for absence of common bile duct stones in patients undergoing laparoscopic cholecystectomy. Surg Endosc. 2008;22(7):1620–4.

13. Al-Jiffry BO, Elfateh A, Chundrigar T, Othman B, Almalki O, Rayza F, et al. Non-invasive assessment of choledocholithiasis in patients with gallstones and abnormal liver function. World J Gastroenterol. 2013;19(35):5877–82.

14. Plaisier PW, van der Hul RL. Surg Endosc 2008;22:1620–1624. Biochemical predictors of common bile duct (CBD) stones. Surg Endosc. 2009;23(4):914. author reply 5.

15. Topal B, Van de Moortel M, Fieuws S, Vanbeckevoort D, Van Steenbergen W, Aerts R, et al. The value of magnetic resonance cholangiopancreatography in predicting common bile duct stones in patients with gallstone disease. Br J Surg. 2003;90(1):42–7.

16. Rickes S, Treiber G, Monkemuller K, Peitz U, Csepregi A, Kahl S, et al. Impact of the operator's experience on value of high-resolution transabdominal ultrasound in the diagnosis of choledocholithiasis: a prospective comparison using endoscopic retrograde cholangiography as the gold standard. Scand J Gastroenterol. 2006;41(7):838–43.

17. Grönroos JM, Haapamäki MM, Gullichsen R. Effect of the diameter of the common bile duct on the incidence of bile duct stones in patients with recurrent attacks of right epigastric pain after cholecystectomy. Eur J Surg. 2001;167(10):767–9.

18. Grande M, Torquati A, Tucci G, Rulli F, Adorisio O, Farinon A. Preoperative risk factors for common bile duct stones: defining the patient at high risk in the laparoscopic cholecystectomy era. J Laparoendosc Adv Surg Tech A. 2004;14(5):281–6.

19. Karincaoglu M, Yildirim B, Seckin Y, Kantarceken B, Aladag M, Hilmioglu F. Common bile duct diameters after endoscopic sphincterotomy in patients with common bile duct stones: ultrasonographic evaluation. Abdom Imaging. 2003;28(4):531–5.

20. Tseng CW, Chen CC, Chen TS, Chang FY, Lin HC, Lee SD. Can computed tomography with coronal reconstruction improve the diagnosis of choledocholithiasis? J Gastroenterol Hepatol. 2008;23(10):1586–9.

21. Lee JK, Kim TK, Byun JH, Kim AY, Ha HK, Kim PN, et al. Diagnosis of intrahepatic and common duct stones: combined unenhanced and contrast-enhanced helical CT in 1090 patients. Abdom Imaging. 2006;31(4):425–32.

22. Soto JA, Alvarez O, Múnera F, Velez SM, Valencia J, Ramírez N. Diagnosing bile duct stones. Am J Roentgenol. 2000;175(4):1127–34.

23. Boraschi P, Giqoni R, Braccini G, Lamacchia M, Rossi M, Falaschi F. Detection of common bile duct stones before laparoscopic cholecystectomy. Acta Radiol. 2002;43(6):593–8.

24. Raval B, Kramer L. Advances in the imaging of common duct stones using magnetic resonance cholangiography, endoscopic ultrasonography, and laparoscopic ultrasonography. Semin Laparosc Surg. 2000;7(4):232–6.

25. Stiris M, Tennøe B, Aadland E, Lunde OC. Cholangiopancreaticography and endoscopic retrograde cholangiopancreaticography in patients with suspected common bile duct stones. Acta Radiol. 2000;41:269–72.

26. Kejriwal R, Liang J, Andrewson G, Hill A. Magnetic resonance imaging of the common bile duct to exclude choledocholithiasis. ANZ J Surg. 2004;74(8):619–21.

27. Schmidt S, Chevallier P, Novellas S, Gelsi E, Vanbiervliet G, Tran A, Schnyder P, Bruneton JN. Choledocholithiasis: repetitive thick-slab single-shot projection magnetic resonance cholangiopancreaticography versus endoscopic ultrasonography. Eur Radiol. 2007;17(1):241–50.

28. Mendler MH, Bouillet P, Sautereau D, Chaumerliac P, Cessot F, Le Sidaner A, et al. Value of MR cholangiography in the diagnosis of obstructive diseases of the biliary tree: a study of 58 cases. Am J Gastroenterol. 1998;93(12):2482–90.

29. Sharma SK, Larson KA, Adler Z, Goldfarb MA. Role of endoscopic retrograde cholangiopancreatography in the management of suspected choledocholithiasis. Surg Endosc. 2003;17(6):868–71.

30. Kubota Y, Takaoka M, Yamamoto S, Shibatani N, Shimatani M, Takamido S, et al. Diagnosis of common bile duct calculi with intraductal ultrasonography during endoscopic biliary cannulation. J Gastroenterol Hepatol. 2002;17(6):708–12.

31. Urbach DR, Khajanchee YS, Jobe BA, Standage BA, Hansen PD, Swanstrom LL. Cost-effective management of common bile duct stones: a decision analysis of the use of endoscopic retrograde cholangiopancre-

atography (ERCP), intraoperative cholangiography, and laparoscopic bile duct exploration. Surg Endosc. 2001;15(1):4–13.

32. Fanelli RD, Gersin KS. Laparoscopic endobiliary stenting: a simplified approach to the management of occult common bile duct stones. J Gastrointest Surg. 2001;5(1):74–80.

33. Fanelli RD, Gersin KS, Mainella MT. Laparoscopic endobiliary stenting significantly improves success of postoperative endoscopic retrograde cholangiopancreatography in low-volume centers. Surg Endosc. 2002;16(3):487–91.

34. Gersin KS, Fanelli RD. Laparoscopic endobiliary stenting as an adjunct to common bile duct exploration. Surg Endosc. 1998;12(4):301–4.

35. Petelin JB. Laparoscopic common bile duct exploration. Surg Endosc. 2003;17(11):1705–15.

36. Petrov MS, Savides TJ. Systematic review of endoscopic ultrasonography versus endoscopic retrograde cholangiopancreatography for suspected choledocholithiasis. Br J Surg. 2009;96(9):967–74.

37. Patel AP, Lokey JS, Harris JB, Sticca RP, McGill ES, Arrillaga A, Miller RS, Kopelman TR. Current management of common bile duct stones in a teaching community hospital. Am Surg. 2003;69(7):555–60.

38. Aljebreen A, Azzam N, Eloubeidi MA. Prospective study of endoscopic ultrasound performance in suspected choledocholithiasis. J Gastroenterol Hepatol. 2008;23(5):741–5.

39. Ang TL, Teo EK, Fock KM. Endosonography- vs. endoscopic retrograde cholangiopancreatography-based strategies in the evaluation of suspected common bile duct stones in patients with normal transabdominal imaging. Aliment Pharmacol Ther. 2007;26(8):1163–70.

40. Lee YT, Chan FKL, Leung WK, Chan HLY, Wu JCY, Yung MY, et al. Comparison of EUS and ERCP in the investigation with suspected biliary obstruction caused by choledocholithiasis: a randomized study. Gastrointest Endosc. 2008;67(4):660–8.

41. Tseng LJ, Jao YT, Mo LR, Lin RC. Over-the-wire US catheter probe as an adjunct to ERCP in the detection of choledocholithiasis. Gastrointest Endosc. 2001;54(6):720–3.

42. Das A, Isenberg G, Wong RC, Sivak Jr MV, Chak A. Wire-guided intraductal US: an adjunct to ERCP in the management of bile duct stones. Gastrointest Endosc. 2001;54(1):31–6.

43. Shah A, Gilmour J, Bransom C, Jones R, Blackett R. Routine on-table cholangiography during laparoscopic cholecystectomy is well worthwhile. Internet J Surg. 2006;12(1):1–4.

44. Rothlin MA, Schlumpf R, Largiader F. Laparoscopic sonography. An alternative to routine intraoperative cholangiography? Arch Surg (Chicago, IL: 1960). 1994;129(7):694–700.

45. Catheline J, Rizk N, Champault G. A comparison of laparoscopic ultrasound versus cholangiography in the evaluation of the biliary tree during laparoscopic cholecystectomy. Eur J Ultrasound. 1999;10(1): 1–9.

46. Fanelli RD. The likelihood of predicting the presence of CBD stones. Presentation given at the 2014 the Society of American Gastrointestinal and Endoscopic Surgeons Annual Meeting. CBD Stones Postgraduate Course. 2014. http://www.sages.org/video/likelihood-predicting-presence-cbd-stones/. Accessed 4 Sep 2014.

47. Dalton SJ, Balupuri S, Guest J. Routine magnetic resonance cholangiopancreatography and intraoperative cholangiogram in the evaluation of common bile duct stones. Ann R Coll Surg Engl. 2005;87(6):469–70.

48. Horwood J, Akbar F, Davis K, Morgan R. Prospective evaluation of a selective approach to cholangiography for suspected common bile duct stones. Ann R Coll Surg Engl. 2010;92(3):206–10.

49. Flum DR, Flowers C, Veenstra DL. A cost-effectiveness analysis of intraoperative cholangiography in the prevention of bile duct injury during laparoscopic cholecystectomy. J Am Coll Surg. 2003;196(3):385–93.

50. Machi J, Tateishi T, Oishi AJ, Furumoto NL, Oishi RH, Uchida S, et al. Laparoscopic ultrasonography versus operative cholangiography during laparoscopic cholecystectomy: review of the literature and a comparison with open intraoperative ultrasonography. J Am Coll Surg. 1999;188(4):360–7.

51. Pucher PH, Brunt LM, Fanelli RD, Asbun HJ, Aggarwal R. SAGES expert Delphi consensus: critical factors for safe surgical practice in laparoscopic cholecystectomy. Surg Endosc. 11 Feb 2015. [Epub ahead of print].

52. Tranter SE, Thompson MH. Potential of laparoscopic ultrasonography as an alternative to operative cholangiography in the detection of bile duct stones. Br J Surg. 2001;88(1):65–9.

53. Tsitouridis I, Lazaraki G, Papastergiou C, Pagalos E, Germanidis G. Low conjunction of the cystic duct with the common bile duct: does it correlate with the formation of common bile duct stones? Surg Endosc. 2007;21(1):48–52.

54. Strnad P, von Figura G, Gruss R, Jareis KM, Stiehl A, Kulaksiz H. Oblique bile duct predisposes to the recurrence of bile duct stones. PLoS One. 2013;8(1):e54601.

55. Kim CW, Chang JH, Kim JH, Kim TH, Lee IS, Han SW. Size and type of periampullary duodenal diverticula are associated with bile duct diameter and recurrence of bile duct stones. J Gastroenterol Hepatol. 2013;28(5):893–8.

56. Sarli L, Costi R, Gobbi S, Iusco D, Sgobba G, Roncoroni L. Scoring system to predict asymptomatic choledocholithiasis before laparoscopic cholecystectomy. A matched case-control study. Surg Endosc. 2003;17(9):1396–403.

Bill S. Majdalany and James Spain

Introduction

Percutaneous biliary access for cholangiography or drainage is within the armamentarium of the Interventional Radiologist and has gained widespread acceptance since initial development of the procedure in the 1970s. However, refinements in ultrasound technology, magnetic resonance imaging (MRI), and computed tomography (CT) coupled with the wide availability of these exams allow rapid, accurate, and noninvasive assessments of the liver and associated structures. In particular, magnetic resonance cholangiopancreatography (MRCP) produces detailed images of the hepatobiliary and pancreatic systems, including the liver, gallbladder, bile ducts, pancreas, and pancreatic ducts. Moreover, as endoscopic techniques, specifically endoscopic retrograde cholangiopancreatography (ERCP), have improved, many

minimally invasive procedures which were historically approached percutaneously can now be performed internally. ERCP has been shown to be particularly successful in managing common hepatic duct or common bile duct pathologies. However, despite the advances in imaging studies and endoscopic therapy, percutaneous biliary access maintains a role in patients who have intrahepatic or hilar biliary disease, have altered surgical anatomy, have failed endoscopic approaches, or cannot be adequately imaged by noninvasive means.

Normal Biliary Anatomy

The liver is comprised of right and left lobes, and within each lobe the hepatic architecture is further characterized by the Couinaud classification, dividing the liver into eight functional segments (Fig. 6.1). Segments II, III, and IV are in the left hepatic lobe and their respective segmental biliary ducts join together forming a horizontally oriented left hepatic duct. Segments VI and VII form the right posterior duct, while segments V and VIII form the right anterior duct [1]. The right anterior duct courses vertically, while the right posterior duct courses horizontally. Together they form the right hepatic duct. Drainage of segment I is variable and is typically through several ducts joining both the right and left hepatic ducts close to their confluence, which forms the

B.S. Majdalany, M.D. (✉)
Department of Radiology, University of Michigan,
201S. 1st Street, Apt. #420, Ann Arbor,
MI 48104, USA
e-mail: bmajdala@med.umich.edu

J. Spain, M.D.
Department of Radiology, The Ohio State University
Wexner Medical Center, Columbus, OH, USA
e-mail: James.Spain@osumc.edu

© Springer International Publishing Switzerland 2016
J.W. Hazey et al. (eds.), *Multidisciplinary Management of Common Bile Duct Stones*,
DOI 10.1007/978-3-319-22765-8_6

Fig. 6.1 Normal
MRCP: The bile ducts
are smoothly contoured
and nearly symmetric
throughout the liver with
the right hepatic duct
(*arrow*) joining with the
left hepatic duct
(*arrowhead*) to form the
common hepatic duct
near the hepatic hilum.
The common hepatic
duct joins with the cystic
duct to form the
common bile duct
(*curved arrow*)

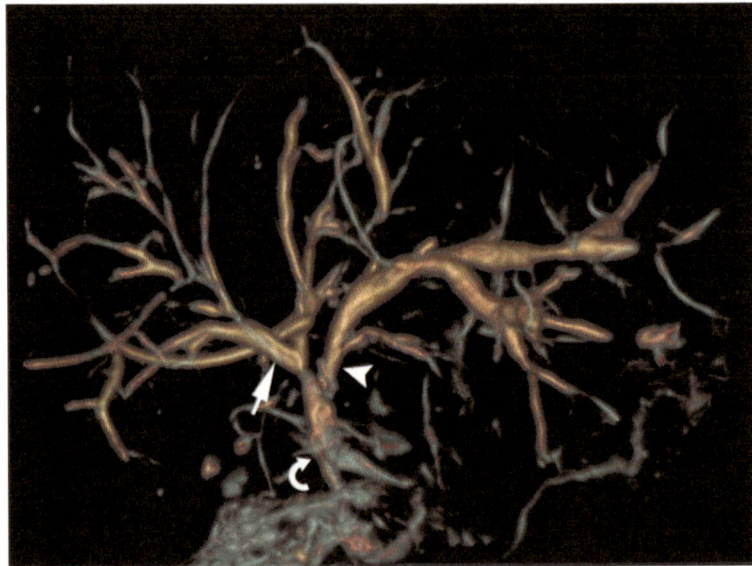

common hepatic duct (CHD). The CHD exits at the hepatic hilum in conjunction with the portal vein and hepatic artery. The cystic duct joins the common hepatic duct, with great variability, to delineate the origin of the common bile duct (CBD). The CBD courses through the hepatoduodenal ligament, where it joins the pancreatic duct and empties into the Ampulla of Vater through the Sphincter of Oddi. This marks the transition from the embryologic foregut, supplied by the celiac axis, to the midgut, supplied by the superior mesenteric artery [2].

Some variability of standard biliary anatomy occurs in approximately 40 % of the population. The most commonly noted variants are at the insertions of segment IV with the left hepatic duct (18 % of individuals), the insertion of the right posterior duct (25 % of individuals), or the convergence of the right and left hepatic ducts to form the CHD (32 % of individuals) [3].

Indications and Contraindications

Percutaneous transhepatic cholangiography (PTC) and percutaneous transhepatic drainage (PTD) are safe and effective, but are secondary examinations generally performed if noninvasive

imaging tests and endoscopic approaches are insufficient for diagnosis and treatment.

PTC is performed by sequentially inserting a thin needle into a peripheral bile duct, injecting contrast, and then acquiring radiographs. Biliary anatomy, luminal abnormalities, and obstructive problems can all be diagnosed. PTD is a therapeutic procedure which requires needle targeting of a biliary radical, wire manipulation within the tree, and placement of a tube or stent, thus potentially providing continuous access to the biliary tree. Common indications for drainage include relieving the symptoms of biliary obstruction, optimizing bilirubin levels to allow for chemotherapy,assisting in the treatment of cholangitis, diverting bile from a site of bile duct injury, and providing a secure access for endobiliary manipulation [4, 5].

There are few absolute contraindications to performing PTC. Given the rich vascularity of the liver, uncorrectable coagulopathy could preclude procedural safety. Correcting the International Normalized Ratio (INR) to approach 1.5 and the platelet count to 50,000 per cubic millimeter or higher, is suggested. Multifocal segmental obstruction, whether from congenital, inflammatory, or neoplastic conditions, can render drainage ineffective. Large volume ascites should be drained prior to attempting biliary access in an effort to prevent bile peritonitis or bleeding complications. Further, it is suggested, in the presence of ascites, to approach the biliary tree from the left, anti-dependent segments of the liver, to minimize peri-catheter leakage [4].

Procedural Preparation

Imaging

Pre-procedural imaging can evaluate for the presence of biliary ductal dilatation, the level of obstruction, the presence and differentiation of hepatic masses or metastases, and the presence of ascites. Both CT and MRI/MRCP (Figs. 6.2, 6.3, and 6.4) provide global imaging of liver anatomy and can help determine the feasibility, safety, and necessity of the procedure in addition to helping facilitate procedural planning. For example, elevated bilirubin in the setting of diffuse hepatic metastases may be functional as opposed to

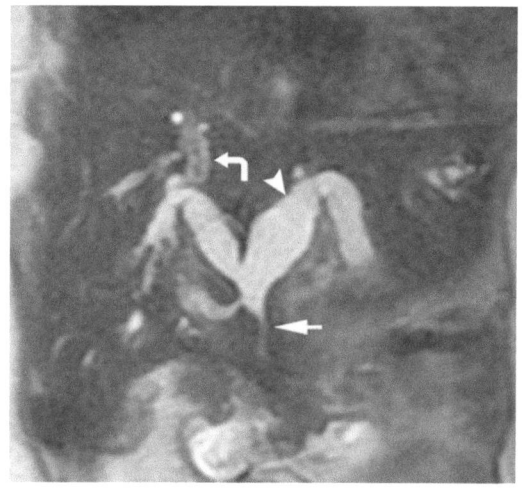

Fig. 6.3 Coronal T2 MRI image of the liver: MRI has better soft tissue characterization than CT and delineates fluid filled structures accurately. Diffuse biliary dilatation is noted in this image with the right superior ducts (*curved arrow*) coalescing centrally to join markedly dilated left hepatic ducts (*arrowhead*) to drain in a tapering common hepatic duct (*arrow*). Below this level a high grade stricture obstructs the biliary tree. For comparison, Fig. 6.2 is of the same patient with CT technique

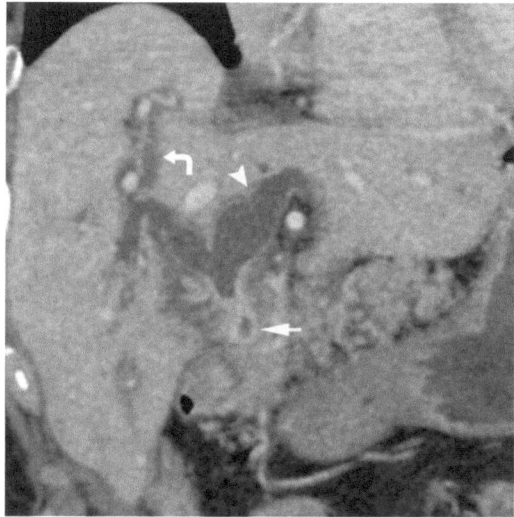

Fig. 6.2 Coronal CT image of the liver, post contrast: CT allows rapid, accurate, and reproducible imaging. Diffuse biliary dilatation is noted in this image with the right superior ducts (*curved arrow*) coalescing centrally to join markedly dilated left hepatic ducts (*arrowhead*) to drain in a tapering common hepatic duct (*arrow*). Below this level a high grade stricture obstructs the biliary tree. For comparison, Fig. 6.3 is of the same patient with MRI/MRCP technique

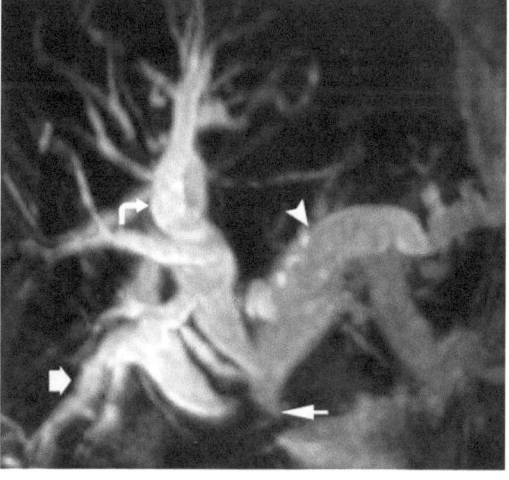

Fig. 6.4 Volume Rendered MRCP: Multiple MRI images are stacked to form 3D volume images of the biliary tree. These images can be rotated to help define branch points, strictures, and abnormal findings with a greater degree of sensitivity. Again, diffuse biliary dilatation is noted in this image with the right superior ducts (*curved arrow*) coalescing centrally to join markedly dilated left hepatic ducts (*arrowhead*) and the right inferior ducts (*block arrow*) to drain in a tapering common hepatic duct (*arrow*)

obstructive. Ultrasound imaging may also be helpful, but can be limited by patient body habitus, operator experience, and may not be able to fully image all pertinent structures [5].

Antibiotics

In its physiologic state, bile is sterile. However, in the setting of biliary disease or prior instrumentation, contamination or colonization can occur with pathogens directly ascending the biliary tree. Enteroccocus, Candida, *Escherichia coli*, Clostridial species, and other gram-negative aerobes are the most common pathogens [6]. In the presence of biliary ductal calculi, Klebsiella, Pseudomonas, and Bacteroides species are frequently present [7].

When the biliary tree is obstructed, elevated bile ductal pressure increases the likelihood of intravasating organisms into the blood stream during cholangiography through the adjacent vascular structures and which can rapidly lead to sepsis and shock. Alternative mechanisms of biliary colonization can include portal venous seeding from gastrointestinal infection or inflammation. Cultures from initial biliary drainage are 60 % positive for organisms, rising to 85 % at 24 h post drain placement, and essentially 100 % during catheter exchanges [8].

The Society of Interventional Radiology endorses routine prophylaxis for biliary procedures without a clear consensus on a first choice antibiotic. Typical regimens include third generation cephalosporins such as ceftriaxone 1 g intravenous (IV), piperacillin-tazobactam 3.375–4.5 g IV, fluoroquinolones such as ciprofloxacin 400 mg IV, ampicillin and gentamicin 1.5–3 g IV and 80 mg IV, respectively, and ampicillin-sulbactam 1.5–3 g IV, among others [9]. The optimal choice is based on institutional antibiograms to provide adequate coverage for the most commonly encountered pathogens.

Sedation

While cholangiography can technically be performed with local lidocaine injection, in many cases this will not suffice for patient comfort especially if biliary drainage is required. The standard approach to analgesia is intravenous conscious sedation (IVCS), which is achieved with a combination of an opiate analog such as fentanyl, morphine, or hydromorphone in combination with a short to moderate duration benzodiazepine such as midazolam or lorazepam [5, 10]. Though more resource intensive and occasionally more difficult to organize, general anesthesia (GA) may be helpful if not necessary in de novo biliary access. GA is particularly useful in helping gain access into a non-dilated biliary tree, in complex procedures expected to span several hours, in patients meeting systemic inflammatory response syndrome (SIRS) criteria to control the hemodynamics of the patient, in procedures requiring large access (>12 French) into the biliary tree, and in cases where a patient cannot tolerate IVCS [11].

Technical Considerations

Right vs Left Approach and Imaging Guidance

Biliary access and drainage may be safely performed from the right, left or both sides of the peripheral biliary tree. When the disease process or the needs of the patient do not present a compelling indication for laterality, then the choice may be arbitrary. In a subset of diseases, particularly if hilar or multifocal, bilateral biliary access will be needed and operators should have the skill set to perform both if necessary. Herein, the advantages and disadvantages of right and left sided approaches are discussed.

A right sided access is typically performed from a mid-axillary skin entry, preferably through a subcostal location but through no more superior location than the tenth intercostal space and with the needle directed one vertebral body superior to the level of entry. Commonly, the approach courses over a rib and through an intercostal space. Uncommonly, the pleura may be traversed at lower thoracic levels. This traditional approach decreases the direct radiation exposure to the operator and allows visualization and drainage of a larger proportion of the hepatic parenchyma and biliary tree. However, potential pleural complications, pain and sensitivity associated with the rib periosteum, and decreased ability for the patient to self care for the access site are potential drawbacks [12].

Left hepatic access is approached in the epigastrium and can usually be visualized with ultrasound without concern for shadowing from ribs. While this position may expose the operator's hands to the radiation beam and scatter, this hazard can be minimized by fluoroscopic angulation and collimation. Because the entry site is near midline and in front of the patient, it is easily visualized and maintained by the patient. Moreover, given that the intercostal space is not transgressed, pulmonary complications and irritation of the rib periosteum does not occur. However, a lesser degree of the hepatic parenchyma is drained, and the approach may not be technically feasible if there are interposed structures anterior to the liver or if the left lobe is behind the xiphoid process [12].

Opinions on approach vary widely and ultimately the decision should be tailored to the patient's needs.

Cholangiography

Percutaneous transhepatic cholangiography (PTC) can accurately delineate biliary anatomy, diagnose biliary abnormalities, and define the level of obstruction, leakage, or biliary injury. To perform cholangiography, first the approach is planned as previously discussed. The skin in the mid-axillary line between T10 and L1, for a right approach, or in the epigastrium for a left approach is deeply infiltrated with lidocaine. When traversing an intercostal space, care must be taken to guide the needle along the superior surface of the rib to avoid involvement of the intercostal artery, vein and nerve. A small incision is made in the skin to facilitate passage of a 21 or 22 gauge × 15–20 cm long needle with inner stylet (Fig. 6.5). When there is intrahepatic biliary ductal dilatation, ultrasound can be used to guide the needle into the bile duct. In the absence of intrahepatic biliary ductal dilatation, some operators will still use ultrasound to direct the needle centrally, but in a manner to avoid large vessels. Angulation of needle advancement is slightly cephalad from the right, with the needle tip approaching, but not crossing the spine. When possible, an obtuse angle between the needle trajectory and targeted bile duct is preferred. The inner stylet is removed and under fluoroscopic guidance, a small aliquot of iodinated contrast is injected, while the needle is simultaneously withdrawn, until a bile duct is opacified. When no bile duct is seen and the needle is nearly at the liver capsule, the inner style is replaced, the needle is

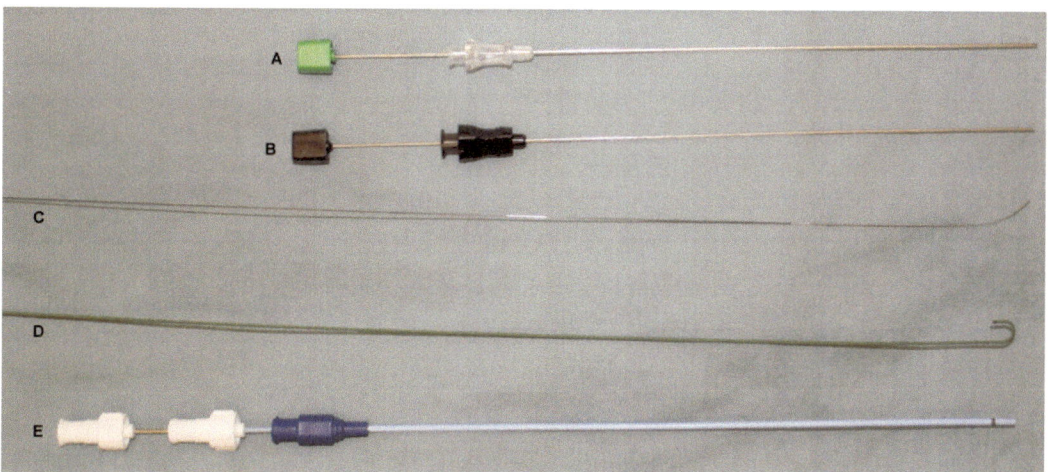

Fig. 6.5 Sample Cholangiography Inventory: While inventory is largely dependent on operator preference and familiarity, some of these are consistently used and can be found in prepackaged commercial kits. (*A*) 21 gauge × 15 cm needle. (*B*) 22 gauge × 15 cm needle. (*C*) Angled tip 0.018″ wire. (*D*) 0.035″ curved tip wire. (*E*) Coaxial dilator with inner metal stiffener

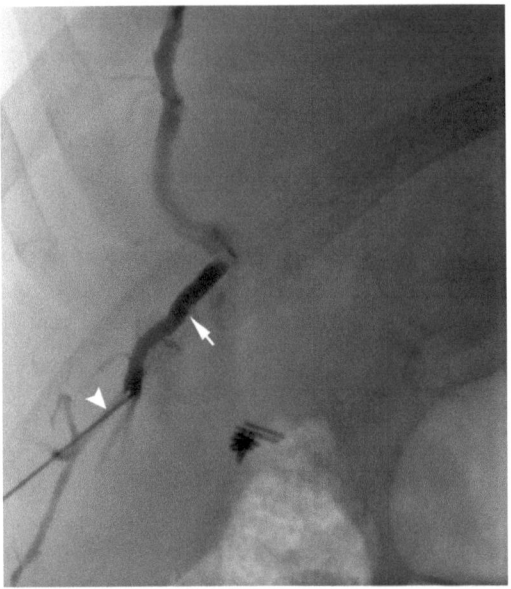

Fig. 6.6 Opacification of a Bile Duct: As the 22 gauge needle (*arrowhead*) was withdrawn from the liver, while simultaneously injecting contrast, a bile duct (*arrow*) was opacified. Gentle injection of contrast and multiple oblique spot radiographs were taken

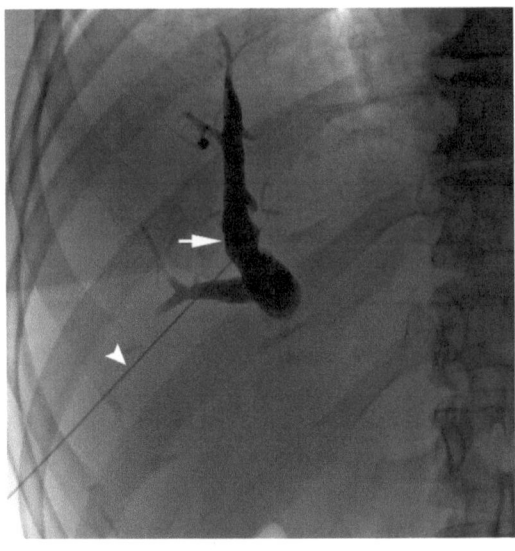

Fig. 6.7 Needle Cholangiography: Contrast was injected through a 22 gauge needle (*arrowhead*) opacifying a segment VIII biliary radical which was markedly dilated (*arrow*). The angulation between the needle and the bile duct would not be optimal for placement of a drain as generally an obtuse angle will be more favorable

re-advanced in a different trajectory (anteroposterior and/or craniocaudad), and the process of slowly injecting contrast with simultaneous withdrawal of the needle is repeated [5, 12].

Upon opacifying a bile duct, bile is aspirated, and an equal amount of contrast is injected to opacify the biliary tree (Figs. 6.6 and 6.7). It is important to avoid over-distension of the biliary tree, as increased pressure, especially in an obstructed patient, can result in sepsis. Multiple spot radiographs are taken in oblique and anterior–posterior projections as contrast fills the biliary tree (Figs. 6.8, 6.9, and 6.10). If drainage is not necessary, then the needle is simply removed [5, 12].

Biliary Drainage

After opacifying the biliary tree and performing cholangiography, a decision can be made whether the currently accessed bile duct is suitable for catheterization and drain placement. Most often, the opacified duct can serve as the definitive access point for drain placement. Occasionally, the needle trajectory can be manipulated, if it is only partially in the bile

duct or at an acute angulation with the biliary radical, to facilitate passage of a 0.018″ wire (Fig. 6.11). If the access is into a larger central biliary duct, the operator should be cognizant that the adjacent vasculature is similarly larger and placement of a drain through a central access route increases the risk of a hemorrhagic complication. In cases where the opacified duct cannot be catheterized due to acute angulation, the first needle is partially withdrawn and reoriented or it is left in place to ensure the ability to opacify the biliary tree and a second puncture is made with a similarly sized needle under fluoroscopic triangulation (Fig. 6.12) [5, 12].

With a suitable bile duct successfully accessed with a needle, a 0.018″ guidewire is advanced into the central biliary tree and if possible into the small bowel. The needle is then removed and over-the-wire, coaxial dilators are placed (Fig. 6.13). The inner dilator accepts a 0.018″ wire and the outer dilator accepts a 0.035″ wire (Fig. 6.14). The inner dilator is removed and, after placing a 0.035″ wire, serial dilation of the tract can be performed to facilitate passage of the definitive multi-side hole biliary drainage catheter, typically ranging from 8 to 10 French in size

Fig. 6.8 Filling the Biliary Tree: Additional contrast was injected through the needle opacifying the right hepatic duct (*arrow*) and left hepatic duct (*arrowhead*), which communicate

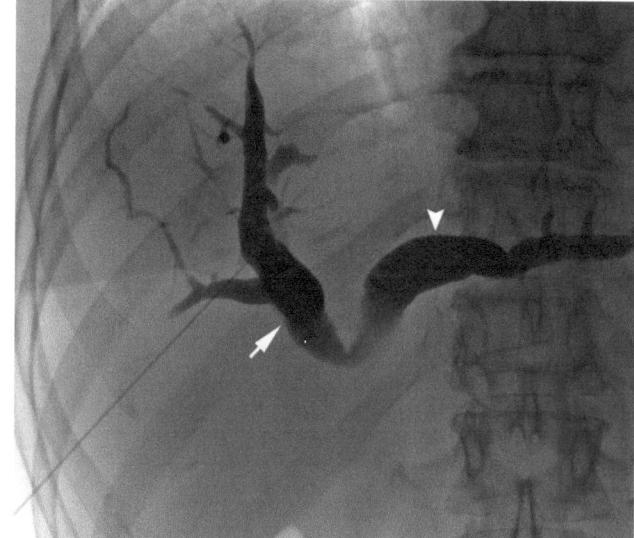

Fig. 6.9 Common Hepatic Duct Stricture: With further contrast filling of the biliary tree, a long segment common hepatic duct stricture is identified (*arrow*). A small volume of contrast opacifies the small bowel (*arrowhead*)

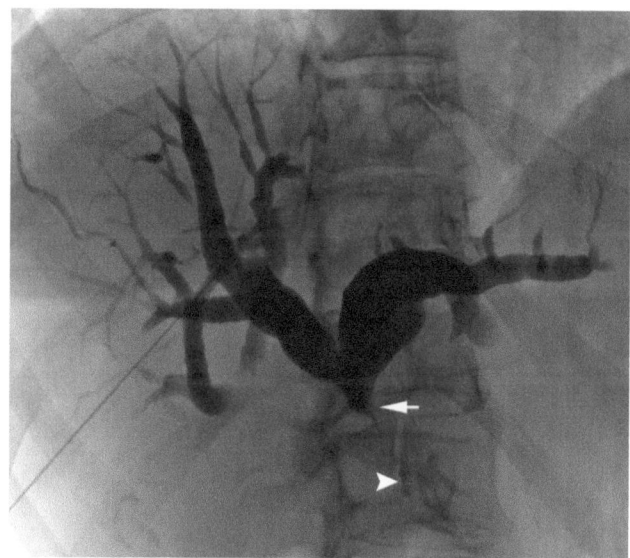

on initial placement (Fig. 6.15). Percutaneous biliary drainage can be achieved with external drain if the wire has not reached the small bowel or with an internal-external drain if it has. When an external biliary drain is placed, the patient usually returns in a matter of days to 2 weeks for another attempt at internalization of the drain. Biliary drains should be flushed with 5–10 mL of normal saline at least daily to maintain patency. While biliary drainage can be performed indefinitely, routine maintenance exchange of the drain is generally required at 6–12 week intervals to preserve patency of the drain [5, 12].

Nondilated and Nontraditional Biliary Access

Occasionally, a non-dilated or decompressed biliary system is encountered and requires transhepatic evaluation and treatment. Challenging scenarios are present, particularly in diffuse inflammatory conditions or iatrogenic biliary leak, among other clinical conditions. Despite the difficulties inherent to this procedure, the potential for benefit for the patient to both define the anatomy and to ameliorate or treat the underlying condition warrants a concerted effort to succeed. Patience

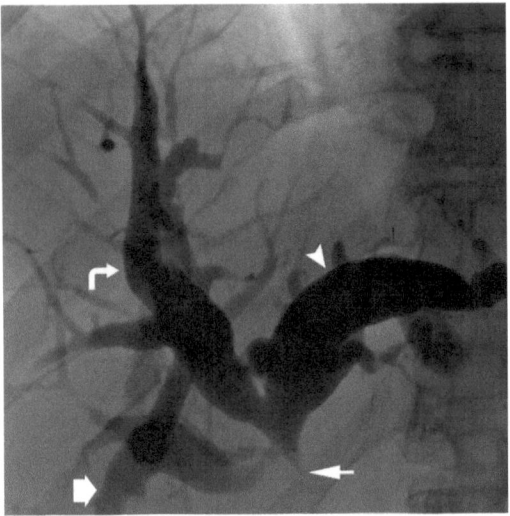

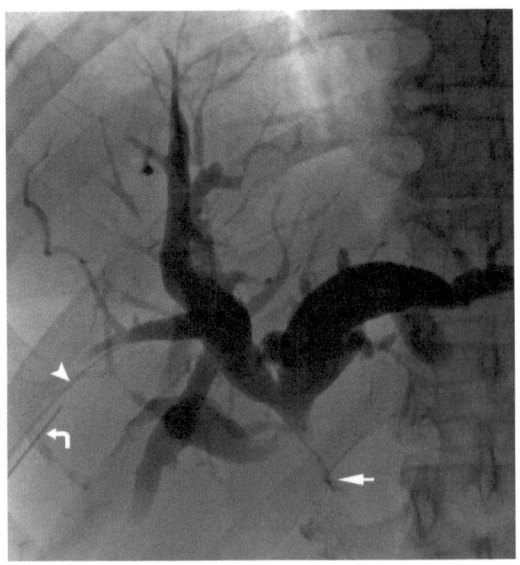

Fig. 6.10 Full Cholangiogram: Diffuse biliary dilatation is noted again in this image with the right superior ducts (*curved arrow*) coalescing centrally to join markedly dilated left hepatic ducts (*arrowhead*) and the right inferior ducts (*block arrow*) to drain in a tapering common hepatic duct (*arrow*). This image can be compared with the CT, MRI, and MRCP images (Figs. 6.2, 6.3, and 6.4) to highlight the technical differences as all are from the same patient within a span of 2 weeks

Fig. 6.12 Definitive Biliary Access: Adjacent to the first needle (*curved arrow*), a second needle (*arrowhead*) was used to puncture a more peripheral duct, and a wire was passed centrally. Over the wire, the inner dilator of the coaxial dilator set was advanced to inject contrast and confirm position (*arrow*)

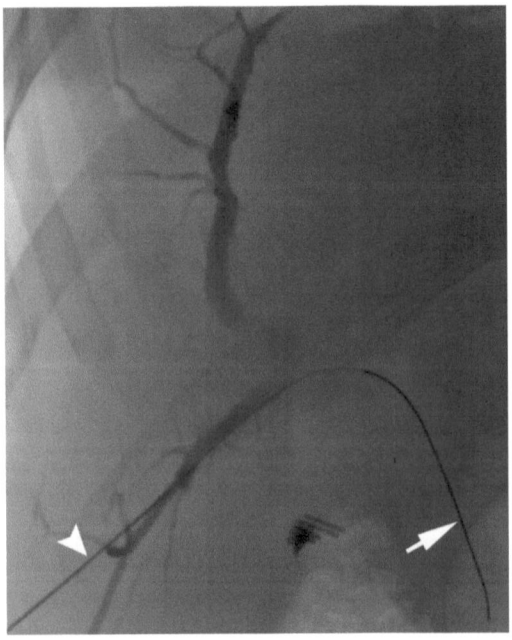

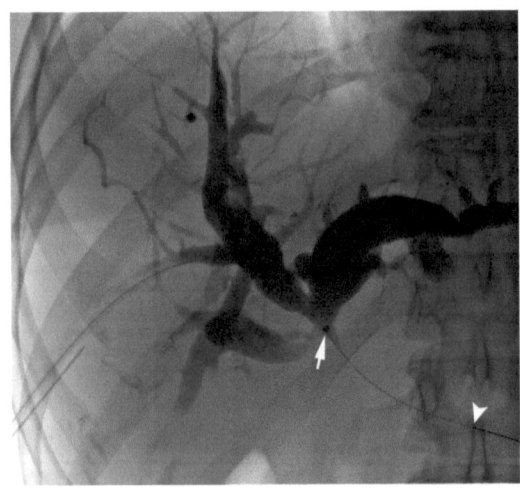

Fig. 6.11 Passage of a 0.018″ wire: The opacified bile duct from Fig. 6.6 was deemed suitable for access and a 0.018″ wire (*arrow*) was passed through the needle (*arrowhead*)

Fig. 6.13 Crossing the Common Hepatic Duct with a wire: The coaxial dilators were then re-advanced over the wire with the outer dilator positioned centrally (*arrow*). A 0.018″ wire was able to cross into the small bowel (*arrowhead*)

Fig. 6.14 Crossing the Common Hepatic Duct with a catheter: Through the dilator, a 4 French catheter (*arrow*) was then used to maintain position within the small bowel (*arrowhead*), and facilitate the upsizing of the wire and eventual drainage catheter placement

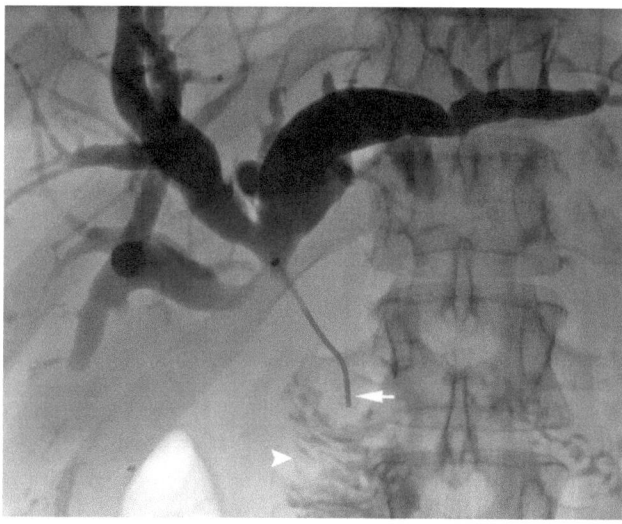

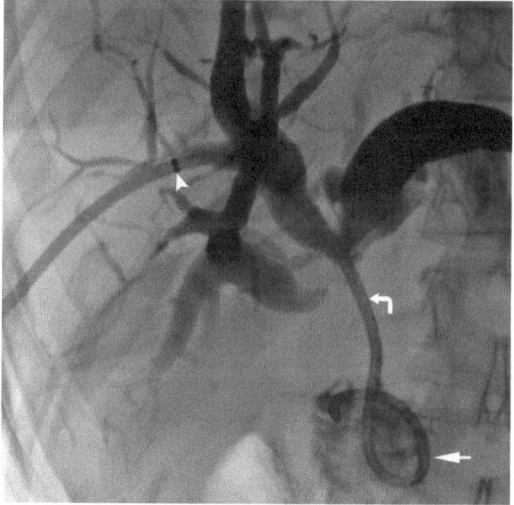

Fig. 6.15 Placement of Internal/External Drainage Catheter: After dilation of the transhepatic tract over the wire, a multi-side hole drainage catheter was passed. The loop retention was formed in the small bowel (*arrow*). Along its length, multiple holes are present (*curved arrow*) from the loop retention to the radiopaque band (*arrowhead*)

system in retrograde fashion. If a more specific injection is required, coaxial placement of a diagnostic catheter can be performed. Moreover, the drain may be removed over the wire and a diagnostic catheter can be introduced to probe the area with contrast or a wire in an attempt to cannulate the biliary tree [13].

When the gallbladder is present, and if the cystic duct is not obstructed, it can be punctured and filled with contrast. With a patent cystic duct, the flow of contrast will continue into the common hepatic and common bile ducts. Alternatively, direct puncture of the central biliary tree, common bile duct, or pre-existing biliary stent can be performed with a 22 gauge needle to opacify the biliary tree and provide a transhepatic target. Trendelenburg positioning of the patient will help the contrast flow in retrograde fashion and fill the intrahepatic ducts [13, 14].

Crossing Strictures/Obstruction

and persistence are necessary, and with repeated attempts success can be realized. Several strategies to opacify and access the biliary tree are discussed with the assumption that the aforementioned techniques were unsuccessful. Once the biliary system is opacified with contrast, then percutaneous targeting can be performed in standard fashion.

If existing drainage catheters are in place, and particularly if bilious drainage is present, they can be injected in attempts to opacify the biliary

Neoplastic, inflammatory, and ischemic strictures or calculi can result in obstruction throughout the biliary tree. If a high grade stricture or obstructive lesion is present, then the primary intent is to gain access beyond the blockage and place an internal–external biliary drain. After stable access into the biliary tree is achieved, a shaped diagnostic catheter and hydrophilic wire are introduced through the access and manipulated beyond the lesion and into the small bowel. When difficulty is encountered, a sheath may be placed to support the catheter and wire and provide stability. However, unnecessary prolonged manipulation of the biliary tree at the time of initial placement may be deleterious to the patient and precipitate an infectious complication. The anatomy of an obstructed biliary tree may be distorted. In this instance, most operators will place a temporary external drain to immediately relieve the biliary obstruction and reattempt internalization within a few weeks after the patient has convalesced and the biliary tree has decompressed.

Results and Complications

Results

Historically, Mueller et al. noted greater than 90 % success rate for cholangiography. More recently, Funaki et al. reported 90 % success rate for cholangiography and biliary drainage in the non-dilated biliary tree. Generally, in the setting of biliary ductal dilatation, cholangiography and biliary drainage can be routinely performed in nearly all patients [15, 16]. The Society of Interventional Radiology Clinical Practice Guideline (SIR-CPG) suggests at least a 95 % and 65 % technical success rate for percutaneous transhepatic cholangiography of dilated and non-dilated ducts, respectively [4]. Regarding biliary drainage, the SIR-CPG reports a 95 % and 70 % success rate for dilated and non-dilated ducts, respectively. Generally, success will mirror the number of passes the operator is willing to make to opacify a biliary radical, though with increasing number of needle passes, the risk of complication also increases [17].

Complications

As for any procedure, cholangiography and drainage are associated with a variety of minor and major intra- and post-procedural complications. The spectrum of complications is similar for each procedure, with drainage resulting in a higher reported rate. Of note, the complication rate with malignant disease has been noted to be higher than benign processes for several reasons including differences in patient age, length of drainage, and overall health [18]. Complication rates are dependent on patient selection and have a wide range in the published literature.

Minor complications can include pain, fever and chills, bile leak, and minor hemobilia. De novo biliary drain placement is associated with pain and irritation, which can originate from the skin entry, traversed tissue, or the liver capsule. Most often, these symptoms are self limited and resolve in a few days. If the drain has been placed along the inferior surface of a rib, pain may be unrelenting due to irritation of the intercostal nerve. The skin entry site should be inspected for irritation from bile and possible tract infection. If the cause is attributable to bile leakage, the drain may have been retracted or obstructed. The drain can be replaced, repositioned, or upsized to minimize bile leakage. Fever and chills are likely a result of transient bacteremia and occurs in less than 5 % of patients. As discussed earlier, prophylaxis with antibiotics is strongly recommended prior to any biliary procedure. If infectious symptoms are noted, it is paramount that they be quickly diagnosed and managed aggressively to prevent septicemia. Additional antibiotics should be administered intravenously to broaden the spectrum of coverage, intravenous hydration should be continued to maintain blood pressure, and the procedure should be completed as expeditiously as possible. Minor hemobilia is not uncommon given the proximity of vessels with the biliary tree. Hemobilia will clear after initial placement within a few days and occasional hemobilia is inconsequential particularly if the drain has been pulled or if the drain is in a location subject to respiratory motion. Generally, as the tract matures minor hemobilia will resolve. The side holes of the drain may become dislodged into an adjacent vein. Drain replacement or upsizing will typically tamponade the bleeding.

Major complications can include sepsis, significant hemobilia, and death with each occurring in less than 5 % of patients. If fever and chills progress to include rigors and hemodynamic instability, aggressive management for septicemia should be implemented. In addition to fluid resuscitation and broadening of the antibiotic spectrum, intravenous meperidine and oxygen should be administered and complete drainage should be performed. The patient will likely require close monitoring and elevation of inpatient care to the intensive care unit [19]. Significant hemobilia, whether persistent or remote from the initial drain placement, can occur if a central access has been created or if an arterial injury has occurred (Fig. 6.16a). Contrast injection of the tract can be performed over the

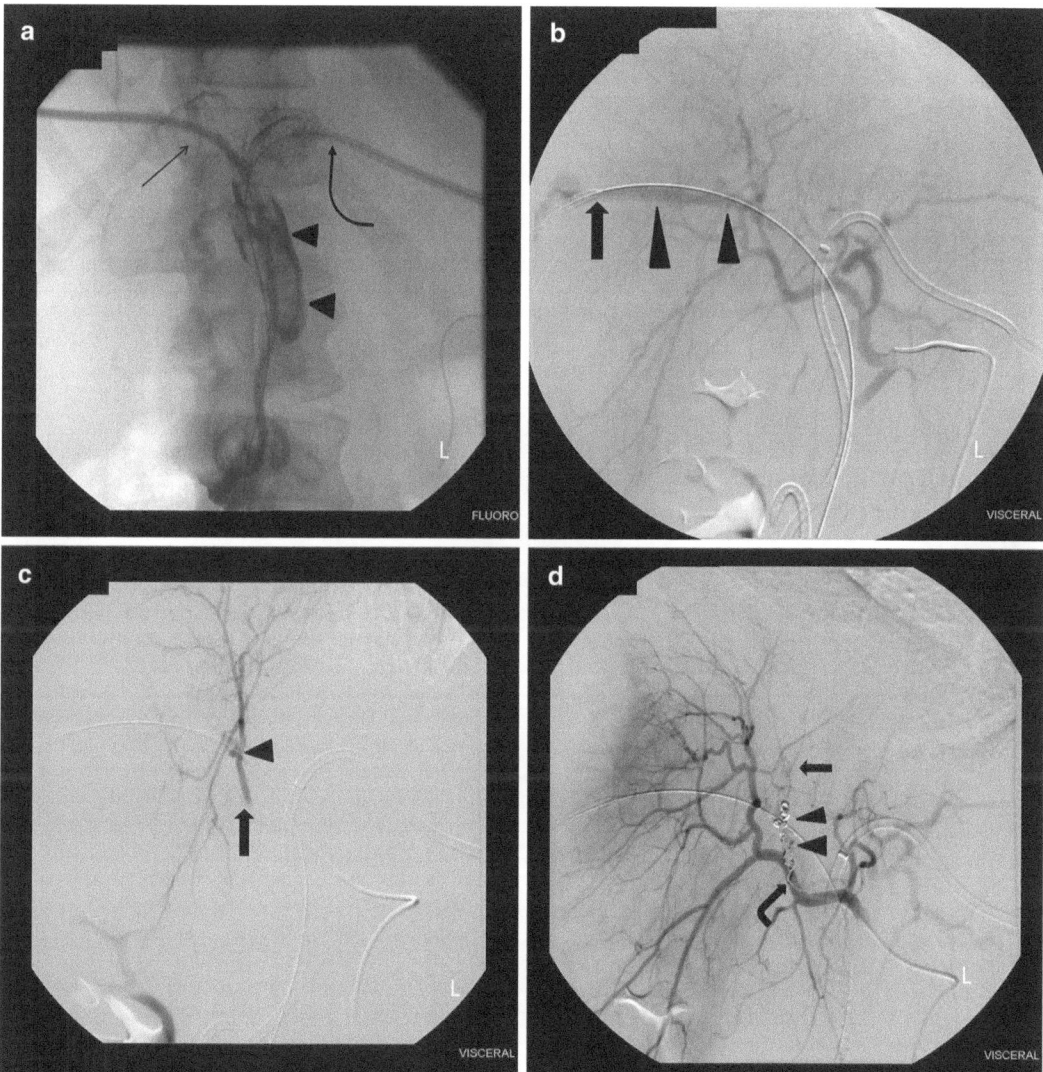

Fig. 6.16 (**a**) Images from a left percutaneous transhepatic biliary drain placement in a 52-year-old male with a provisional diagnosis of pancreatic adenocarcinoma and presenting with persistently elevated liver enzymes and hemobilia after a right biliary drain placement. There are filling defects (*arrowheads*) in the common bile duct, consistent with blood clot. The right drain (*arrow*) is in good position and is patent. The left drain (*curved arrow*) is being inserted. (**b**) Subtracted image from a common hepatic arteriogram with the right biliary drain removed over a wire and a new right drain (*arrow*) partially inserted in the tract. Contrast extravasates along the transhepatic tract (*arrowheads*), indicating direct arterial communica-tion with the tract. (**c**) Subtracted images from a superselective segmental right hepatic arterial injection through a microcatheter (*arrow*). A pseudoaneurysm (*arrowhead*) and the affected hepatic arterial branch were identified. (**d**) Subtracted images from a common hepatic arterial injection after coil embolization of the injured right hepatic arterial branch. A series of microcoils (*arrowheads*) have been placed distal to and proximal to the pseudoaneurysm, resulting in occlusion of that segment. Smaller right hepatic arterial branches distal to the site of occlusion were already being reconstituted (*arrow*) via intrahepatic arterial collaterals. Some coils inadvertently prolapsed into the right hepatic artery (*curved arrow*)

wire to delineate the source of injury. If the portal vein is involved, typically there is dark red non-pulsatile blood, and the tract can be embolized with Gelfoam after establishment of an alternative biliary drain tract. If a hepatic artery has been traversed, this will usually manifest as bright red pulsatile blood and should be treated immediately. Hepatic arteriography should be performed with the drain slightly pulled back over a wire (Fig. 6.16b), to help find the site of bleeding. In the event that an arterial injury is found, superselective coil embolization (Fig. 6.16c, d) is performed across the injury, distal to proximal [19, 20]. Death is uncommon and is frequently the result of preexisting comorbidities as opposed to the procedure related mortality.

Aside from direct procedural complications, sporadic small case series and case reports have documented metastatic implantation along biliary catheter tracts. In these cases, the prognosis is usually poor but surgical excision can be attempted [21–27].

References

1. Couinaud C. Le foie. Etudes anatomiques et chirurgicales. Paris: Masson; 1957. p. 530.
2. Gazelle GS, Lee MJ, Mueller PR. Cholangiographic segmental anatomy of the liver. Radiographics. 1994; 14:1005–13.
3. Castaing D. Surgical anatomy of the biliary tract. HPB (Oxford). 2008;10(2):72–6.
4. Saad WE, Wallace MJ, Wojak JC, Kundu S, Cardella JF. Quality improvement guidelines for percutaneous transhepatic cholangiography, biliary drainage, and percutaneous cholecystostomy. J Vasc Interv Radiol. 2010;21(6):789–95.
5. Covey AM, Brown KT. Percutaneous transhepatic biliary drainage. Tech Vasc Interv Rad. 2008;11:14–20.
6. Clark CD, Picus D, Dunagan WC. Bloodstream infections after interventional procedures in the biliary tract. Radiology. 1994;191(2):495–9.
7. Sheen-Chen S, Chen W, Eng H, et al. Bacteriology and antimicrobial choice in hepatolithiasis. Am J Infect Control. 2000;28(4):298–301.
8. Rösch T, Triptrap A, Born P, et al. Bacteriobilia in percutaneous transhepatic biliary drainage: occurrence over time and clinical sequelae. A prospective observational study. Scand J Gastroenterol. 2003; 38(11):1162–8.
9. Venkatesan AM, Kundu S, Sacks D, et al. Practice guideline for adult antibiotic prophylaxis during vascular and interventional radiology procedures. J Vasc Interv Radiol. 2010;21:1611–30.
10. Mueller PR, Wittenberg KH, Kaufman JA, Lee MJ. Patterns of anesthesia and nursing care for interventional radiology procedures: a national survey of physician practices and preferences. Radiology. 1997; 202:339–43.
11. Lee MJ, Mueller PR, Saini S, et al. Percutaneous dilatation of benign biliary strictures: single session therapy with general anesthesia. Am J Roentgenol. 1991;157:1263.
12. Saad WEA. Transhepatic techniques for accessing the biliary tract. Tech Vasc Interv Rad. 2008;11:21–42.
13. Kim HS, Lund GG, Venbrux AC. Advanced percutaneous transhepatic biliary access. Tech Vasc Interv Rad. 2001;3:153–71.
14. Ginat D, Saad WEA. Cholecystostomy and transcholecystic biliary access. Tech Vasc Interv Rad. 2008; 11:2–13.
15. Mueller PR, Harbin WP, Ferrucci Jr JT, Wittenberg J, vanSonnenberg E. Fine-needle transhepatic cholangiography: reflections after 450 cases. Am J Roentgenol. 1981;136(1):85–90.
16. Funaki B, Zaleski GX, Straus CA, et al. Percutaneous biliary drainage in patients with nondilated intrahepatic bile ducts. Am J Roentgenol. 1999;173: 1541–4.
17. Jaques PF, Mauro MA, Scatliff JH. The failed transhepatic cholangiogram. Radiology. 1980;134(1):33–5.
18. Yee ACN, Ho C. Complications of percutaneous biliary drainage: benign vs malignant disease. Am J Roentgenol. 1987;148:1207–9.
19. Winick AB, Waybill PN, Venbrux AC. Complications of percutaneous transhepatic biliary interventions. Tech Vasc Interv Rad. 2001;3:200–6.
20. Saad WEA, Davies MG, Darcy MD. Management of bleeding after percutaneous cholangiography or transhepatic biliary drain placement. Tech Vasc Interv Rad. 2008;11:60–71.
21. Chapman WC, Sharp KW, Weaver F, Sawyers JL. Tumor seeding from percutaneous biliary catheters. Ann Surg. 1989;209:708–13. discussion 713–15.
22. Inagaki M, Yabuki H, Hashimoto M, Maguchi M, Kino S, Sawa M, Ojima H, Tokusashi Y, Miyokawa N, Kusano M, Kasai S. Metastatic seeding of bile duct carcinoma in the transhepatic catheter tract: report of a case. Surg Today. 1999;29:1260–3.
23. Sakata J, Shirai Y, Wakai T, Nomura T, Sakata E, Hatakeyama K. Catheter tract implantation metastases associated with percutaneous biliary drainage for extrahepatic cholangiocarcinoma. World J Gastroenterol. 2005;11(44):7024–7.
24. Shimizu Y, Yasui K, Kato T, Yamamura Y, Hirai T, Kodera Y, Kanemitsu Y, Ito S, Shibata N, Yamao K, Ohhashi K. Implantation metastasis along the percutaneous transhepatic biliary drainage sinus tract. Hepatogastroenterology. 2004;51:365–7.
25. Tersigni R, Rossi P, Bochicchio O, Cavallini M, Ambrogi C, Bufalini G, Alessandroni L, Arena L,

Armeni O, Miraglia F, Stipa S. Tumor extension along percutaneous transhepatic biliary drainage tracts. Eur J Radiol. 1986;6:280–2.

26. Oleaga JA, Ring EJ, Freiman DB, McLean GK, Rosen RJ. Extension of neoplasm along the tract of a transhepatic tube. Am J Roentgenol. 1980;135: 841–2.

27. Kim WS, Barth KH, Zinner M. Seeding of pancreatic carcinoma along the transhepatic catheter tract. Radiology. 1982;143:427–8.

Veeral M. Oza and Marty M. Meyer

Acute Gallstone Pancreatitis

The most common cause of acute pancreatitis (AP) in the Western Hemisphere is gallstones [1]. Some studies have reported recovery of gallstones in stool from 85 to 90 % of patients with AP [2]. Mortality in AP is approximately 5 % among all patients and has been reported to be as high as 30 % in severe cases [3]. Gallstone pancreatitis occurs when a CBDS travels distally and obstructs the ampulla and/or compresses the septum between the distal CBD and pancreatic duct. These processes lead to reflux of bile into the pancreas and increased pressure within the pancreatic duct. The net result is pancreatic ductal injury with release of proteolytic enzymes into the pancreatic interstitium leading to autodigestion and inflammation [2, 4–6]. Given such high mortality rates of AP, resolution of the ongoing insult to the pancreas is paramount in trying to start the healing process.

V.M. Oza, M.D. • M.M. Meyer, M.D. (✉)
Division of Gastroenterology, Hepatology
and Nutrition, Department of Internal Medicine,
The Ohio State University Wexner Medical Center,
395 W. 12th Avenue, 2nd Floor, Columbus,
OH 43210, USA
e-mail: veerubhai@gmail.com;
marty.meyer@osumc.edu

The role and timing of endoscopic intervention, namely endoscopic retrograde cholangiopancreatography (ERCP), in gallstone-mediated AP is controversial, with some studies showing benefit of early intervention and others showing no benefit and possibly even a worse outcome [7–14]. In the absence of cholangitis and biliary obstruction, the current consensus recommends conservative measures prior to attempting ERCP for acute gallstone-mediated pancreatitis, as ERCP within 24–72 h of presentation does not lead to any reduction in mortality [7].

Acute Cholangitis/Sepsis

Unlike gallstone-mediated pancreatitis, there is strong data to support urgent ERCP in patients with cholangitis. The indication for ERCP in patients with concern of cholangitis includes fever, jaundice, and sepsis. A conjugated bilirubin level greater than 5 mg/dl and presence of a persistent biliary obstruction or those patients who have worsening clinical status, e.g., worsening leukocytosis, signs of decompensation such as hypotension, and rising liver transaminases all support a clinical diagnosis of cholangitis.

Early antibiotic therapy is warranted in cases of suspected cholangitis. In those patients that do

© Springer International Publishing Switzerland 2016
J.W. Hazey et al. (eds.), *Multidisciplinary Management of Common Bile Duct Stones*,
DOI 10.1007/978-3-319-22765-8_7

not respond to antibiotic therapy, urgent biliary decompression should be pursued [15]. If a patient is medically unstable, or if an attempt at endoscopic drainage has failed, a percutaneous transhepatic cholangiography (PTC) with biliary drainage is recommended [15]. The specific interventions of a successful ERCP procedure, including the role of sphincterotomy and stent placement, are discussed in other chapters of this book.

Postsurgical Anatomy

Successful ERCP is dependent on the ability to advance the side-viewing duodenoscope to the level of the ampulla. In addition, it is equally important that the duodenoscope maintains an optimal and stable position. Due to rising rates of obesity across the world, more patients are undergoing bariatric surgery, leading to altered anatomy of the upper and mid gastrointestinal tract. This has led to increased utilitization of novel techniques to endoscopically visualize the ampulla.

In patients with either a Roux-en-Y gastrojejunostomy or Billroth II gastrectomy (distal antrectomy) the duodenum drains through a distal afferent limb to the gastric remnant via an end-to-side gastrojejunostomy, although in Billroth II the gastric pouch has a more proximal anastomosis with the jejunum [16, 17]. Due to this altered anatomy, accessing the duodenum with a standard technique is challenging and a balloon enteroscopy is often performed. The success rate in such cases where the papilla is visualized with a forward-viewing endoscope is estimated to be about 60–80 % [18–20].

In addition to using balloon enteroscopy to reach the ampulla, a combined surgical and endoscopic approach has recently been developed with excellent success rates. Usually performed in the operating room, it involves placement of a trocar in the bypassed stomach under direct visualization. The duodenoscope can then be introduced through this port and the duodenum can be accessed with ease. This procedure is known as the laparoscopic transgastric endoscopic approach. In one series, the technical success rate in the transgastric method was 100 % versus 59 % for balloon-assisted enteroscopy technique [19]. It should be noted that despite the high technical success rate of the combined surgical/endoscopic approach, this is an invasive approach and requires a sterile environment, a skilled endoscopist and good communication amongst all providers [16, 17].

"Difficult Stones"

In patients that are post-cholecystectomy with evidence of retained CBDS, or evidence of multiple stones within the duct, ERCP is considered first-line therapy due to the low morbidity and mortality when compared to surgical approaches (discussed in other chapters of this book). ERCP with sphincterotomy and balloon extraction should be attempted as the first modality to remove CBDS. If stone extraction fails, a sphincterotomy with macrodilation of the sphincter of Oddi can be performed [21]. If clearance attempts still fail, a biliary stent should be left in place and the procedure can be reattempted in 4–6 weeks. If endoscopic access of the papilla fails, a PTC drain may be placed to achieve biliary decompression.

Endoscopic Therapy in Anticoagulated Patients

Patients presenting with cholangitis or with gallstone-mediated AP commonly take therapeutic anticoagulation, using agents such as enoxaparin or warfarin, or an antiplatelet medication such as clopidogrel. Given the increased risk of bleeding associated with these agents, one needs to weigh the likelihood of bleeding against the dangers of delaying endoscopic therapy.

The patients at highest risk for clinically significant hemorrhage include those taking therapeutic anticoagulation, clopidogrel or other hematologic disorders resulting in a platelet count less than $50,000K/\mu L$ or INR greater than 2.5. To reduce bleeding risk in such cases, ERCP without sphincterotomy should be performed and a plastic biliary stent should be placed. Once the coagulation parameters have been corrected, the

ERCP can be repeated and a sphincterotomy with removal of the CBDS can be done. With the exception of emergencies, the sphincterotomy can be delayed as outlined above.

In patients in whom coagulation parameters cannot be corrected, one can perform a 'classic' biliary dilation—a dilation of up to 10 mm—at the sphincter of Oddi. The balloon sphincter dilation technique minimizes the risk of bleeding due to a lesser degree of mucosal disruption. However this also exposes the patient to complications of post-ERCP AP and cholecystitis [22–24]. These risks should be discussed while obtaining the informed consent.

Ideally the INR should be less than 1.5 prior to a sphincterotomy. This intervention is considered safe in patients on aspirin [15]. In those patients using clopidogrel, it is recommended by the American Society of Gastrointestinal Endoscopy to hold it for 7–10 days prior to intervention. To further mitigate the risk of bleeding, endoscopists should use a blend of coagulation and cutting current for the sphincterotomy [15].

Conclusion

Over the last decade there has been a rise of CBDS and the associated complications. The challenge presented by the rising obesity epidemic has been countered by new technology and devices as well as novel procedures, especially for patients who have had bariatric surgery. Anticoagulated patients should have their coagulopathy reversed, unless the risk from this delay is greater than then likelihood of bleeding from ERCP. An endoscopic approach is safe and should always be considered as the first-line therapeutic approach. Surgical and interventional radiology techniques can be definitive and are reserved for cases where endoscopic treatment fails.

References

1. Attasaranya S, Fogel EL, Lehman GA. Choledocholithiasis, ascending cholangitis, and gallstone pancreatitis. Med Clin North Am. 2008;92(4):925–60. x.

2. Acosta JM, Ledesma CL. Gallstone migration as a cause of acute pancreatitis. N Engl J Med. 1974; 290(9):484–7.

3. Pitchumoni CS, Patel NM, Shah P. Factors influencing mortality in acute pancreatitis: can we alter them? J Clin Gastroenterol. 2005;39(9):798–814.

4. Acosta JM, Pellegrini CA, Skinner DB. Etiology and pathogenesis of acute biliary pancreatitis. Surgery. 1980;88(1):118–25.

5. Lightner AM, Kirkwood KS. Pathophysiology of gallstone pancreatitis. Front Biosci. 2001;6:E66–76.

6. Wang GJ, et al. Acute pancreatitis: etiology and common pathogenesis. World J Gastroenterol. 2009;15(12): 1427–30.

7. Fogel EL, Sherman S. ERCP for gallstone pancreatitis. N Engl J Med. 2014;370(2):150–7.

8. Chen P, et al. Pilot study of urgent endoscopic intervention without fluoroscopy on patients with severe acute biliary pancreatitis in the intensive care unit. Pancreas. 2010;39(3):398–402.

9. Fan ST, et al. Early treatment of acute biliary pancreatitis by endoscopic papillotomy. N Engl J Med. 1993;328(4):228–32.

10. Folsch UR, et al. Early ERCP and papillotomy compared with conservative treatment for acute biliary pancreatitis. The German Study Group on Acute Biliary Pancreatitis. N Engl J Med. 1997;336(4): 237–42.

11. Neoptolemos JP, et al. Controlled trial of urgent endoscopic retrograde cholangiopancreatography and endoscopic sphincterotomy versus conservative treatment for acute pancreatitis due to gallstones. Lancet. 1988;2(8618):979–83.

12. Nowak A, Nowakowska-Dulawa E, Marek TA, Rybicka J. Final results of the prospective, randomized, controlled study on endoscopic sphincterotomy versus conventional management in acute biliary pancreatitis. Gastroenterology. 1995;108:A380.

13. Oria A, et al. Early endoscopic intervention versus early conservative management in patients with acute gallstone pancreatitis and biliopancreatic obstruction: a randomized clinical trial. Ann Surg. 2007;245(1): 10–7.

14. Zhou MQ, Li NP, Lu RD. Duodenoscopy in treatment of acute gallstone pancreatitis. Hepatobiliary Pancreat Dis Int. 2002;1(4):608–10.

15. Williams EJ, et al. Guidelines on the management of common bile duct stones (CBDS). Gut. 2008;57(7): 1004–21.

16. Moreels TG. Altered anatomy: enteroscopy and ERCP procedure. Best Pract Res Clin Gastroenterol. 2012;26(3):347–57.

17. Moreels TG. ERCP in the patient with surgically altered anatomy. Curr Gastroenterol Rep. 2013;15(9): 343.

18. Cho S, et al. 'Short' double-balloon enteroscope endoscopic retrograde cholangiopancreatography in patients with a surgically altered upper gastrointestinal tract. Can J Gastroenterol. 2011;25(11):615–9.

19. Schreiner MA, et al. Laparoscopy-assisted versus balloon enteroscopy-assisted ERCP in bariatric post-Roux-en-Y gastric bypass patients. Gastrointest Endosc. 2012;75(4):748–56.

20. Yamauchi H, et al. Short-type single balloon enteroscope for endoscopic retrograde cholangio-pancreatography with altered gastrointestinal anatomy. World J Gastroenterol. 2013;19(11): 1728–35.

21. Karsenti D. Endoscopic management of bile duct stones: residual bile duct stones after surgery, cholangitis, and "difficult stones". J Visc Surg. 2013;150(3 Suppl):S39–46.

22. Baron TH, Harewood GC. Endoscopic balloon dilation of the biliary sphincter compared to endoscopic biliary sphincterotomy for removal of common bile duct stones during ERCP: a metaanalysis of randomized, controlled trials. Am J Gastroenterol. 2004;99(8):1455–60.

23. Bergman JJ, et al. Randomised trial of endoscopic balloon dilation versus endoscopic sphincterotomy for removal of bileduct stones. Lancet. 1997;349(9059):1124–9.

24. Park DH, et al. Endoscopic sphincterotomy vs. endoscopic papillary balloon dilation for choledocholithiasis in patients with liver cirrhosis and coagulopathy. Gastrointest Endosc. 2004;60(2):180–5.

Special Considerations for the Surgeon

Michael Paul Meara

Introduction

Significant advances in minimally invasive surgery and endoscopic techniques have redefined the management of common bile duct stones. Disease processes, which would keep patients hospitalized for protracted periods of time, have migrated to outpatient or overnight stays. Despite this, it is important in the management of these issues that special consideration be lent to resource management, physiologic considerations, previous and current anatomic issues, and ultimately specific surgical planning should operative intervention be required. While the move to minimally invasive and endoscopic techniques has lessened the need for operative intervention, it has not diminished its importance and the vital role it serves in the care of these patients. It is in this vein that we must consider the experience young surgeons emerging from training have and their comfort operating in this anatomic area.

M.P. Meara, MD, MBA (✉)
Division of General and Gastrointestinal Surgery,
The Ohio State University Wexner Medical Center,
University Hospital East, 11th Floor Tower, 1492 E
Broad St Ste 1102, Columbus, OH 43205-1546, USA
e-mail: Michael.Meara@osumc.edu

Resources and Limitations

In the management of common bile duct stones, a wide "tool box" of both resources and technical expertise is required for the many presentations in which stones can occur. The physician must recognize the expertise required in all fields responsible for management of these issues. This includes expertise in advanced endoscopy and the various techniques available for common bile duct stone management. In the event of endoscopic failure, other expertise may be required. A specific working knowledge of both open and laparoscopic techniques to address these issues is furthermore important. A further adjunct which may be required is the expertise of a well-trained interventional radiologist who may be able to assist with percutaneous access of the biliary system or abdominal drainage in the postoperative management of the patient [1].

The first consideration of common bile duct stones it to be aware of the resources available at your specific institution. Adequate resources can be a vague term, but consideration of some the following items is important for treatment of the patient's with common bile duct stones. A working knowledge of these resources is essential to operative planning and for definitive disposition of the patient. Supplied with this knowledge, the treating physician should be able to decide where the patient's needs will be best served. If this is a patient who can be treated at the presenting institution, they should be admitted and cared for without delay or detriment to the patient [2].

The treating physician must consider the nature of the intervention required for the patient. If the patient is presenting hemodynamically stable, the resources required may simply include an available endoscopy suite and an endoscopist to perform the appropriate procedure. If the stones ultimately prove too large to address endoscopically, resources should include a surgeon and operative suite ready to address the patient's specific disease. This may be amenable to being addressed either laparoscopically or in an open operative fashion. Specific attention should be lent to the patient's comorbidities and their ability to tolerate specific anesthetics as well. These considerations can largely be readily assessed at bedside in the emergency department and the decision to provide definitive care addressed immediately [3, 4].

With specific respect to open operative considerations, it is expected that a hospital with inpatient surgical services will have standard open operating equipment available as well as anesthesia support should the patient require emergent surgical intervention. In the event of a patient who is decompensating from overwhelming biliary sepsis who needs emergent decompression, these may be the only tools you require, though supportive postoperative care is equally important. Ensuring that the operative suite has specialized tools and instruments that may be required for biliary surgery is also important. Preparation for this potential is best performed in an elective setting prior to their operative need [4].

For the laparoscopic setting, laparoscopic cholecystectomy as an emerging technology in the 1990s found rapid penetrance in the field of surgery. Its benefits were quickly recognized and the supporting technology worked diligently to keep pace with its emergence. In a relatively small amount of time, laparoscopic cholecystectomy overtook open cholecystectomy and has become the gold standard for management of benign biliary disease. Correlating with this emergence was the acceptance of this technology and its introduction into surgical training. As this technology took its place in the surgical field, the resources

necessary to support its wide spread prevalence were equally quickly adopted from large urban centers to even the most rural environments. After addressing the common bile duct stones, should laparoscopic cholecystectomy be required, this should be readily available at most institutions for definitive treatment of cholelithiasis that has transitioned to choledocholithiasis [4].

Lastly, it is important to know when the needs of the patient will outstrip the resources specifically available at your institution. At this junction, a working knowledge of the referral patterns and regional services available to your institution is important to provide rapid disposition to the patient. Regardless of the approach you may take to treat the patient, if the patient presents with hemodynamic instability or overwhelming sepsis, the patient may require admission to an intensive care unit for monitoring and resuscitation. If these resources are unavailable at the presenting institution, transfer is required for timely care of the patient. It is also important to remember that the needs and resources of the patient can change dramatically during their stay in the hospital. For example, if benign common bile duct stones transform to acute or necrotizing pancreatitis, a patient who is originally appropriate for a primary care center may require transfer to a tertiary care facility for management. Plans should also be in place for transfer should complications arise from an endoscopic or operative procedure and the post-procedural care for these patients is not available. Support again may entail ICU monitoring and care, as well as adjuncts including interventional radiology [5].

As an aside, specific regional systems may become overburdened at times and leave patient's waiting for hours or even days in extreme cases. Backup plans and nonstandard referral patterns may be required to disposition the patient who needs urgent endoscopic or operative intervention [2].

Physiologic Considerations

Assessing the physiology of a patient who presents with common bile duct stones and related disease is important to assist in the preoperative workup, intraoperative management, and postoperative care.

The physiologic status and impact of a patient cannot be understated. The physiologic status of a patient can be broken down into two settings. The first is the acute changes that have developed as a result of the discovered bile duct stones. The second is the physiologic derangements related to their chronic medical comorbidities. These include derangements to the hepatic, respiratory, and cardiovascular systems among other issues.

Acutely, when excretion of bile into the enteral system has been impeded, there is a subsequent buildup of bilirubin in the blood stream. This ultimately results in the clinical manifestation of jaundice. Similarly, the patient may manifest scleral icterus, which is an additional manifestation. Total bilirubin ranges from 0.2 to 14 mg/dL, but jaundice and icterus may not become present until values exceed 3 mg/dL. Dark urine may be observed and bilirubin can be detected in the urine as well. Because of the lack of bile excreted into the gastrointestinal tract, pale stools may also be observed [6].

With regards to the hepatic system, biliary obstruction can result in a wide variety of issues from minimal insult to the system to complete and devastating hepatic failure. Much of this level of impact has to do with the duration of which biliary obstruction goes untreated. Obstruction can result in ongoing injury on the hepatocellular level leading to liver function derangements. Complications of biliary obstruction include derangements in the coagulation pathway and subsequent coagulopathy. This can be supportively treated with fresh frozen plasma and vitamin K in parallel with timely assessment of the biliary obstruction [7].

Further physiologic issues primarily result from the resulting cholangitis. Obstruction of the biliary system can predispose the patient to bacterial translocation. This results from a buildup for bacteria in the biliary system secondary to the inability to adequately drain. This inability to drain has several infectious consequences. Hepatic abscesses can readily form in the presence of obstruction. Furthermore, bacteria can then more readily translate into the circulatory system on the hepatocellular level. Bacterial isolates are commonly *Escherichia coli*, Klebsiella, Proteus, and Pseudomonas species. Treatment with antibiotics is essential, but only moderately effective until the underlying obstruction has been treated. The concomitant presence of endotoxin in the blood in addition to bacteremia may lead to overwhelming circulatory collapse [7].

Overwhelming sepsis and circulatory collapse can predispose the patient to severe, overwhelming multisystem organ failure. Renal failure can result from direct insult from circulating endotoxin, secondary to bodily fluid derangements, and decreased renal blood flow secondary to sepsis. The presence of renal failure is an ominous sign in the patient with obstructive jaundice. Supportive care when sepsis is present is essential to survival, but ultimate relief of the obstruction the key to patient survival [7].

The wide breadth of chronic patient ailments can all be affected to some degree by resulting biliary obstruction from common bile duct stones. The impact of this can vary based on their degree of chronic disease and degree of insult resulting from the patient's obstruction. All of the discussed physiologic changes must be carefully assess and treated in the appropriate setting. Consideration of the pre-procedural, peri-procedural, and post-procedural changes the patient will experience is important in the care of the patient and the setting in which the patient will be managed.

Anatomic Considerations

The ductal anatomy can be extremely variable when surgically approaching biliary disease. This remark was made by Eisendrath in 1918, repeated by Hayes 40 years later, and found its way into text books to follow, "In no area of the human body are the relationships as described in the text books of anatomy more misleading as to constancy than the region encompassing the extrahepatic biliary ducts" [8]. Despite this, we as medical professionals continue to learn the simplistic view that is the anatomy of the porta hepatis. This involves the exiting of a duct from each of the lobes of the liver coming to a confluence to form the common hepatic duct. This travels for a short course till it is joined by the cystic duct to form the common bile duct. This extends for 6–8 cm until finally being joined briefly by the pancreatic duct and terminating at the ampulla of Vater as it empties into the duodenum. Despite traditional teaching, notable, highly variable changes can occur.

The variably of hepatic ducts primarily is derived from the drainage of the right anterior and right posterior segments of the liver. These two segments are drained by independent ducts which typically join to form the right hepatic duct. The right and left hepatic duct join to form the common hepatic duct. Variability stems from configuration of the joining of the anterior and posterior segments. Either may join with the left hepatic duct with the remaining duct becoming the sole right hepatic. This variability can be further influenced by the presence of aberrant ducts. Aberrant ducts have been described from 1 to 30 % of cases. A working knowledge of common variants and the ability to interpret cholangiography, both endoscopic and intraoperative, can help avoid subsequent complications (Figs. 8.1, 8.2, 8.3, 8.4, 8.5, and 8.6) [8].

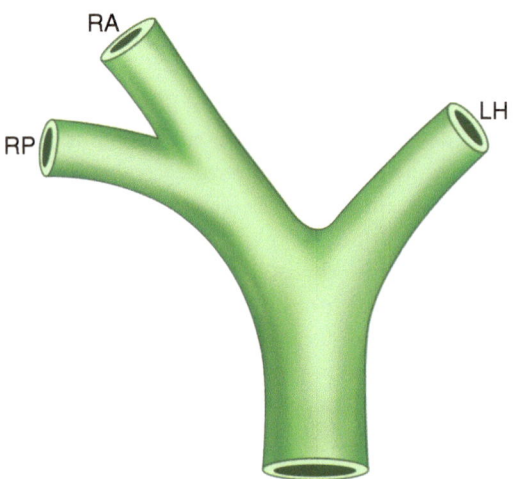

Fig. 8.1 Typical hepatic duct anatomy

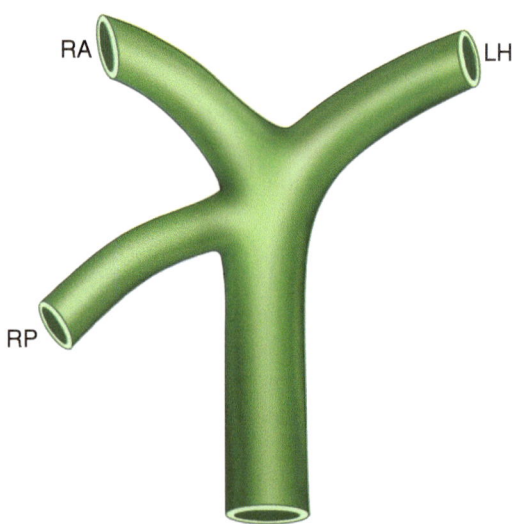

Fig. 8.3 Ectopic insertion of the right posterior into the common hepatic (Variant 01)

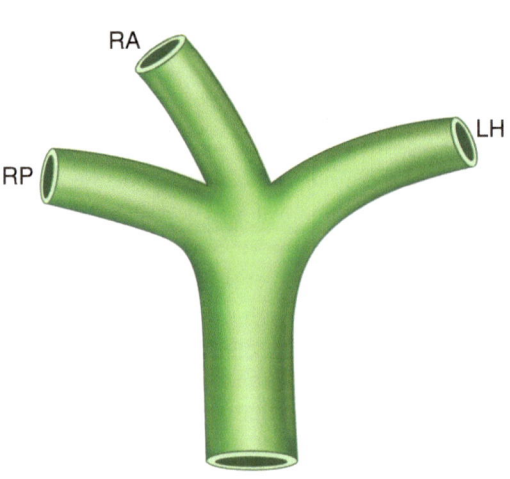

Fig. 8.2 Triple confluence

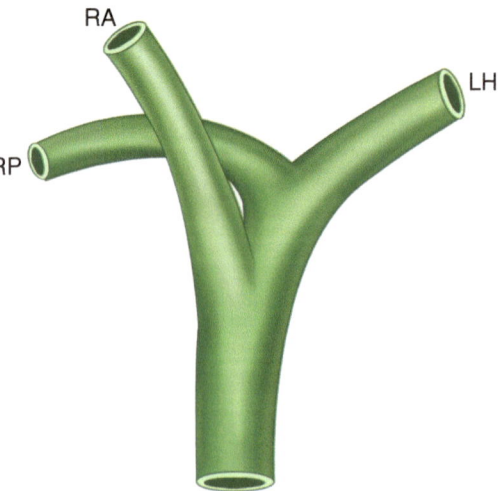

Fig. 8.4 Ectopic insertion of the right posterior into the common hepatic (Variant 02)

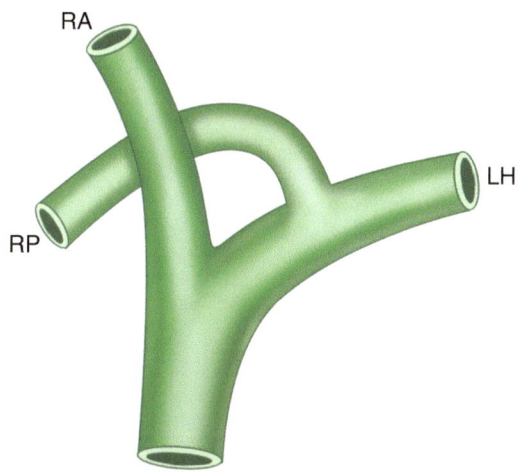

Fig. 8.5 Ectopic insertion of the right posterior into the left hepatic (Variant 01)

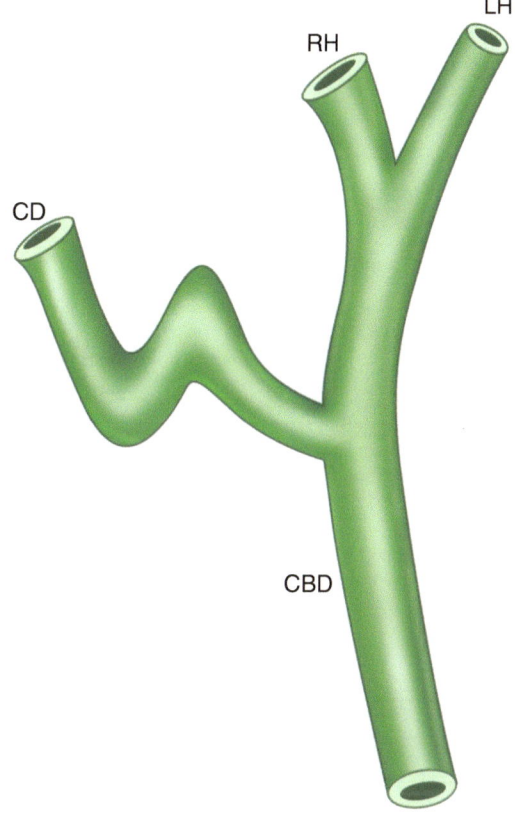

Fig. 8.7 Variations in cystic duct anatomy—typical anatomy 75 %

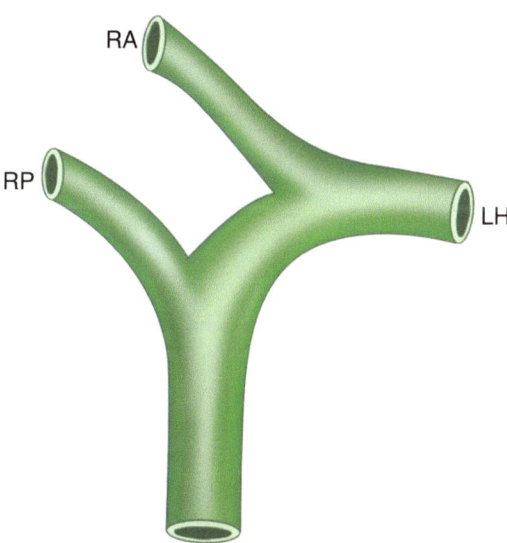

Fig. 8.6 Ectopic insertion of the right anterior into the left hepatic (Variant 02)

The cystic duct anatomy can be equally variable. Traditionally, the cystic duct exits the gallbladder and joins the common hepatic duct to form the common bile duct after traveling a length of approximately 4 cm. The anatomy of the cystic duct can be highly variable beyond this standard description. The duct can be entirely absent, with the base of the gallbladder joining directly with the common hepatic duct. The cystic duct can be short from that standpoint, or variably long, traveling anterior or posterior to the common hepatic duct itself. It can also join directly with the right hepatic duct. It is this high variability that lends itself to the incidence of common bile duct injury during laparoscopic cholecystectomy. Injuries to the common duct are estimated to occur 0.1–0.25 % of the time during open cholecystectomy and 0.6 % of the time during laparoscopic cholecystectomy. The ability to appreciate and identify variable anatomy is essential to avoidance or recognition of this complication (Figs. 8.7, 8.8, and 8.9).

In the event of operative intervention, beyond knowledge of the biliary anatomy and its various aberrations, one should also be familiar with the arterial anatomy, which can be equally varied. The typical arterial anatomy to the gallbladder originates from the celiac axis. The celiac artery

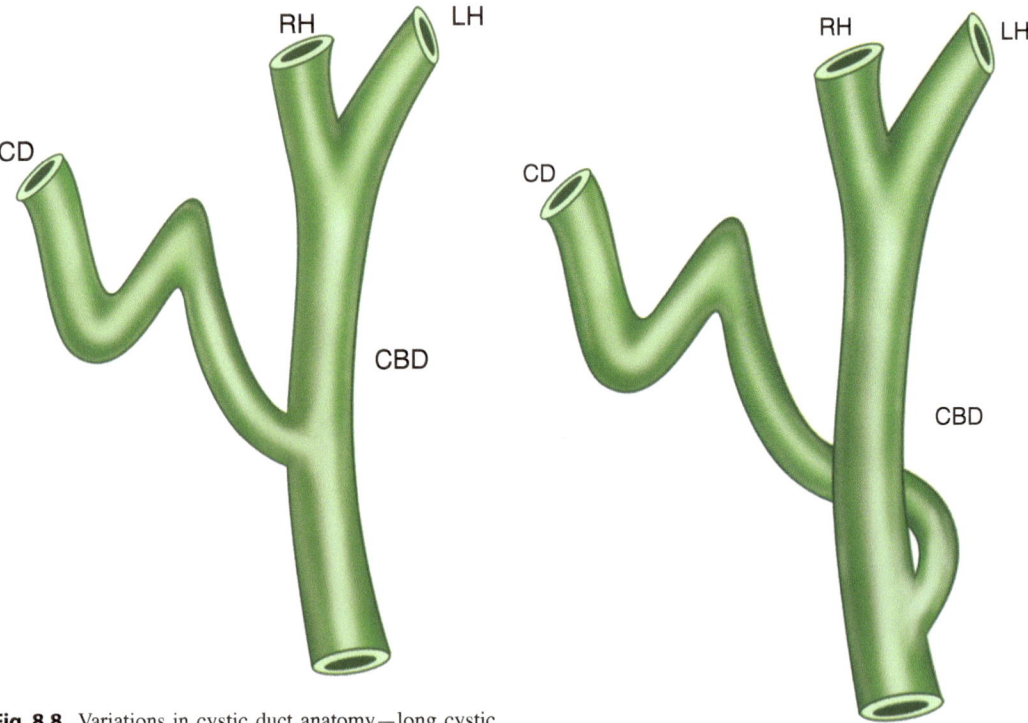

Fig. 8.8 Variations in cystic duct anatomy—long cystic duct 20 %

Fig. 8.9 Variations in cystic duct anatomy—posterior cystic duct 5 %

arises from the aorta and provides the origin for three vessels, the left gastric artery, the splenic artery, and the common hepatic artery. The common hepatic artery should lie posterior and medial to the common bile duct. Traditionally, the common hepatic artery should bifurcate to a right and left hepatic artery. The cystic artery normally derives from the right hepatic artery prior to the right hepatic entering the right lobe of the liver. Variations of the right hepatic artery traditional anatomy are the most common changes appreciated during gallbladder and bile duct surgery. The variations are defined as replaced arteries or accessory arteries. Replaced arteries represent a substituted artery, whereas an accessory vessel is defined as an additional artery. Both variations should be appreciated. We know from autopsy studies that up to one quarter of patients will have some form of aberrant anatomy. Of this one quarter, 70 % of aberrations are replaced right hepatic arteries, while the

remaining 30 % are accessory vessels [8]. In reference to replaced right hepatic artery, the most common origin is the superior mesenteric artery, and less commonly from other vessels such as the aorta, gastroduodenal artery, or one of the pancreatic vessels (Figs. 8.10, 8.11, and 8.12).

A working knowledge of the anatomic relationship between the biliary anatomy and the arterial anatomy is essential for surgical management of biliary disease. Typically, the cystic artery arises laterally to the bile duct and courses anteriorly towards the gallbladder. If the cystic artery has an aberrant origin (which it may in up to 20 % of cases), it may need to course anteriorly or posterior to the bile duct prior to its supply to the gallbladder. Delineating its course can be particularly important in common bile duct exploration. In a rare, but described situation, two cystic arteries may supply the gallbladder. Dependent on their anatomic origins, they may course anteriorly or posteriorly to the bile duct.

Fig. 8.10 Hepatic artery abnormalities— typical anatomy

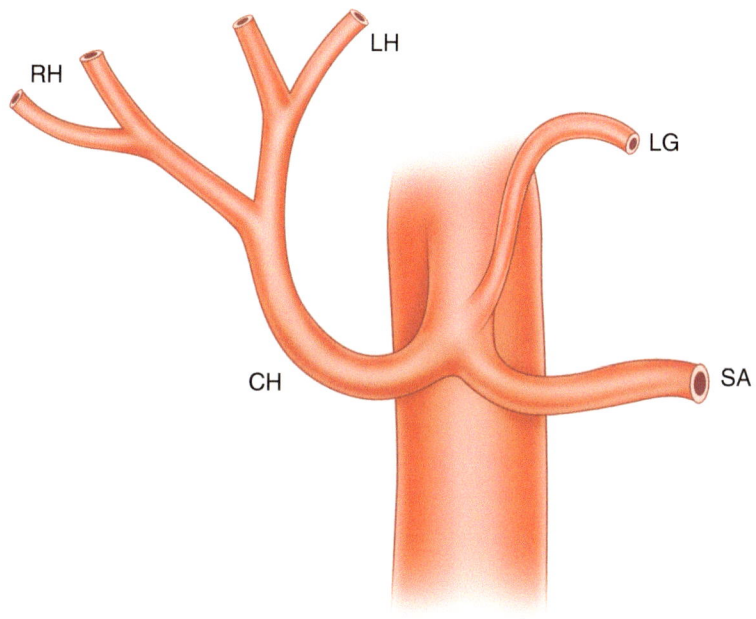

Fig. 8.11 Hepatic artery abnormalities— accessory right hepatic artery

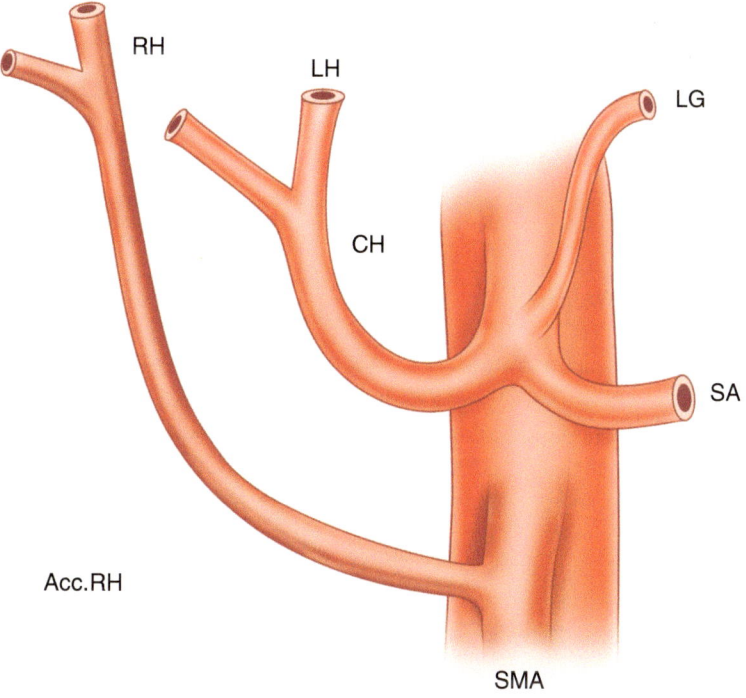

Fig. 8.12 Hepatic artery abnormalities—replaced right hepatic artery

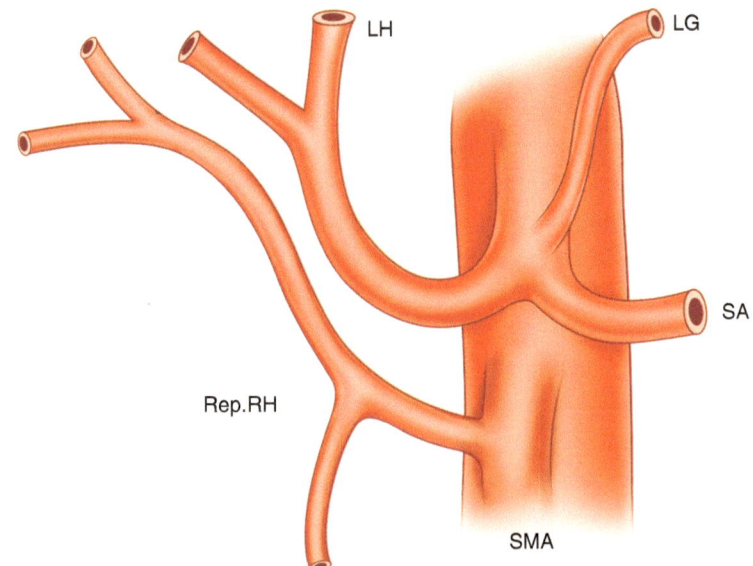

In the event of a common bile duct exploration, careful identification and control of these vessels in warranted [8].

Anatomically, variations of anatomy of the biliary system and its associated anatomy are the expectation, not the exception. When embarking on laparoscopic or open exploration, a working knowledge of these variations is key for prevention of injury or the recognition and control of injury when one does occur [8].

Surgical Training

As the advent of laparoscopic and minimally invasive surgery has changed the face of modern surgical practices, so has surgical residency training been changed. This change has been multifaceted and not solely related to changes in operative approach. Changes have been attributed to duty hour restrictions, the increasing frequency of surgical residency pursuing postgraduate fellowships, as well as the increase in laparoscopy negating the need for open cholecystectomy. This has further been underscored by endoscopic

techniques curtailing the need for open and transcystic common bile duct exploration. Regardless of the etiology, young surgeons have less experience with this anatomy and frequently of the operations required [9].

Implementation of the 80 h work-week has had multiple impacts in both case volume and case breadth [10]. A systematic review of the ACGME case log database has demonstrated a decrease in total case volume, both during the chief resident year as well as throughout surgical training. A decrease in case volume has lead to the popularization of specialized fellowships after residency training. Many of these changes have lead to a narrowing of case breadth, with many of the complex surgeries falling outside of training which was previously referred to as "chief level" cases. Lack of experience in these fields can lend to discomfort managing these issues and necessitating transfer to management of a disease process at a "high volume" institution [11].

The increasing specialization in General surgery has also impacted case volume and surgeons comfort levels. In a survey which was distributed to chief residents, only 18 % of respondents reported feeling comfortable performing a common bile duct exploration [12]. It's not unreasonable to conclude that these cases would fall to individuals with increasing sub-specialization including those entering hepatobiliary or surgical oncology fellowships. This lack of comfort in the general surgery community limits the options available to patients as well as diminishes locations where these procedures maybe available.

Lastly, with the increase in minimally invasive transcystic and endoscopic interventions for common bile duct management, open surgical considerations for these issues are becoming less frequently taught [13, 14]. It is not rare that graduating chief residents emerging from training haven't seen a dearth of these cases. Individual practice patterns within training institutions may severely limit resident experience. Young surgeons emerging from residency may bear with them the practices and prejudices which they have earned at their training institution.

Conclusion

Multiple issues must be accounted for when surgically managing common bile duct stones. The resources available at your institution must be adequate, and if not, prompt recognition of this fact and transfer is imperative. Knowledge of the biliary anatomy, its numerous variations, and the physiologic derangements inherent to its obstruction must be accounted for when surgical intervention is going to be undertaken. Lastly, it is important to realize that young surgeons without specialized training may be uncomfortable or even unprepared in the setting of recent changes in residency training.

References

1. Marks J, Dunkin B. Principles of flexible endoscopy for surgeons. New York, NY: Springer; 2013.
2. Shelton J, Kummerow K, Phillips S, Griffin M, Holzman M, Nealon W, et al. An urban-rural blight? Choledocholithiasis presentation and treatment. J Surg Res. 2012;173(2):193–7.
3. Greenberger N. Current diagnosis & treatment gastroenterology, hepatology, & endoscopy. New York, NY: McGraw Hill Medical; 2012.
4. Brunicardi F, Andersen D, Billiar T, Dunn D, Hunter J. Schwartz's principles of surgery. New York, NY: McGraw-Hill Education; 2014.
5. Costi R. Diagnosis and management of choledocholithiasis in the golden age of imaging, endoscopy and laparoscopy. World J Gastroenterol. 2014;20(37): 13382.
6. Harrison T, Longo D, Kasper D, Jameson J, Fauci A, Hauser S, et al. Harrison's principles of internal medicine. New York, NY: McGraw-Hill; 2012.
7. Wang L, Yu W. Obstructive jaundice and perioperative management. Acta Anaesthesiol Taiwan. 2014; 52(1):22–9.
8. Berci G, Cuschieri A. Bile ducts and bile duct stones. Philadelphia, PA: W.B. Saunders; 1997.
9. Chung R, Wojtasik L, Pham Q, Chari V, Chen P. The decline of training in open biliary surgery. Surg Endosc. 2003;17(2):338–40.
10. Jamal M, Wong S, Whalen T. Effects of the reduction of surgical residents work hours and implications for surgical residency programs: a narrative review. BMC Med Educ. 2014;14 Suppl 1:S14.
11. Drake F, Horvath K, Goldin A, Gow K. The general surgery chief resident operative experience. JAMA Surg. 2013;148(9):841.
12. Fonseca A, Reddy V, Longo W, Gusberg R. Graduating general surgery resident operative confidence: perspective from a national survey. J Surg Res. 2014; 190(2):419–28.
13. Tutton M, Pawa N, Arulampalam T, Motson R. Training higher surgical trainees in laparoscopic common bile duct exploration. World J Surg. 2010; 34(3):569–73.
14. Richards M, McAteer J, Drake F, Goldin A, Khandelwal S, Gow K. A national review of the frequency of minimally invasive surgery among general surgery residents. JAMA Surg. 2015;150(2):169.

Percutaneous Methods of Common Bile Duct Stone Retrieval

Joshua D. Dowell, Jeffrey Weinstein, Annie Lim, and Gregory E. Guy

Abbreviations

ERCP   Endoscopic retrograde cholangiopancreatography
PTGB-RV Percutaneous transgallbladder rendezvous technique

Introduction

The role of percutaneous access for the treatment of symptomatic bile duct stones dates back to the 1960s and 1970s in which stones were removed by forceps through the postoperative sinus tract or expulsed into the duodenum through the T-tube tract [1–4]. As endoscopic retrograde cholangiopancreatography (ERCP) [5, 6] has now emerged as the first choice treatment of biliary stones, percutaneous approaches to symptomatic choledocholithiasis today are reserved for cases in which ERCP has failed or is not possible due to prior surgical or anatomic considerations. Many percutaneous techniques have been described for such cases or in collaboration with ERCP in the form of rendezvous procedures. In this chapter, the percutaneous approaches to bile duct stones will be explored, including indications and procedural considerations particularly for patients in which ERCP may be challenging or not possible.

Trans T-tube Techniques

In 1972 Burhenne [1, 2] initially described the fluoroscopically guided extraction of retained stones through a T-tube mature sinus tract. In this technique, 5–8 weeks are allowed following the surgical placement of the T-tube for maturation of the tract. Using local anesthesia-, the T-tube is then removed over guide wire and access to the biliary system is obtained via advancing a directional catheter over a wire. Contrast cholangiography is performed to visualize the anatomy and the location of the retained biliary stones. The

J.D. Dowell, M.D., Ph.D. (✉) • A. Lim, D.O.
Division of Vascular and Interventional Radiology,
Department of Radiology, Wexner Medical Center,
The Ohio State University, 395 W 12th Ave.,
Suite 424, Columbus, OH 43210, USA
e-mail: Joshua.Dowell@osumc.edu;
annie.lim@osumc.edu

J. Weinstein, M.D.
Division of Vascular and Interventional Radiology,
Department of Radiology, Einstein Medical Center,
Philadelphia, PA, USA
e-mail: weinstej@Einstein.edu

G.E. Guy, M.D.
Division of Vascular and Interventional Radiology,
Department of Radiology, The Ohio State University
Wexner Medical Center, 395 W 12th Ave., 4th Floor,
Columbus, OH 43210, USA
e-mail: gregory.guy@osumc.edu

© Springer International Publishing Switzerland 2016
J.W. Hazey et al. (eds.), *Multidisciplinary Management of Common Bile Duct Stones*,
DOI 10.1007/978-3-319-22765-8_9

guide wire can then be advanced to the duodenum to facilitate drainage catheter insertion if necessary following stone extraction. A stone basket is delivered through the catheter or sheath and advanced adjacent to or immediately distal to a biliary stone. The basket is used to engage the stone and then withdrawn to extract the stone.

In this technique, the basket is not routinely closed as it may fragment or disengage the stone prior to its removal. However, dependent upon its size, stone fragmentation may be necessary for retrieval through the sinus tract. Large stones up to 8 mm may be removed through the sinus tract of a 14–16 F T-tube [7]. Those stones exceeding 8 mm in diameter should be fragmented prior to extraction. Once fragmented, the smaller stones, measuring less than 3 mm in diameter, usually pass spontaneously through the ampulla into the duodenum. Saline, contrast media, heparin, and monooctanoin have been reported to aid in passing these smaller stones through the ducts [7]. The mature sinus tract, even within 24 h of inadvertent T-tube removal, may be recannulated to facilitate stone extraction or expulsion [1, 2].

The technical success rate of stone extraction through a T-tube tract is 95 % with a complication rate of approximately 5 % [8]. Failure of stone extraction is often related to larger or impacted stones or the presence of a tortuous sinus tract. Procedural complications include fever, sepsis, tract perforation, cholangitis, bile peritonitis, bile collections, and pancreatitis [7]. Reported alternatives to this technique include the use of an immature tract [9]. Tracts approximately 2 weeks after surgical T-tube placement have been successfully utilized [9]. Additionally, 7 F sheaths have been advanced through the T-tube to facilitate stone expulsion using an angioplasty balloon without the removal of the T-tube [7].

Transhepatic Papillary Balloon Dilation

Bile duct stone extraction through a percutaneous transhepatic approach may cause parenchymal damage to the liver. Therefore, several strategies have been devised to facilitate percutaneous treatment by expulsion techniques through the papilla rather than through extraction (Fig. 9.1). These techniques include mechanical or chemical fragmentation of stones to reduce their size, such as with monooctanoin, as well as techniques to chemically relax or actively stretch the sphincter of Oddi through balloon dilation [8, 10–12].

Percutaneous balloon dilation of the sphincter of Oddi for stone removal was initially described by Centola et al. in 1981 [10]. In this technique, percutaneous transhepatic cholangiography with drain placement is performed a few days prior to stone removal by standard protocol [13] using ultrasound and fluoroscopic guidance for decompression of the biliary system. External biliary drainage for a few days prior to stone removal also allows biliary and sphincter wall edema to resolve. Cholangiography is again performed to clarify anatomy and stone position. The drainage catheter is then removed over wire and a hydrophilic guide wire with directional catheter is utilized to access through the papilla and into the duodenum, beyond the obstructing stones. A 6–9 F vascular sheath is advanced over wire immediately proximal to the stone. An angioplasty balloon is inserted over the wire, through the sheath, and across the papilla. Balloon diameter for papillary dilation is determined by the largest diameter of the stone and not to exceed 12 mm [7, 10, 13]. Those stones exceeding 12 mm may be fragmented within the common bile duct using either a basket or lithotripsy instrument. The sphincter is dilated using the balloon until the waist disappears at 6–8 atm pressure for 1–3 min [7, 10, 13]. The balloon is then deflated and pulled back to a position proximal to the obstructing stone. The angioplasty balloon or a Fogarty balloon is inflated and advanced over wire to, with the support of the vascular sheath, push the stone into the duodenum through the dilated sphincter. An alternative method utilizes a small choledochoscope (usually through a 12 French or larger sheath) for direct visualization of the stone during passage to the duodenum. Following stone expulsion, cholangiography with contrast is again performed to confirm stone passage and evaluate for any complication. A drainage catheter is again placed in the biliary

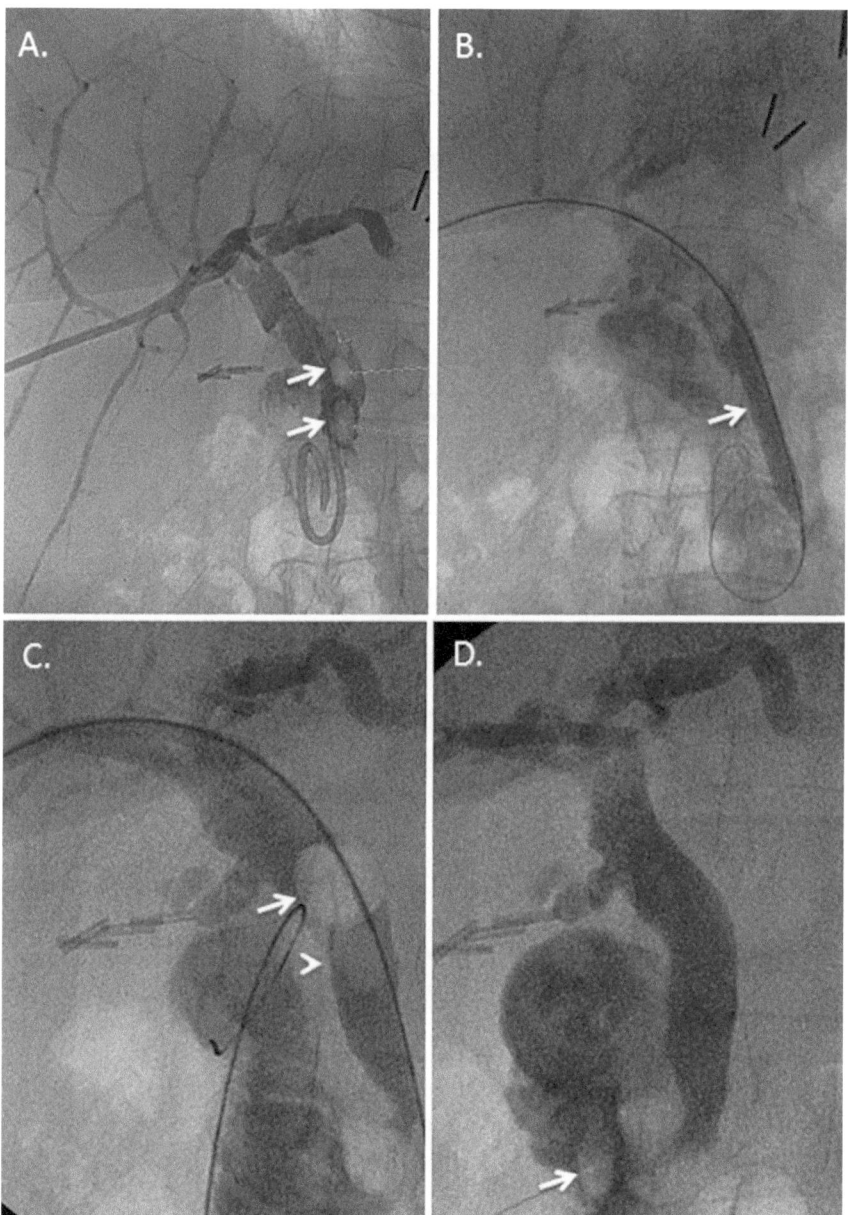

Fig. 9.1 (**a**) Contrast cholangiogram through the existing percutaneous internal–external biliary drain of a 65-year-old female with several filling defects (*arrow*) representing stones within the common bile duct. (**b**) Balloon dilatation of the papillary duct using a 10 mm angioplasty balloon (*arrow*). (**c**) Pushing the stone (*arrowhead*) with a Fogarty balloon (*arrow*) toward the duodenum and (**d**) final cholangiogram showing patency of the common bile duct with the stone in the duodenum (*arrow*)

system for at least 1–3 days. The catheter may be removed once free flow of contrast passes to the duodenum with no filling defects to suggest residual biliary stones. Angiographic occlusion balloons can also be used to clear bile duct stones [7]. The benefit of this procedure is that the balloon catheter is useful for cases with anastomotic strictures as well as stone formation.

The technical success rate for percutaneous transhepatic papillary balloon dilation and stone expulsion is dependent upon radiologist experience and technique. Gil et al. [14] reported successful stone expulsion in 36 of 38 patients using percutaneous transhepatic papillary balloon dilation. Further, transduodenal biliary stone removal with a modified Dormia basket using a transhepatic percutaneous approach was successful in all 34 patients [11]. More recently, Kint et al. [13] reported total stone clearance of the common bile duct in 104 of 110 patients using percutaneous transhepatic balloon dilation. In this study, if stone size exceeded 10 mm, mechanical lithotripsy was performed. Stones were then removed by percutaneous extraction or evacuation into the duodenum. An additional study by Ozcan et al. [15] found a similar success rate of 95.7 % in their retrospective review of 261 patients. In these cases, balloon dilation of the papilla was done using 8–12 mm balloons. In case of failure with stone expulsion, dilation may be repeated with a larger balloon (2 mm larger than the diameter of the first one), not exceeding 20 mm in diameter [15]. In a prospective study on large stones greater than 10 mm in size, percutaneous papillary large balloon dilation (12–20 mm) during percutaneous cholangioscopic lithotripsy has also been shown to be successful [16].

Balloon dilation is mostly well tolerated by patients. Mild abdominal pain following the procedure is expected to resolve within a few hours from the procedure [17]. Further, the transient adverse effects such as nausea, vomiting, and abdominal pain have been noted to respond to analgesic and antiemetic drugs following the procedure [15]. In a large series by Kint et al., complications were reported in 10.9 % of patients [13]. Minor complications (in 6 of 110 patients) included small liver abscesses, pleural empyema, hemobilia, and mild fever. Major complications included hypoxia ($n=1$), sepsis ($n=4$), and death ($n=1$) [13]. All patients should receive prophylactic broad-spectrum antibiotics (cephalosporin) immediately prior to this procedure. A similar complication rate was reported by Ozcan et al. in review of 261 patients [15]. In this series, major complications were encountered in 6.8 % [15].

Anatomic or Surgical Consideration

ERCP is more challenging or impossible in patients with Billroth II gastrectomy compared to those patients with normal anatomy [18]. In patients with Roux-en-Y reconstruction, the increased length of the afferent and efferent limbs makes it difficult to reach the papilla [19]. Although single- or double-balloon enteroscopy has allowed deep insertion into the small bowel, successful biliary cannulation is still challenging. Further, the maneuverability of the enteroscope is poor if there is loop formation. Although the ampulla is reached in over 90 % of cases, the success rate of diagnostic endoscopic cholangiography in these surgical cases with altered anatomy is 48–70 % [20–22]. For this reason, patients with variant anatomy or surgically altered anatomy may require a percutaneous approach for treatment of obstructing bile stones. Percutaneous transhepatic choledochoscopic lithotomy or papillary balloon dilation may be performed as described above in these patients. Jeong et al. [23] reported complete stone removal in 20 patients post Billroth II gastrectomy in which ERCP had failed. Minor complications including fever, hemobilia, hyperamylasemia, and wound pain were encountered in 5 of 20 patients. No major complications were reported [23]. Choledocholithiasis indeed is a possible complication following gastrectomy. In these cases, a percutaneous approach for treatment may therefore be helpful, particularly in elderly patients, patients whose papilla cannot be detected by ERCP due to Billroth II gastrectomy, and those patients who refuse a surgical approach [18].

In patients with surgically altered anatomy, a percutaneous approach may be attempted either using the intrahepatic ducts or gallbladder. The former is preferred in cases of intrahepatic biliary ductal dilatation; however, the latter may be attempted in cases of a non-dilated or minimally dilated biliary system. Percutaneous transgallbladder rendezvous technique (PTGB-RV) has been reported in patients with both normal and surgically altered anatomy [24]. In PTG-RV, a cholecystostomy tube is initially placed by standard protocol [24] under ultrasound and fluoroscopic guidance. PTGB-RV is attempted 1–2 weeks following cholecystostomy tube placement. The tube is removed over a guide wire, and a directional catheter with a hydrophilic directional guide wire is used to navigate through the gallbladder, cystic duct, common bile duct, and to the duodenum. The enteroscope is then inserted to the papilla and the guide wire is grasped using forceps. Biliary cannulation can then be accomplished by guiding the ERCP cannula over the antegrade-placed guide wire. The common bile duct stones are retrieved using a basket catheter, retrieval balloon catheter, or fragmented after endoscopic papillary balloon dilation. Following the procedure, a drainage catheter is placed again in the gallbladder and which may be removed in 1–2 weeks if no residual stones are identified on contrast cholangiography.

Additionally, percutaneous transhepatic management of common bile duct stones may be helpful following laparoscopic gastric bypass surgery or in high-risk elderly patients. Patients with morbid obesity have a higher incidence of gallstones [19]. The altered anatomy following laparoscopic gastric bypass surgery does not allow conventional ERCP. Although double balloon enteroscope-assisted ERCP, laparoscopic transgastric ERCP, and laparoscopic or open biliary surgery are options, percutaneous transhepatic cholangiography with papillary balloon dilation and stone expulsion can also be attempted [19]. In high-risk elderly patients, percutaneous transhepatic small-caliber choledochoscopic lithotomy, using electrohydraulic lithotripsy, has been show safe and effective in a prospective study of 65 patients [25]. In this study, a choledochoscope was advanced from a transhepatic approach and stones up to 45 mm in diameter were fragmented with electrohydraulic shock waves and pushed through to the duodenum with the choledochoscope. Biliary bleeding was encountered in eight of 65 patients; however, no major complications were reported. These studies delineate the safety of percutaneous transhepatic stone removal in an otherwise challenging patient population due to patient anatomy, surgical history, or comorbidities.

Discussion

ERCP is the treatment of choice for bile duct stones and yields a technical success rate ranging from 76 to 95 % [15, 26–29]. Treatment failures are most commonly due to duodenal diverticulum, duodenal stenosis, ampullary stenosis, variant biliary anatomy, prior gastrointestinal surgery, large stones exceeding 15 mm in diameter, or elderly patients [7, 30–33]. In these cases, percutaneous transhepatic approaches may be entertained as alternative treatment for stone removal.

Since its introduction in 1962 [34], percutaneous treatment of bile duct stones has allowed patients to avoid the challenges associated with surgery through its minimally invasive approach. Initially described through use of the mature sinus tract from a T-tube, percutaneous approaches for stone removal were expanded by Burhenne by using baskets in the early 1970s [1, 2]. These approaches continued to advance alongside their endoscopic counterpart and percutaneous transhepatic stone expulsion into the duodenum was described in 1979 [35, 36]. Over the next several decades numerous percutaneous techniques have been attempted to treat obstructing bile stones. These techniques have included the use of baskets and forceps as well as balloons to extract or expulse the stones. Although contact chemolitholysis is no longer recommended given its high rate of side-effects, including nausea, vomiting, and diarrhea in up to 50 % of patients, which requires cessation of therapy in 9 % [37, 38], adaptations of many of these other transhepatic percutaneous approaches remain useful for patients with obstructing calculi. As stone extraction through the percutaneous transhepatic approach may cause parenchymal liver damage, stone expulsion into the duodenum through the papilla is the most widely used percutaneous approach [7, 10, 14].

Percutaneous transhepatic stone removal, most commonly by expulsion into the duodenum through the papilla, is an effective and safe alternative to surgery particularly when endoscopic stone extraction has failed or is not possible. In specific patient populations, such as following Billroth II gastrectomy or laparoscopic Roux-en-Y gastric bypass, percutaneous approaches may be the best option for patients with symptomatic choledocholithiasis. With the increase in global obesity, the need for bariatric surgery will continue to incline in the future. Given the association of gallstones in bariatric patients following surgery, an increasing number of patients with surgically altered anatomy will require management for symptomatic stones. Therefore, an understanding of transhepatic percutaneous approaches is important to provide optimal care for these patients and those that are not candidates for ERCP.

The authors report no conflicts of interest

References

1. Burhenne HJ. Extraktion von residual steinen der gallenwege ohne reoperation. RöFo. 1972;117:425–8.
2. Burhenne HJ. Nonoperative retained biliary tract stone extraction: a new roentgenologic technique. Am J Roentgenol. 1973;117:388–99.
3. Mueller PR. Biliary interventions: a historical perspective. Semin Interv Rad. 1996;13:197–200.
4. Fennessy JJ, You KD. A method for the expulsion of stones retained in the common bile duct. Am J Roentgenol. 1970;110:256–9.
5. Kawai K, Akasaka Y, Murakami K, et al. Endoscopic sphincterotomy of the ampulla of Vater. Gastrointest Endosc. 1974;20:148–51.
6. Classen M, Demling L. Endoscopische Sphinkerotomie der papilla vateri and steinextraction aus dem ductus choledochus. Dtsch Med Wochenschr. 1974;99:496–7.
7. Ilgit E, Gürel K, Önal B. Percutaneous management of bile duct stones. Eur J Radiol. 2002;43(3):237–45.
8. Burhenne HJ. Percutaneous extraction of retained biliary tract stones: 661 patients. Am J Roentgenol. 1980;134:888–98.
9. Muchart J, Perendreu J, Casas JD, et al. Balloon catheter sphincteroplasty and biliary stone expulsion into the duodenum in patients with an indwelling T tube. Abdom Imaging. 1999;24:69–71.
10. Centola CAP, Jander HP, Stauffer A, et al. Balloon dilatation of the papilla of Vater to allow biliary stone passage. Am J Roentgenol. 1981;136:613–4.
11. Clouse ME, Stokes KR, Lee RGL, et al. Bile duct stones: percutaneous transhepatic removal. Radiology. 1986;160:525–9.
12. Minami A, Maeta T, Kohi F, et al. Endoscopic papillary dilation by balloon and isosorbid dinitrate

13. Kint J, Ven den Bergh J, Van Gelder R, et al. Percutaneous treatment of common bile duct stones: results and complications in 110 consecutive patients. Dig Surg. 2015;32(1):9–15.
14. Gil S, Iglesia P, Verdu JF, et al. Effectiveness and safety of balloon dilation of the papilla and the use of an occlusion balloon for clearance of bile duct calculi. Am J Roentgenol. 2000;174:1455–60.
15. Ozcan N, Kahriman G, Mavili E. Percutaneous transhepatic removal of bile duct stones: results of 261 patients. Cardiovasc Intervent Radiol. 2012;35(3):621–7.
16. Han J, Jeong S, Lee D. Percutaneous papillary large balloon dilation during percutaneous cholangioscopic lithotripsy for the treatment of large bile-duct stones: a feasibility study. J Korean Med Sci. 2015;30(3):278–82.
17. Komatsu Y, Kawabe T, Toda N, et al. Endoscopic papillary dilation (EPD) for the treatment of common bile duct stones and papillary stenosis. Endoscopy. 1983;30:12–7.
18. Shirai N, Hanai H, Kajimura M, et al. Successful treatment of percutaneous transhepatic papillary dilation in patients with obstructive jaundice due to common bile duct stones after Billroth II gastrectomy: report of two emergent cases. J Clin Gastroenterol. 2000;30(1):91–3.
19. Milella M, Alfa-Wali M, Leuratti L, et al. Percutaneous transhepatic cholangiography for choledocholithiasis after laparoscopic gastric bypass surgery. Int J Surg Case Rep. 2014;5(5):249–52.
20. Saleem A, Baron TH, Gostout CJ, et al. Endoscopic retrograde cholangiopancreatography using a single-balloon enteroscope in patients with altered Roux-en-Y anatomy. Endoscopy. 2010;42:656–60.
21. Itoi T, Ishii K, Sofuni A, et al. Long- and short-type double-balloon enteroscopy-assisted therapeutic ERCP for intact papilla in patients with a Roux-en-Y anastomosis. Surg Endosc. 2011;25:713–21.
22. Lennon AM, Kapoor S, Khashab M, et al. Spiral assisted ERCP is equivalent to single balloon assisted ERCP in patients with Roux-en-Y anatomy. Dig Dis Sci. 2012;57:1391–8.
23. Jeong E, Kang D, Kim D, et al. Percutaneous transhepatic choledochoscopic lithotomy as a rescue therapy for removal of bile duct stones in Billroth II gastrectomy patients who are difficult to perform ERCP. Eur J Gastroenterol Hepatol. 2009;21(12):1358–62.
24. Okuno M, Iwashita T, Yasuda I, et al. Percutaneous transgallbladder rendezvous for enteroscopic management of choledocholithiasis in patients with surgically altered anatomy. Scand J Gastroenterol. 2013;48(8):974–8.
25. Ogawa K, Ohkubo H, Abe W, et al. Percutaneous transhepatic small-caliber choledochoscopic lithotomy: a safe and effective technique for percutaneous

transhepatic common bile duct exploration in high-risk elderly patients. J Hepatobiliary Pancreat Surg. 2002;9(2):213–7.

26. Prachayakul V, Aswakul P. Endoscopic ultrasound-guided biliary drainage as an alternative to percutaneous drainage and surgical bypass. World J Gastrointest Endosc. 2015;7(1):37–44.

27. Freeman ML, Nelson DB, Sherman S, et al. Complications of endoscopic biliary sphincterotomy. N Engl J Med. 1996;335:909–18.

28. Vaira D, D'Anna L, Ainley C, et al. Endoscopic sphincterotomy in 1000 consecutive patients. Lancet. 1989;2(8660):431–4.

29. Neoptolemos JP, Carr-Locke DL, Fraser I, et al. The management of common bile duct calculi by endoscopic sphincterotomy in patient with gallbladders in situ. Br J Surg. 1984;71:69–71.

30. Ozcan N, Erdogan N, Baskol M. Common bile duct stones detected after cholecystectomy: advancement into the duodenum via the percutaneous route. Cardiovasc Intervent Radiol. 2003;26:150–3.

31. Huang SM, Wu CW, Chau GY, et al. An alternative approach of choledocholithotomy via laparoscopic choledochotomy. Arch Surg. 1996;131:407–11.

32. Miller BM, Kozarek RA, Ryan Jr JA, et al. Surgical versus endoscopic management of common bile duct stones. Ann Surg. 1988;207:135–41.

33. Merzane SG, Stein EJ, Burke DR, et al. Removal of retained common bile duct stones with angiographic occlusion balloons. AJR Am J Roentgenol. 1986; 146:383–5.

34. Mondet AF. Technic of blood extraction of calculi in residual lithiasis of the choledochus. Bol Trab Soc Cir B Aires. 1962;46:278–90.

35. Perez MR, Oleaga JA, Freiman DB, et al. Removal of a distal common bile duct stone through percutaneous transhepatic catheterization. Arch Surg. 1979;114: 107–9.

36. Dotter CT, Bilbao MK, Katon RM. Percutaneous transhepatic gallstone removal by needle tract. Radiology. 1979;133:242–3.

37. Haskin PH, Teplick SK, Sammon JK, et al. Monooctanoin infusion and stone removal through the transparenchymal tract: use in 17 patients. AJR Am J Roentgenol. 1987;148:185–8.

38. Kelly E, Williams JD, Organ CH, et al. A history of the dissolution of retained choledocholithiasis. Am J Surg. 2000;180:86–98.

Mohammad H. Shakhatreh and J. Royce Groce

Introduction

The management of common bile duct stones has dramatically transformed in the last 50 years. What used to involve laparotomy with common bile duct exploration now has evolved into a much less invasive endoscopic treatment. The endoscopic management of common bile duct stones involves removing the stones or bypassing the obstruction caused by the stones and achieving transpapillary biliary drainage. Both of these techniques usually require sphincterotomy or sphincteroplasty to increase the size of the biliary orifice and allow for stone extraction. Stone extraction can be achieved using different techniques and tools; the decision is largely based on the size and location of the stones (Fig. 10.1). Wire baskets or balloon catheters are adequate in stone extraction in more than 80–90 % of all patients with CBD stones [1], other techniques can be used for larger or difficult to remove stones such as mechanical lithotripsy, electrohydraulic lithotripsy, and laser lithotripsy.

M.H. Shakhatreh, M.D., M.P.H. • J.R. Groce, M.D. (✉)
Division of Gastroenterology, Hepatology, and
Nutrition, Department of Internal Medicine,
The Ohio State University Wexner Medical Clinic,
395 W. 12th Avenue, Columbus, OH 43210-1228, USA
e-mail: J.Royce.Groce@osumc.edu;
mhshakhatreh@carilionclinic.org

Endoscopic Sphincterotomy

The advent of endoscopic sphincterotomy (ES) in 1974 [2] has decreased the need for common bile duct exploration with its associated complications (Fig. 10.2). In a cohort of 134 patients undergoing ERCP for choledocholithiasis, 129 patients (96 %) successfully underwent ES, and among this group, the bile duct was cleared of stones in 119 patients (92.5 % of patients with successful ES) [3]. After ES, stones passed spontaneously in 78 cases (65.5 %) and by instrumental extraction in 41 (34.5 %). An early prospective study [4] comparing 50 patients undergoing ES to 102 patients undergoing common bile duct exploration (CBDE) for choledocholithiasis, after excluding patients with acute cholecystitis, idiopathic pancreatitis, sphincter of Oddi dysfunction (SOD), and malignant disease found that complications were much fewer in patients undergoing ES vs. patients undergoing CBDE (15 % vs. 41 %, $p < 0.025$) in patients with a prior cholecystectomy.

Although ES is a safe alternative to surgery, patients can still develop early and late complications related to the procedure. In a review of prospective studies between 1977 and 2006 involving 16,855 patients [5], ERCP-related complications such as pancreatitis, infections (cholecystitis, cholangitis), bleeding, perforations and cardiopulmonary and miscellaneous complications were analyzed. Although there was no restriction to procedures with ES, the overall complication rates were low; 3.47 % (95 %CI 3.19–3.75), 1.44 % (95 %CI 1.26–1.62), 1.34 % (95 %CI 1.16–1.52), 0.60 % (95 %CI 0.48–0.72), and 1.33 % (95 %CI 1.13–1.53), respectively. A retrospective study [6] of 80 patients (93.4 % Caucasian) who underwent ES for management of CBD stones and followed up

for a mean duration of 7.75 years (range: 5–14 years) found that eight patients (10 %) developed late-occurring biliary events related to ES; these included abdominal pain, pancreatitis, recurrent stones, and papillary stenosis. In a Japanese cohort study evaluating long-term complications of ES [7], 262 patients who underwent ES were followed up for a mean of 61.6 months. These patients were split into four groups; (A) 28 patients with prior cholecystectomy, (B) 129 patients who underwent cholecystectomy following ES, (C) 46 patients with gallstones and an intact gallbladder, and (D) 69 patients with an acalculous gallbladder. Recurrence of CBD stones occurred in 29 patients (11.1 %); the recurrence rates were higher in group C (17.4 %) than in group B (7.8 %) ($p < 0.05$) and higher in group A (22.7 %) than in group D (10.1 %) ($p < 0.01$). Most recurrences were managed by endoscopic transpapillary stone extraction. Earlier studies have demonstrated that after adequate sphincterotomy, most stones pass spontaneously within 1 week [8]. However, due to the risks involved with leaving stones in the common bile duct (obstruction and cholangitis), most endoscopists attempt stone removal at the time of ES.

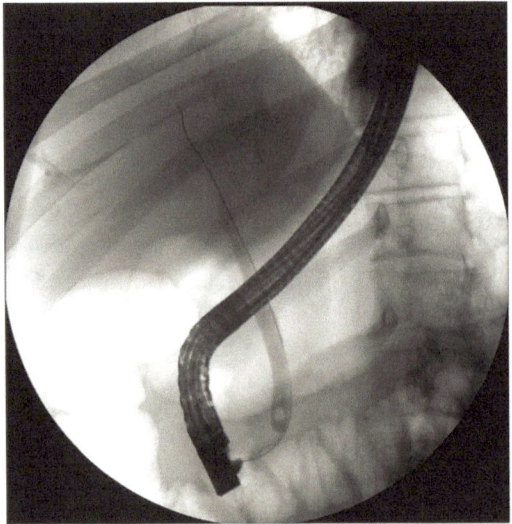

Fig. 10.1 Common bile duct stone

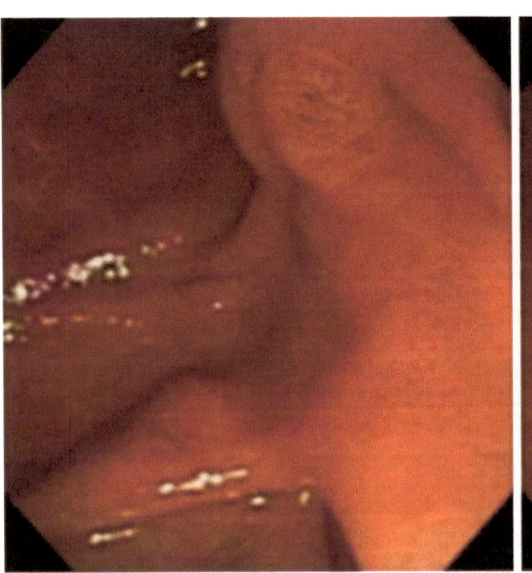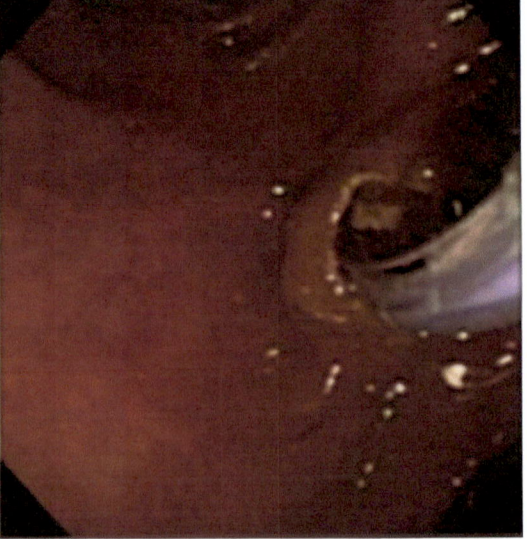

Fig. 10.2 The papilla before and after sphincterotomy

Endoscopic Sphincteroplasty (Endoscopic Papillary Balloon Dilation [EPBD])

The concept of dilating the papillary orifice instead of cutting the muscle around the papilla to allow for stone removal was first introduced in 1982 [9]. Since then, it has gained wide acceptance, especially in patients with coagulopathy and those with abnormal anatomy (periampullary diveritcula, Billroth II, etc.).

EPBD has a similar efficacy to ES in removal of CBD stones (Fig. 10.3). A meta-analysis of eight prospective, randomized trials comparing EPBD with ES [10] found the overall success rate for stone removal (94.3 % vs. 96.5 %, $p=0.2$, respectively) and overall complications (10.5 % vs. 10.3 %, $p=0.9$, respectively) were not statistically different between the two techniques. However, in 23 % of patients undergoing EPBD, ES was needed as a 'rescue' procedure to extract the stones, and this contributed to the overall success rate. Bleeding occurred less frequently with EPBD (0 % vs. 2.0 %, $p=0.001$), but pancreatitis was more common with EPBD (7.4 % vs. 4.3 %, $p=0.05$). Rates of infection (2.7 % for EPBD vs. 3.6 % for ES, $p=0.3$) and perforation (0.4 % vs. 0.4 %, $p=1.0$) were similar between the two treatment modalities. Mechanical lithotripsy was needed more often in patients undergoing EPBD than in patient undergoing ES (20.9 % vs. 14.8 %, $p=0.01$, respectively).

Multiple or large stones usually require ES. A small randomized controlled trial [11] comparing long-term outcomes after EPBD vs. ES in 32 patients with common bile duct stones reported similar success rates, but higher recurrence rates in the EPBD group (25 % in EPBD vs. 6.3 % in ES) at the mid-term evaluation (<1 year). However, over the long term, patients who underwent ES had higher recurrence rates than those who underwent EPBD (26.7 % vs. 6.3 %, respectively), this, however, was not statistically significant when analyzed with the log-rank test ($p=0.12$). EPBD was more successful when patients had three stones or less and with stones smaller than 15 mm.

In patients with large stones and failed extraction after adequate ES, removal of stones can be accomplished by dilating the biliary orifice using large-diameter balloons. In a retrospective analysis of 58 patients in whom ES and balloon/basket extraction were unsuccessful [12], the biliary orifice was dilated using 12–18 mm esophageal/pyloric balloons in patients with a tapered bile duct or 15–20 mm esophageal/pyloric balloons in patients with square, barrel-shaped and/or large (>15 mm) stones during the same session.

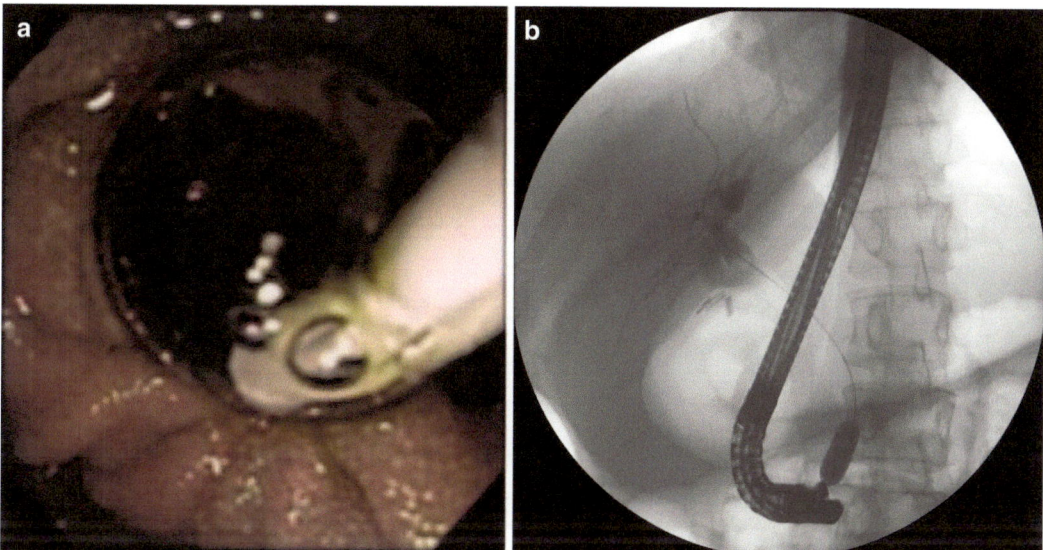

Fig. 10.3 (a, b) Endoscopic papillary balloon dilation (EPBD)

Stone clearance was completed in 88 % of these patients with a complication rate of 15.5 % (mild cholangitis in two patients, mild pancreatitis in two patients, and bleeding in five patients). More bleeding was noted in those with a tapered bile duct group (33 % vs. 7.5 %, $p < 0.05$). Mechanical lithotripsy was only required in a minority of cases (7 %). A review of multiple studies examining the efficacy of endoscopic papillary large-balloon dilation (EPLBD) reported success rates of 72–100 % during the first ERCP and 95–100 % after multiple ERCPs [13].

Mechanical Lithotripsy

Mechanical lithotripsy has become the international standard after ES for the treatment of non-extractable bile duct stones, particularly those smaller than 2.8 cm [14], although EPLBD has been gaining acceptance as an alternative in the gastroenterology community (see above). Mechanical lithotripsy uses physical force to break stones into smaller pieces, facilitating extraction (Fig. 10.4). The success rate of ES and mechanical lithotripsy is 90–97 % if the stone can be captured by the basket [1]. Reasons for failure of mechanical lithotripsy include inability to grasp the stone, minimal fragmentation, abnormal bile duct configuration, and mis-shapen baskets or failure to deploy the basket

[15]. Other uncommon reasons for failure include breakage of the basket inside the bile duct and inability to break the stone. Currently, baskets with built-in breaking points are used to avoid basket impaction/trapping inside the common bile duct. A retrospective review of 643 cases of biliary mechanical lithotripsy done in seven expert centers reported a complication rate of 3.6 % [16]. Most of the complications were managed endoscopically, and only one patient required surgery.

Electrohydraulic Lithotripsy (EHL)

EHL systems consist of a bipolar probe and a charge generator. When a charge is transmitted across the electrodes at the tip of the probe, a spark is created. This induces expansion of the surrounding fluid and an oscillating spherical shock wave of adequate pressure to fragment the stone [17]. The procedure is usually done using direct choledochoscopy to avoid damage to surrounding biliary mucosa and biliary perforation (Fig. 10.5). Once the stone is fragmented, extraction is done using standard techniques of baskets/balloons. The reported success rate of EHL is 95–100 %, with failures primarily due to inability to make contact between the fiber and the stone, malfunctioning of the fiber or bleeding that precludes stone visualization [15].

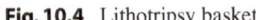

Fig. 10.4 Lithotripsy basket

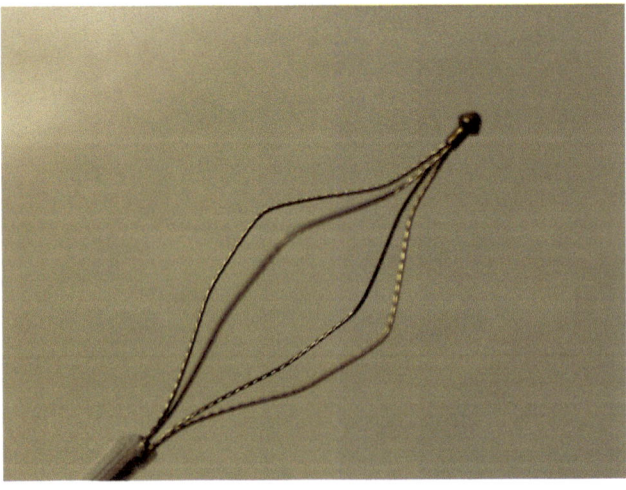

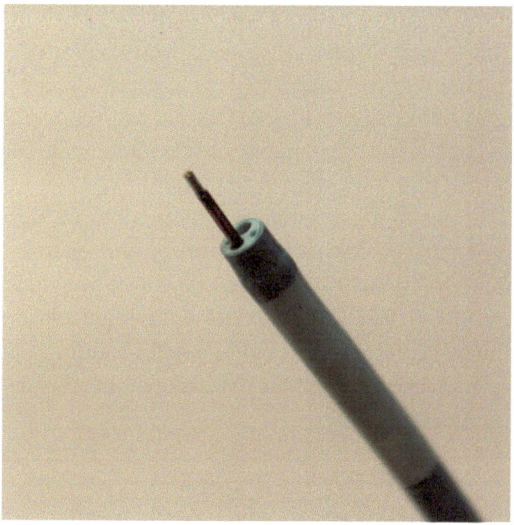

Fig. 10.5 EHL probe through Spyglass™ (Boston-Scientific) cholangioscope

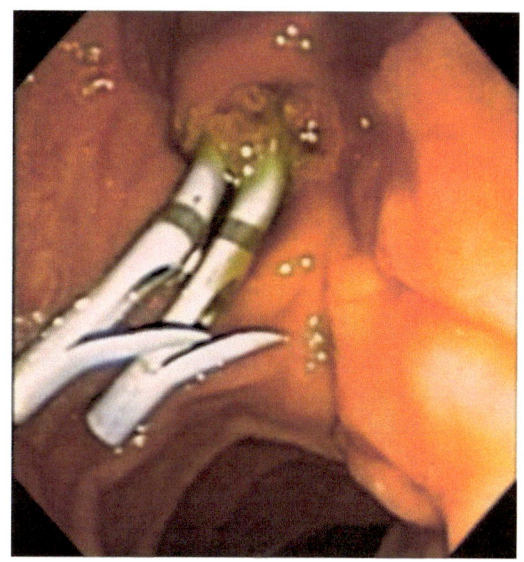

Fig. 10.6 Biliary stents

Laser Lithotripsy

Focusing laser light of a high-power density on the surface of a stone creates a plasma composed of a gaseous collection of ions and free electrons. This plasma bubble oscillates and induces cavitation with tensile and compressive waves that shatter the stone surface [17]. Several commercially available and FDA cleared systems are available; these systems use Holmium:yttrium aluminum garnet (YAG) or the frequency-doubled, double-pulse neodymium:YAG (FREDDY) lasers. An important development in laser lithotripsy has been that of the stone tissue detection system, which provides laser systems with a "feedback" mechanism to avoid accidental laser radiation to the bile duct wall [15]. When in contact with the bile duct, the laser pulse is automatically turned off, thus minimizing the amount of laser energy that is in contact with the bile duct. Studies using laser lithotripsy showed effective fragmentation of bile duct stones in 92 % of patients, with complete clearance of the bile duct in 64–97 % of patients [18]. Reported

complications included hemobilia and cholangitis, which occurred in 7 % of patients. EHL and laser lithotripsy are considered comparable in terms of efficacy, however laser systems are less portable and considerably more expensive.

Biliary Stenting

In patients with large biliary stones and failed stone extraction, or in patients with high-risks for complications such as bleeding, placing a stent into the biliary tree to overcome the obstruction caused by the stone(s) is a viable alternative and can be a bridge to stone extraction at a later date (Fig. 10.6). Several studies have looked into the effect of placing a plastic biliary stent on the fragmentation and reduction in size of difficult common bile duct stones. In a prospective cohort study, 64 patients who failed conventional stone retrieval underwent biliary plastic stent placement [19]. Six months later follow-up ERCPs showed a decrease in stone size in 83 % of patients and stone fragmentation was observed in 72 % of patients, which allowed for complete stone removal in 40 patients (62.5 %) and incomplete removal in 24 patients (37.5 %). Another study evaluating the effect of biliary stent placement among 40 patients with large (≥ 20 mm) or multiple (≥ 3) stones 2 months later found the median number of stones decreased from 4.0 to 2.0 ($p < 0.0001$) [20]. In addition, larger stones became smaller and small stones disappeared. Stone clearance was achieved in 93 % of patients at the second ERCP. Similarly, a plastic biliary stent was placed in 45 patients with large common bile duct stones (≥ 16 mm) or difficult to remove stones with conventional therapy [21]. An ERCP was repeated 3–6 months later, and a decrease in stone size or fragmentation of the stones was noted in 73 % of patients (median size from 23.1 to 15.4 mm, $p < 0.05$), while the stones disappeared completely or changed into sludge in 22 %. Only 2 patients (4 %) had no change in size or number of stones. In 96 % of patients, the stones were removed completely.

Outcomes

ERCP is a high risk procedure; the main complications arising from it include perforation, bleeding, and pancreatitis. Several national cohort studies have looked into the relationship between center volume, endoscopists' volume, and ERCP outcomes. In a national Swedish study evaluating 12,695 ERCPs performed for benign biliary disease [22], the authors found an increase in the incidence of failed ERCP in centers with low procedure volume (≤ 87 ERCPs/year) compared to centers with high procedure volume (>87 ERCPs/year) with an OR of 2.72 for low-volume vs. high volume, $p = 0.007$. In a retrospective cohort study of 15,514 ERCPs performed in the state of Indiana between 2001 and 2011 the failure rate was higher among low volume (9.5 %) compared with high volume (5.7 %) providers ($p < 0.001$) [23]. The authors concluded that with each additional ERCP performed per year, the odds of having a failed procedure decreased by 3.3 % (95 %CI 1.6–5.0 %). A national Austrian cohort study examined 22 % (3,132) of all ERCPs done nationally and compared the outcomes between high volume

(>50 ERCPs/year) and low volume (<50 ERCPs/year) endoscopists [24]. The study reported a higher success rate in high volume endoscopists (86.9 % vs. 80.3 %, $p < 0.001$) and a lower overall complication rate among high volume endoscopists (10.2 % vs. 13.6 %, $p = 0.007$).

Despite the differences in definitions of high-volume and low-volume centers and endoscopists, the conclusion that can be drawn from these results is that ERCP should be thought of as a high-risk procedure, but adequate training and experience decrease the overall complication and failure rates.

References

1. Hochberger J, Tex S, Maiss J, Hahn EG. Management of difficult common bile duct stones. Gastrointest Endosc Clin N Am. 2003;13(4):623–34.
2. Demling L, Koch H, Classen M, Belohlavek D, Schaffner O, Schwamberger K, et al. Endoscopic papillotomy and removal of gall-stones: animal experiments and first clinical results (author's transl). Dtsch Med Wochenschr. 1974;99(45):2255–7.
3. Cotton PB. Non-operative removal of bile duct stones by duodenoscopic sphincterotomy. Br J Surg. 1980;67(1):1–5.
4. Worthley CS, Watts JM, Toouli J. Common duct exploration or endoscopic sphincterotomy for choledocholithiasis? Aust N Z J Surg. 1989;59(3): 209–15.
5. Andriulli A, Loperfido S, Napolitano G, Niro G, Valvano MR, Spirito F, et al. Incidence rates of post-ERCP complications: a systematic survey of prospective studies. Am J Gastroenterol. 2007;102(8): 1781–8.
6. Folkers MT, Disario JA, Adler DG. Long-term complications of endoscopic biliary sphincterotomy for choledocholithiasis: a North-American perspective. Am J Gastroenterol. 2009;104(11):2868–9.
7. Kageoka M, Watanabe F, Maruyama Y, Nagata K, Ohata A, Noda Y, et al. Long-term prognosis of patients after endoscopic sphincterotomy for choledocholithiasis. Dig Endosc. 2009;21(3):170–5.
8. Cotton PB. ERCP. Gut. 1977;18(4):316–41.
9. Staritz M, Ewe K, Meyer zum Buschenfelde KH. Endoscopic papillary dilatation, a possible alternative to endoscopic papillotomy. Lancet. 1982; 1(8284):1306–7.
10. Baron TH, Harewood GC. Endoscopic balloon dilation of the biliary sphincter compared to endoscopic biliary sphincterotomy for removal of common bile duct stones during ERCP: a metaanalysis of randomized, controlled trials. Am J Gastroenterol. 2004;99(8): 1455–60.

11. Tanaka S, Sawayama T, Yoshioka T. Endoscopic papillary balloon dilation and endoscopic sphincterotomy for bile duct stones: long-term outcomes in a prospective randomized controlled trial. Gastrointest Endosc. 2004;59(6):614–8.

12. Ersoz G, Tekesin O, Ozutemiz AO, Gunsar F. Biliary sphincterotomy plus dilation with a large balloon for bile duct stones that are difficult to extract. Gastrointest Endosc. 2003;57(2):156–9.

13. Chung JW, Chung JB. Endoscopic papillary balloon dilation for removal of choledocholithiasis: indications, advantages, complications, and long-term follow-up results. Gut Liver. 2011;5(1):1–14.

14. Cipolletta L, Costamagna G, Bianco MA, Rotondano G, Piscopo R, Mutignani M, et al. Endoscopic mechanical lithotripsy of difficult common bile duct stones. Br J Surg. 1997;84(10):1407–9.

15. Raijman I. Intracorporeal lithotripsy in the management of biliary stone disease. Semin Laparosc Surg. 2000;7(4):295–301.

16. Thomas M, Howell DA, Carr-Locke D, Mel Wilcox C, Chak A, Raijman I, et al. Mechanical lithotripsy of pancreatic and biliary stones: complications and available treatment options collected from expert centers. Am J Gastroenterol. 2007;102(9):1896–902.

17. DiSario J, Chuttani R, Croffie J, Liu J, Mishkin D, Shah R, et al. Biliary and pancreatic lithotripsy devices. Gastrointest Endosc. 2007;65(6):750–6.

18. Yasuda I, Itoi T. Recent advances in endoscopic management of difficult bile duct stones. Dig Endosc. 2013;25(4):376–85.

19. Aslan F, Arabul M, Celik M, Alper E, Unsal B. The effect of biliary stenting on difficult common bile duct stones. Prz Gastroenterol. 2014;9(2):109–15.

20. Horiuchi A, Nakayama Y, Kajiyama M, Kato N, Kamijima T, Graham DY, et al. Biliary stenting in the management of large or multiple common bile duct stones. Gastrointest Endosc. 2010;71(7):1200–1203.e2.

21. Fan Z, Hawes R, Lawrence C, Zhang X, Zhang X, Lv W. Analysis of plastic stents in the treatment of large common bile duct stones in 45 patients. Dig Endosc. 2011;23(1):86–90.

22. Kalaitzakis E, Toth E. Hospital volume status is related to technical failure and all-cause mortality following ERCP for benign disease. Dig Dis Sci. 2015;60:1793.

23. Cote GA, Imler TD, Xu H, Teal E, French DD, Imperiale TF, et al. Lower provider volume is associated with higher failure rates for endoscopic retrograde cholangiopancreatography. Med Care. 2013;51(12):1040–7.

24. Kapral C, Duller C, Wewalka F, Kerstan E, Vogel W, Schreiber F. Case volume and outcome of endoscopic retrograde cholangiopancreatography: results of a nationwide Austrian benchmarking project. Endoscopy. 2008;40(8):625–30.

Surgical Treatment and Outcomes

Ashwini Kumar and Jose M. Martinez

Introduction

The incidence of choledocholithiasis in patients undergoing cholecystectomy is estimated to be 10 %. The presence of common bile duct stones is associated with several known complications including cholangitis, gallstone pancreatitis, obstructive jaundice, and hepatic abscess. Making the diagnosis early and prompt management is crucial. Traditionally, when choledocholithiasis is identified with intraoperative cholangiography during the cholecystectomy, it has been managed surgically by open choledochotomy and placement of a T-tube. This open surgical approach has a morbidity rate of 10–15 %, mortality rate of <1 %, with a <6 % incidence of retained stones [1]. Led by improvements in imaging technology like magnetic resonance cholangiopancreatography (MRCP) and minimally invasive techniques like endoscopic retrograde cholangiopancreatography (ERCP), endoscopic ultrasound (EUS), and lapa-roscopy, the morbidity of managing choledocholithiasis has reduced.

Currently, different treatment options include preoperative or postoperative ERCP with endoscopic biliary stone extraction, and laparoscopic or open surgical bile duct clearance. Other options can be used if needed and available, such as percutaneous transhepatic cholangiography (PTC), electrohydraulic lithotripsy (EHL), extracorporeal shockwave lithotripsy (ESWL), laser lithotripsy, and dissolving solutions. These options may be useful in patients who are not appropriate surgical candidates. Patients who fail endoscopic retrieval of CBD stones, as well as cases in which an endoscopic approach is not appropriate, should be explored surgically.

Intraoperative Cholangiography

Intraoperative cholangiogram (IOC) is imaging of bile duct during the surgery by injecting contrast into the biliary system. IOC is performed for proper identification if the anatomy is unclear, and for recognition of any calculus or other obstructing pathology. It also allows for verification of a ductal injury, so that a plan for remediation can be made promptly. Selective, as compared to routine use of IOC minimizes unnecessary biliary instrumentation.

Once the cystic duct has been dissected circumferentially, and a 'critical view' has been

A. Kumar, M.B.B.S., M.D. (✉)
Department of Laparoendoscopic Surgery,
University of Miami, Miami, FL, USA

1202 Walton Ave., Jourdanton, TX 78026, USA
e-mail: ashwinikumarz@yahoo.com

J.M. Martinez, M.D.
Department of Surgery, Miller School of Medicine,
University of Miami, Miami, FL, USA
e-mail: JMartinez4@med.miami.edu

© Springer International Publishing Switzerland 2016
J.W. Hazey et al. (eds.), *Multidisciplinary Management of Common Bile Duct Stones*,
DOI 10.1007/978-3-319-22765-8_11

obtained, a clip is applied across the gallbladder-cystic duct junction. A small vertical ductotomy is created below the clip taking special precaution not to injure the posterior wall of the cystic duct. After milking the contents of the duct toward and out of the ductotomy, a cholangio-catheter is inserted either through the existing laparoscopic port, or a separate stab incision in the right upper quadrant near the midclavicular line. The catheter is passed into the ductotomy in the cystic duct with laparoscopic instruments, and held in place with a balloon, clamp, or clip.

In order to verify the catheter is within the cystic duct and there is no leak present, saline is injected through the catheter into the cystic duct. The contrast and tubing should be free of air bubbles, which can create filling defects and can be confused for biliary stones. Contrast is injected under continuous fluoroscopic visualization with a 1:1 dilution of water-soluble contrast and saline. Fluoroscopy allows real-time imaging of the duct, and reduces radiation dose as well as procedural time in comparison to plane X-ray films used in past. Placement of a hydrophilic guidewire through the cholangiogram catheter facilitates placement of instruments for CBD stone extraction and dilatation of the cystic duct with balloon catheters or mechanical dilators if necessary.

There are a number of key anatomical and fluoroscopic findings that must be identified at time of performing an IOC. It is important to evaluate the IOC images for the size of CBD, right and left hepatic ducts, length of the cystic duct and the junction with the CBD, any filling defects, and flow of contrast into the duodenum. If biliary ducts are visualized, but the contrast does not flow freely into the duodenum, placing the patient into reverse Trendelenburg position, and administration of IV glucagon to relax the sphincter of Oddi can be helpful. On the other hand, administration of morphine sulfate to induce spasm of sphincter of Oddi, and placing the patient in Trendelenburg position can be helpful if right and left hepatic ducts are not visualized. Visualization of filling defects, dilated bile ducts, or failure of contrast to flow into the duodenum is suggestive of choledocholithiasis.

Intraoperative cholangiography (IOC) is recommended, in patients who have not been diagnosed, but are with intermediate or high probability of choledocholithiasis, although opinion varies between providers. Some surgeons perform routine IOC before every cholecystectomy. Others obtain selective IOC based upon findings of elevated liver function tests, a dilated common bile duct, or a history of pancreatitis. No benefits of routine use of IOC have been demonstrated in detecting CBD stones. IOC on the other hand, has added a mean of 16 min to the total operating time [2]. Laparoscopic IOC has a reported sensitivity of 80–92.8 % and specificity of 76.2–97 % for detection of CBD stones [3].

MRCP and EUS have shown preoperative findings concordant with IOC results, and can be used as a screening tool for detection of CBD stones. However, the cost and availability are limiting factors for use of these diagnostic modalities.

Management Options Based on the Risk of Choledocholithiasis

Patients at low risk of choledocholithiasis should undergo cholecystectomy, without any further evaluation, as additional investigations and interventions have associated risks and may not be cost effective. Routine use of IOC or intraoperative ultrasound for this group remains controversial. Patients at intermediate or high risk of harboring common bile duct stones can be managed in a number of ways. Institutional protocol, available expertise, and resources may dictate the approach to the management of patients with suspected choledocholithiasis. Incidence of recurrent symptoms, gallstone pancreatitis, and cholangitis are higher if a diagnosis of choledocholithiasis is missed. Therefore patients with intermediate risk of having choledocholithiasis can undergo either additional evaluation including EUS, MRCP, and ERCP or should be taken to the operating room with laparoscopic IOC or ultrasound. A laparoscopic cholecystectomy should be done if these investigations are negative for choledocholithiasis; if positive, a laparoscopic CBD exploration should be undertaken. In the absence of expertise and resources for CBD exploration, postoperative ERCP should be carried out [4].

Patients at high risk of choledocholithiasis frequently need therapeutic intervention; further evaluation in the form of preoperative ERCP or IOC should be done. Randomized controlled trials comparing two-stage management with ERCP followed by laparoscopic cholecystectomy, and single stage laparoscopic IOC with transcystic, or transductal stone retrieval showed no difference in primary duct clearance rate (88 %), morbidity, or mortality. Intraoperative or postoperative ERCP is also an option if IOC is positive. Preoperative ERCP or, MRCP should be considered for patients who are clinically jaundiced [4].

Preoperative Preparation

Risks and benefits including retained stones, biliary leak, bowel/pancreas/liver injury, and abscess formation should be discussed with the patients while obtaining informed consent. Also, patients should be made aware about the alternatives to surgical exploration.

Common pathogens in biliary tract include enteric gram-negative bacilli, enterococcus, and clostridia, which may lead to cholangitis, and sepsis in cases of choledocholithiasis. It is recommended that preoperatively these patients should receive appropriate antibiotics to cover the above-mentioned pathogens. A first generation cephalosporin (Cephazolin) or second-generation cephalosporin (Cefotetan/Cefoxitin) should be administered within an hour prior to the surgical incision.

Prophylaxis for deep venous thrombosis such as sequential compression dressing according to the institutional protocol should be employed. A surgical timeout including correct patient identity, planned operation, and informed consent should be done.

Laparoscopic CBD Exploration

In early part of 1990s, laparoscopic cholecystectomy quickly became standard of care for treatment of symptomatic gallbladder disease. As the development in laparoscopic techniques and instrumentation evolved, it allowed the explora-

tion of common bile duct at the time of laparoscopic cholecystectomy to popularize. Laparoscopic common bile duct exploration (LCBDE) allows for single stage treatment of gallstone disease, reducing overall hospital stay, improving safety and cost-effectiveness when compared to the two-stage approach of ERCP and laparoscopic cholecystectomy [5]. Bile duct clearance can be confirmed by direct visualization with a choledochoscope. But, before the advent of choledochoscope, bile duct clearance was uncertain, and blind instrumentation of the duct resulted in accentuated edema and inflammation. Due to advancement in instruments, optical magnification, and direct visualization, laparoscopic exploration of the CBD results in fewer traumas to the bile duct. This has led to an increasing tendency to close the duct primarily, reducing the need for placement of T-tubes. Still, laparoscopic bile duct exploration is being done in only a few centers. Apart from the need for special instruments, there is also a significant learning curve to acquire expertise to be able to perform a laparoscopic bile duct surgery.

Morbidity and mortality rates of laparoscopic exploration are comparable to ERCP (2–17 and 1–5 %), and there is no clear difference in primary success rates between the two approaches. However, the endoscopic approach may be preferable for elderly and frail patients, who are at higher risk with surgery. Patients older than 70–80 years of age have a 4–10 % mortality rate with open duct exploration. It may be as high as 20 % in elderly patients undergoing urgent procedures. In comparison, advanced age and comorbidities do not have a significant impact on overall complication rates for ERCP [3].

Intraoperative cholangiogram as described, is indispensable for successful CBD exploration. A C-arm and trained personnel to handle it should be available for fluoroscopy. A flexible choledochoscope, separate light source, monitor, 3–5 French biliary Fogarty catheters, wire baskets, guidewire, balloons, mechanical dilators, and T-tubes should be available.

A success rate of over 90 % has been reported with laparoscopic CBD exploration. Availability of surgical expertise and appropriate equipment affect the success rate of laparoscopic exploration, as does the size, number of the CBD stones, as well as biliary anatomy. Over the years, laparoscopic exploration has become efficient, safe, and cost effective. Complications include CBD laceration, stricture formation, bile leak, abscess, pancreatitis, and retained stones [6].

In cases of failure of laparoscopic CBD exploration, a guidewire or stent can be passed through the cystic duct, common bile duct, and through the ampulla into the duodenum followed by cholecystectomy. This makes the identification and cannulation of the ampulla easier during the postoperative ERCP.

Laparoscopic common bile duct exploration is traditionally performed through a transcystic or transductal approach. The transcystic approach is appropriate under certain circumstances. These include a small stone (<10 mm) located in the CBD, presence of small common bile duct (<6 mm), or if there is poor access to the common duct. The transductal approach is preferable in cases of large stones, stones in proximal ducts (hepatic ducts), large occluding stones in a large duct, presence of multiple stones, or if the cystic duct is small (<4 mm) or tortuous. Contraindications for laparoscopic approach include lack of training, and severe inflammation in the porta hepatis making the exploration difficult and risky.

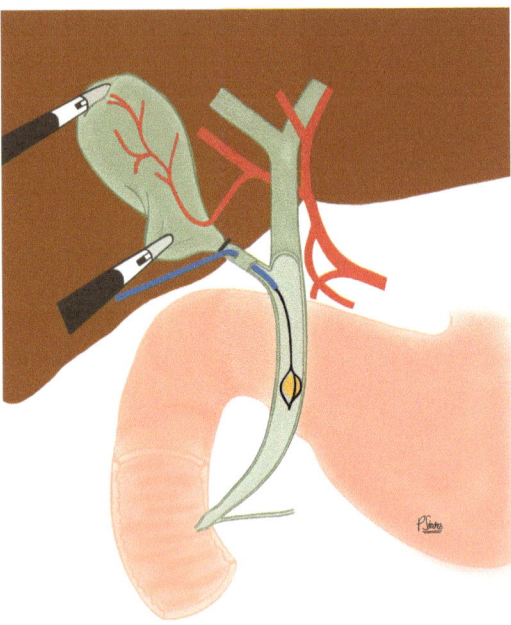

Fig. 11.1 Laparoscopic transcystic choledocholithotomy—ductotomy is made in the cystic duct. A helical basket is passed through the working channel of the choledochoscope, and stone is retrieved through the ductotomy (Courtesy of Priscila Sanchez, University of Miami)

Laparoscopic Transcystic Approach (Fig. 11.1)

In the transcystic approach, the gallbladder is grasped and retracted cephalad to facilitate visualization and manipulation. The ductotomy in the cystic duct made for the IOC can be used to pass the catheter. A saline flush with administration of 1–2 mg of glucagon to relax the sphincter of Oddi may be successful in clearing small stones through the sphincter of Oddi or opening in the cystic duct. If repeated attempts at flushing remains unsuccessful, a basket or biliary balloon catheter can be passed over a guidewire into the bile duct through the cystic duct under fluoroscopic guidance. Balloons should be passed under fluoroscopic guidance into the duodenum through the ampulla. The balloon is inflated in the duodenum and withdrawn until resistance is felt at ampulla. It is then deflated and withdrawn about 1 cm, followed by gentle inflation and withdrawn through the common bile duct into the cystic ductotomy to retrieve the stones. Transcystic use of a biliary balloon catheter should be done carefully, as it can pull the stone in to the common hepatic duct. This can usually be retrieved by ductal irrigation combined with changes in position of the patient; if this is unsuccessful a choledochotomy may be needed or may be managed with a postoperative ERCP.

If use of a balloon or irrigation fails, a 3 mm choledochoscope with a working channel can be passed through the cystic duct. Balloon dilation of the cystic duct may be needed if the stone is larger than the lumen of the cystic duct or advancement of choledochoscope is limited secondary to a small cystic duct size. In general, the cystic duct can be progressively dilated up to

8 mm, but should not be dilated to more than the internal diameter of the CBD.

A choledochoscope can be passed into the peritoneal cavity through a midaxillary port or an extra port and should be passed into the CBD over a guidewire. Better visualization and irrigation of the duct is obtained with isotonic sodium chloride solution injected under high pressure. A helical basket is passed through the working channel of the choledochoscope under direct visualization, and it is opened after advancing it beyond the stone. Stone is captured as the basket is pulled backwards and rotated. Alternatively, the choledochoscope may be used to push CBD stones distally into the duodenum through the ampulla. Conclusive demonstration of clearance of the duct is critical, and therefore a completion IOC should always be performed.

Balloon dilatation of the sphincter of Oddi as well as antegrade sphincterotomy has also been described using the transcystic approach. Balloon dilatation has been associated with significantly lower incidence of bleeding when compared to sphincterotomy. But because of its association with a significantly increased rate of pancreatitis [7], its use should be confined to patients with coagulopathy/cirrhosis or in cases of difficult endoscopic access as in patients with Billroth II gastrectomy, Roux-en-Y anastomosis, or juxtapapillary diverticulum.

At the completion of a transcystic stone retrieval, the cholecystectomy is completed. Following this, the cystic duct stump is secured with clips or an endoloop. A drain placement may be considered if there is a concern for bile leak. The morbidity of laparoscopic common bile duct exploration has been reported to be equivalent to that of a standard laparoscopic cholecystectomy alone [8].

Laparoscopic Transductal Approach (Fig. 11.2)

Laparoscopic choledocholithotomy is technically more challenging and can be utilized in case of failure of the transcystic approach, or in cases which are not appropriate for a transcystic

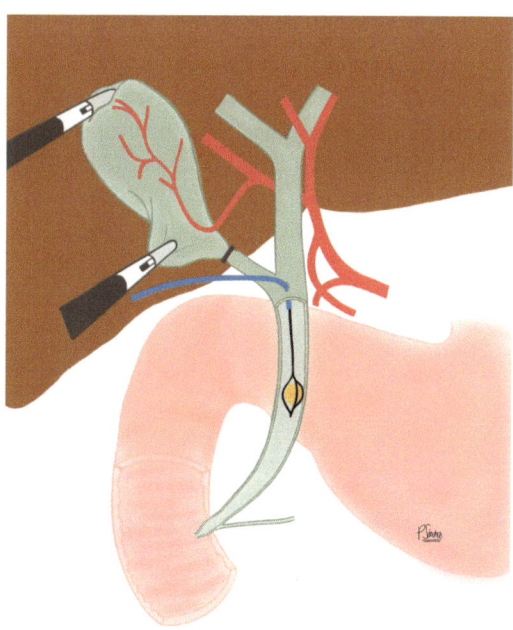

Fig. 11.2 Transductal choledocholithotomy: A longitudinal ductotomy is made on the common bile duct. A helical basket is passed through the working channel of the choledochoscope, and stone is retrieved (Courtesy of Priscila Sanchez, University of Miami)

approach. It can be accomplished with a variety of techniques using basket or balloon catheter with or without fluoroscopic guidance, and choledochoscopic manipulations. The dome of gallbladder is grasped and retracted cephalad for exposure. A 30° scope is used to visualize the supraduodenal CBD. After identification of the junction of cystic duct with the CBD, the anterior surface of the CBD is exposed. Needle aspiration with bile content confirms identification. Stay sutures are placed on the CBD at 3 and 9 o'clock to facilitate traction, manipulation, and provide a seal during choledochoscopy with saline infusion if needed. A longitudinal ductotomy of 1–2 cm is created on the anterior surface of the CBD between stay sutures, using laparoscopic scissors. The ductotomy should be at least the diameter of largest stone, and should be made anteriorly in a longitudinal fashion and not on the sides or transversely. This is done to keep the blood supply of the duct intact.

After accessing the CBD, a catheter is first inserted into the CBD, and saline infusion should be used to clear the duct. This maneuver is generally successful in clearing smaller, non-adherent stones. If the saline infusion fails in clearing the CBD of stones, retrieval using a balloon or wire basket under fluoroscopic guidance should be undertaken. Alternatively a choledochoscope can be passed through the ductotomy. In the transductal approach, a larger size choledochoscope (up to 5 mm) can be used to allow the passage of larger instruments, and provide good direct visualization.

In patients with a dilated CBD, the choledochotomy can be primarily closed with interrupted fine monofilament absorbable suture. Primary closure is associated with shorter operative time and length of hospital stay. Higher patient satisfaction and reduced hospital expenses have been reported [6].

It is still a common practice to close the choledochotomy around a T-tube (14 Fr). It is passed through a laparoscopic port, and into the CBD through the choledochotomy. The horizontal limb of the T-tube can be opened, or up to half of the circumference can be excised depending on personal preferences. Also, some surgeons prefer to leave one end of the horizontal limb long, so that it can be passed through the ampulla as a stent. The choledochotomy is closed with interrupted absorbable suture snugly around the T-tube to prevent a bile leak. A T-tube also provides a route for ductal imaging in the postoperative period and access for removal of any residual CBD stones. A closed suction drain may be placed near the choledochotomy closure. As in transcystic approach, conclusive demonstration of the clearance of the duct is critical, and can be obtained with a completion cholangiogram before closing using the T-tube, specifically looking for any leak at the choledochotomy site, or filling defects. In cases where a T-tube is not placed, a cholangiogram should be done by passing a cholangiogram catheter through the choledochotomy site. Bringing the stay sutures together helps to prevent any contrast leak by approximating the edges of choledochotomy.

Complications due to placement of a T-tube include biliary obstruction, dislodgement or fracture of the tube, bacteremia, bile leak, pancreatitis, and bile duct stricture [9]. They can also act as a foreign body leading to precipitation of bile salts and pigments and may lead to stone recurrence. A cholangiogram should be obtained prior to removal of a T-tube to rule out bile leak and to confirm duct clearance. T-tube can be removed at around 10 days postoperatively. Different authors have suggested removal ranging from 5 to 6 days to 4–5 weeks after surgery. Retained stones can be removed percutaneously following maturation of the T-tube tract. Alternatively, ERCP can be utilized.

Some surgeons prefer closing the choledochotomy primarily with placement of a transcystic biliary drainage catheter instead of a T-tube, as they as easier to place and also allow access to retrieved biliary stones. However, they have been reported to have a significantly higher rate of bile leak compared to T-tubes (14 % versus 3.5 % respectively) [10]. Operative time (97 min versus 75 min), and length of hospital stay (6 days versus 2 days) were found to be significantly longer when performing a laparoscopic choledochotomy versus a transcystic exploration in an observational study. The rate of stone clearance was similar [8, 11].

Open Common Bile Duct Exploration

Traditionally, an open common bile duct exploration was the primary method of managing CBD stones. With the development of less invasive techniques and improved success rates, the open operative approach to CBD exploration is used less frequently. This historical operation is still of significant value and may occasionally be needed in certain circumstances. Open CBD exploration is still the primary approach in remote areas where specialized laparoscopic surgeons, endoscopist or interventional radiologist are not available. Anatomical alterations (often post-surgical), or severe inflammation in the triangle of Calot may decrease the success rate of minimally invasive approaches to the management of CBD stones, and force the surgeon to rely on the open approach to clear the CBD. In cases where both laparoscopic exploration and postoperative ERCP are unsuccessful, or in patients with complications from laparoscopic CBD exploration, the open approach should be undertaken. Patients undergoing open cholecystectomy with verified CBD stones should also have the stones cleared at time of surgery via an open approach.

A right upper quadrant subcostal or midline incision should be used for open common bile duct exploration. The exposure is gained by retracting the liver superiorly, duodenum inferiorly, and the stomach to the left. Medialization of the duodenum allows exposure and manipulation of the distal common bile duct. The proximal cystic duct should be clipped or ligated to prevent gallstones from migrating from the gallbladder into the cystic duct and CBD. The CBD is then opened anteriorly and longitudinally for 1–2 cm after placing the stay sutures as described earlier (Fig. 11.2). The CBD is then manually manipulated to extract the stone through the choledochotomy. If this fails to mobilize the stone, a Fogarty catheter can be passed into the proximal duct followed by the distal duct to retrieve the stones. Alternatively a pituitary scoop or Randall stone forceps can be used. Saline irrigation should be done for removal of debris by flushing. Choledochoscopy with saline infusion under pressure using a pressure pump, intravenous tubing, and three-way stopcock can be done to clear the stone from the CBD. Wire basket retrieval can also be performed through the working channel of a choledochoscope. Electrohydraulic or laser lithotripsy may improve the duct clearance in case of a large or impacted stone. This is done by using an electrohydraulic lithotripsy probe, or laser fiber under direct visualization of the stone with a choledochoscope. Closure of choledochotomy can be done as described with laparoscopic choledochotomy, either primarily with interrupted absorbable sutures in cases of a dilated CBD, or over a 14 Fr T-tube. A completion T-tube cholangiogram should be obtained.

Impacted Stone

Uncommonly, an impacted stone is encountered, which is difficult to remove laparoscopically. Retrieval in these cases may be achieved by choledochoscopically assisted lithotripsy (electrohydraulic or laser), and extracting the smaller fragments laparoscopically.

Duodenotomy with choledocho-enterostomy, or sphincterotomy have been described, but rarely used. If experience in performing a duodenotomy, and choledocho-enterostomy or sphincterotomy or lithotripsy is not available, a T-tube should be placed and cholecystectomy should be completed. Then the patient should be referred to a specialized center where endoscopic or percutaneous removal is usually successful with the use of electrohydraulic or laser lithotripsy in conjunction with sphincterotomy.

Conclusion

With advancement in imaging technology, laparoscopic and endoscopic techniques, management of common bile duct stone has changed drastically in recent years. This has made the treatment of this condition safe and more efficient. Many options are now available to manage this condition, and any particular modality for treatment should be chosen carefully based on the patient related factors, institutional protocol, available expertise, resources, and cost-effectiveness.

References

1. Ko CW, Lee SP. Epidemiology and natural history of common bile duct stones and prediction of disease. Gastrointest Endosc. 2002;56(6 Suppl):S165–9.
2. Ford JA, Soop M, Du J, Loveday BP, Rodgers M. Systematic review of intraoperative cholangiography in cholecystectomy. Br J Surg. 2012;99(2):160–7.
3. Williams EJ, Green J, Beckingham I, Parks R, Martin D, Lombard M, et al. Guidelines on the management of common bile duct stones (CBDS). Gut. 2008;57(7):1004–21.
4. Committee ASoP, Maple JT, Ben-Menachem T, Anderson MA, Appalaneni V, Banerjee S, et al. The role of endoscopy in the evaluation of suspected choledocholithiasis. Gastrointest Endosc. 2010;71(1):1–9.
5. Perissat J, Huibregtse K, Keane FB, Russell RC, Neoptolemos JP. Management of bile duct stones in the era of laparoscopic cholecystectomy. Br J Surg. 1994;81(6):799–810.
6. Petelin JB. Laparoscopic common bile duct exploration. Surg Endosc. 2003;17(11):1705–15.
7. Baron TH, Harewood GC. Endoscopic balloon dilation of the biliary sphincter compared to endoscopic

biliary sphincterotomy for removal of common bile duct stones during ERCP: a metaanalysis of randomized, controlled trials. Am J Gastroenterol. 2004; 99(8):1455–60.

8. Hanif F, Ahmed Z, Samie MA, Nassar AH. Laparoscopic transcystic bile duct exploration: the treatment of first choice for common bile duct stones. Surg Endosc. 2010;24(7):1552–6.

9. Shojaiefard A, Esmaeilzadeh M, Ghafouri A, Mehrabi A. Various techniques for the surgical treatment of common bile duct stones: a meta review. Gastroenterol Res Pract. 2009;2009:840208.

10. Tang CN, Tai CK, Ha JP, Tsui KK, Wong DC, Li MK. Antegrade biliary stenting versus T-tube drainage after laparoscopic choledochotomy--a comparative cohort study. Hepatogastroenterology. 2006; 53(69):330–4.

11. Topal B, Aerts R, Penninckx F. Laparoscopic common bile duct stone clearance with flexible choledochoscopy. Surg Endosc. 2007;21(12):2317–21.

Surgical Procedures to Prevent Recurrence

Edward L. Jones

Introduction

The management of distal common bile duct obstruction is typically done via endoscopic retrograde cholangiopancreatography (ERCP). Up to one fourth of patients who undergo endoscopic treatment for biliary stones will experience a recurrence months to years later [1]. Several risk factors for recurrence have been identified in retrospective studies. These include multiple common bile duct stones (≥ 2), biliary dilatation (≥ 13 mm), open cholecystectomy, lithotripsy, and hepatolithiasis. Additional factors associated with recurrence are those that result in biliary stasis such as a peri-ampullary diverticulum, papillary stenosis, biliary stricture, and angulation of the common bile duct ($\geq 145°$) [2, 3]. These factors are more common in the obese and patients with sudden weight loss (often following bariatric surgery) as well as those of East Asian descent [4, 5].

Patients who fail the initial endoscopic treatment for their stones can undergo repeat ERCP but may also be treated surgically. Surgery should also be considered as the primary treatment in patients at high risk of recurrence and those with altered anatomy such as Roux-en-Y gastric bypass. To achieve wide, unfettered enteric drainage there are three main surgical options: transduodenal sphincteroplasty, choledochoduodenostomy, or hepaticojejunostomy. The specific indications, contraindications, advantages, disadvantages, and outcomes of each procedure will be discussed so that the physician can make a rationale decision as to the best choice for the clinical situation.

Transduodenal Sphincteroplasty

Indications

Transduodenal sphincteroplasty should be considered in those patients who cannot be treated endoscopically due to altered anatomy as well as those with multiple or impacted stones in the ampulla of Vater. Additional indications include recurrent biliary obstruction due to papillary stenosis or sphincter of Oddi dysfunction after endoscopic sphincterotomy. Patients with pancreatitis secondary to pancreas divisum may also benefit from sphincteroplasty of the minor papilla. Transduodenal sphincteroplasty is contraindicated in patients with a common bile duct diameter >2 cm, a long distal common bile duct stricture, a large peri-ampullary diverticulum or severe inflammation of the duodenal wall and pancreatic head. Significant morbidity is <10 %

E.L. Jones, M.D. (✉)
Department of Surgery, Denver VA Medical Center and the University of Colorado, 1055 Clermont St, Denver, CO 80220, USA
e-mail: Edward.Jones@UCDenver.edu

© Springer International Publishing Switzerland 2016
J.W. Hazey et al. (eds.), *Multidisciplinary Management of Common Bile Duct Stones*,
DOI 10.1007/978-3-319-22765-8_12

in recent studies and improvement in pain is achieved in 60–75 % of patients at 2–5 years post procedure [6, 7]. Younger patients with chronic pancreatitis are associated with poorer outcomes regardless of the indication.

Pertinent Anatomy

The common bile duct begins after the cystic duct inserts and travels in the portal triad, posterior to the duodenal bulb and into the pancreatic groove along the posterior surface of the pancreas. It then shares a fibrous layer with the medial wall of the

duodenum for approximately 5 mm before joining the pancreatic duct [8]. This creates the ampulla of Vater which is 2–3 mm in length and lies within the submucosa of the second portion of the duodenum. The pancreatic duct is typically medial to the common bile duct and can have a separate opening into the duodenum in 9 % of patients. Both ducts may also have openings directly at the ampulla in 6 % of patients.

There are four anatomic sphincters associated with the distal common bile duct and pancreatic duct that form the sphincter complex initially described by Oddi (Fig. 12.1). Three interconnected sphincters are located at the distal bile

Fig. 12.1 Sphincter of Oddi Complex. (**a**) Insertion of the distal common bile duct and pancreatic ducts into the second portion of the duodenum. (**b**) Intertwining smooth muscle fibers of the ampulla of Vater. (**c**) The four sphincter mechanisms of the complex. (**d**) Cross section of the ampulla of Vater and the intersphincteric septum

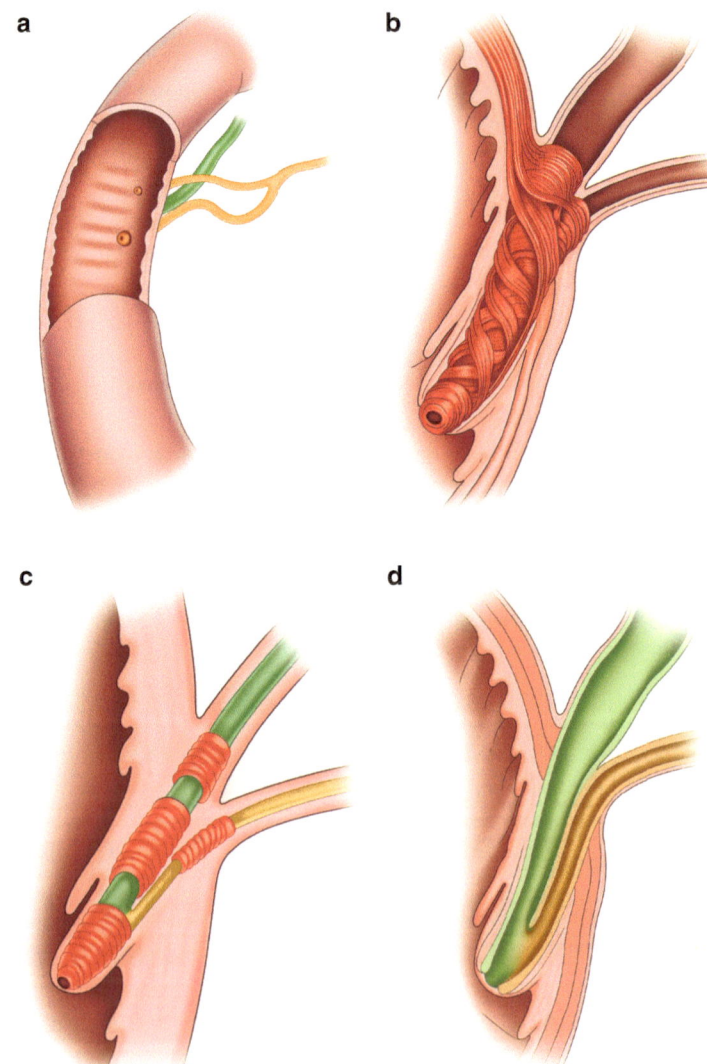

duct with an additional sphincter at the termination of the pancreatic duct. This complex can be as short as 6 mm or as long as 30 mm and generates a basal resistance of approximately 5 mmHg. Phasic contractions (100–150 mmHg) occur every 2–6 min with bile flow during the relaxation phase between contractions. Basal pressures >40 mmHg and phasic contractions >220 mmHg for >8 s at a frequency of >10/min suggest an abnormal sphincter mechanism (sphincter of Oddi dysfunction).

The blood supply to the common bile duct is derived from the celiac access and enters the duct at 3 and 9 o'clock from the following vessels (cranio-caudal): the right hepatic artery, the gastroduodenal artery, the retroduodenal atery and the anterior superior pancreaticoduodenal artery. Significant variation can exist in the arterial (and venous) supply. As the duct passes behind the duodenum, the retroduodenal and superior pancreaticoduodenal arteries create a para-biliary plexus that diffusely supplies the bile duct in contrast to the supraduodenal portion with its supply entering at 3 and 9 o'clock. However, only 10 % of arterial branches enter in the 10–11 o'clock region of the ampulla of Vater [9]. Thus, sphincterotomy (whether endoscopic or open) will result in less arterial bleeding if made in the 10–11 o'clock region of the major papilla.

Surgical Technique

It is important to utilize precise terminology when describing procedures on the sphincter of Oddi. A sphincterotomy is an incision into the sphincter without suturing or further alteration of the anatomy. A sphincteroplasty is an incision into the sphincter of Oddi with suturing of the common bile duct mucosa to the duodenal mucosa. Additional cutting of the septum (septectomy) between the pancreatic duct and the common bile duct may be required in patients with recurrent pancreatitis. This can be done with or without suture reinforcement (septoplasty).

To begin the procedure, access to the right upper quadrant is obtained via a subcostal or midline incision followed by an extended Kocher

maneuver once the gallbladder has been removed. It is often of benefit to utilize a radiolucent operative table in case cholangiography or pancreatography is needed. When kocherizing the duodenum it is important continue mobilization onto the third part of the duodenum to ensure a tension-free closure. The major papilla is located at the lower one-third of the second part of the duodenum and identification can be aided by passing a 4 or 6 French Fogarty catheter through the cystic duct stump (or via a supraduodenal choldochotomy) into the common bile duct and duodenum. Inflation of the balloon allows palpation through the wall of the duodenum and improves the accuracy of the longitudinal duodenotomy.

Once opened, the major papilla should be readily palpable via the Fogarty balloon if it is not immediately visible (Fig. 12.2a). The minor papilla is typically located approximately 2 cm cephalad but may be closer in cases of pancreas divisum. Once these have been identified, retaining sutures are placed in the duodenal wall adjacent to the papillary complex to elevate and expose the ampulla (Fig. 12.2b). Loupe magnification may be of benefit as the goal is to precisely incise the intramural portion of the distal common bile duct and suture the common bile duct mucosa to the duodenal mucosa. The sphincterotomy is started with a 5 mm incision at the 10–11 o'clock with a needle-tip cautery on top of the Fogarty catheter. Absorbable, monofilament 4-0 to 5-0 sutures are then placed every 1–2 mm with slight traction to hold open the bile duct (Fig. 12.3a). A grooved needle director or lacrimal duct probe can be inserted into the common bile duct and the incision and suture is continued for the entire length of the intramural common bile duct, typically extending from 6 mm up to 3 cm in total length.

After completing the initial sphincterotomy it is important to identify the pancreatic duct. The opening is typically between 4 and 6 o'clock on the medial aspect of the newly created opening (Fig. 12.3b). A lacrimal duct probe can be gently placed in the pancreatic duct to avoid unintentional closure of the orifice while placing the medial sutures of the sphincteroplasty. If the duct cannot be identified, intravenous secretin (75 U/kg) can

Fig. 12.2 Identification
and incision of the
ampulla of Vater. (**a**)
Fogarty balloon inserted
and insufflated in the
duodenum can be
palpated to localize the
ampulla of Vater and
optimize the location of
the duodenotomy. (**b**)
The Fogarty catheter can
be used as a guide for
the initial
sphincterotomy

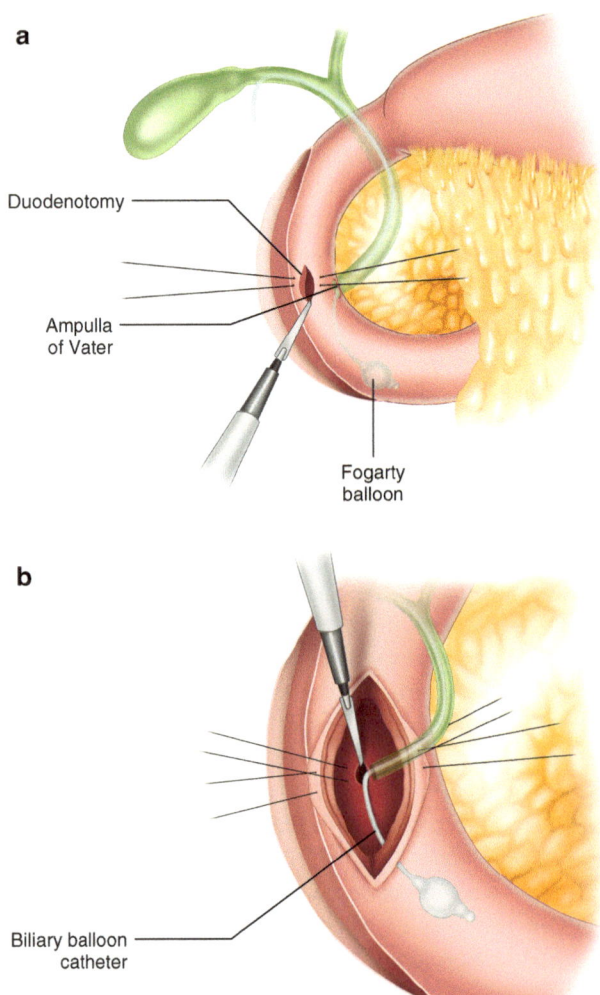

a

Duodenotomy

Ampulla
of Vater

Fogarty
balloon

b

Biliary balloon
catheter

be given to aid in localization. If the pancreatic duct still cannot be identified, avoidance of sutures between 3 and 6 o'clock is recommended as inadvertent closure of the pancreatic duct will result in serious postoperative pancreatitis. Lastly, careful placement of the apex stitch is necessary to secure the common bile duct to the wall of the duodenum at the part where it is most extramural in location and prevent leakage of bile.

Patients who have had recurrent pancreatitis may develop stenosis of the pancreatic duct orifice. Septectomy should be performed by cutting of the septum between the common bile duct and pancreatic duct. This is done by placing a lacrimal duct probe into the duct and carefully incising

over this with the needle-tip electrocautery. Avoidance of the incision into the pancreatic parenchyma is recommended to reduce the incidence of postoperative pancreas but cannot always be avoided. If extension into the gland is done or troublesome bleeding encountered then a septoplasty can be completed with absorbable 4-0 or 5-0 suture in interrupted fashion.

Once the sphincteroplasty is complete the common bile duct can be explored in retrograde fashion with a Fogarty catheter, baskets or a choledochoscope to ensure complete clearance of the obstruction. If preferred, cholangiography and/or pancreatography can also be done with gentle injection of contrast via an appropriately sized

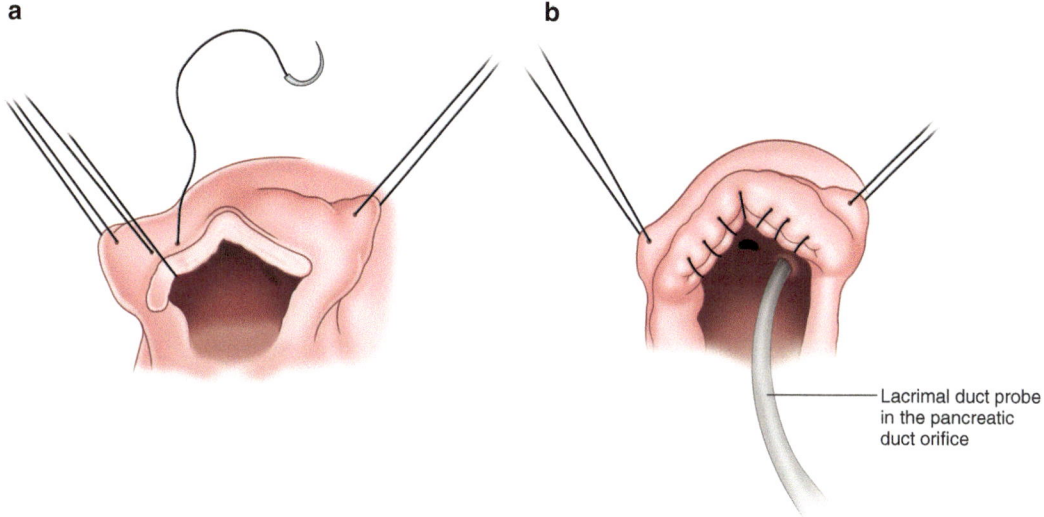

Fig. 12.3 Sphincteroplasty technique and identification of the pancreatic duct. (**a**) Sphincteroplasty sutures begin laterally and are placed in interrupted fashion every 1–2 mm. (**b**) The pancreatic duct orifice is identified medially and protected from inadvertent closure during sphincteroplasty

angiocatheter. Ductal drainage via a T-tube is not typically required unless a significant amount of swelling and edema is expected as can be the case with stone impaction at the ampulla of Vater. Duodenal closure should be done in longitudinal fashion with a single layer of 2-0 or 3-0 suture in Lembert fashion. A closed suction drain is placed posterior to the duodenum and pancreas.

Complications and Postoperative Care

Early complications of transduodenal sphinctero-plasty include acute pancreatitis (0.6 %), bleeding (0.3 %) and leakage from the duodenal suture line (0.6 %). Pancreatitis is managed with prolonged bowel rest and antibiotics if there is evidence of infection. Duodenal leak may require additional drainage if the closed suction drain does not adequately control the leak. Reoperation with diversion and pyloric exclusion may be used as a last resort. Significant bleeding, while rare, should be treated with radiographic embolization of the bleeding vessel. Pneumobilia should be expected (permanently) and indicates a patent

sphincteroplasty but cholangitis should always be ruled out prior to patient discharge. Finally, recurrent stenosis is seen in approximately 2 % of patients and should be confirmed by an upper gastrointestinal barium study. This will demonstrate a *lack* of contrast refluxing into the biliary system due to the stenosis. This can be further evaluated by ERCP or magnetic resonance cholangiopancreatography.

Following surgery, a nasogastric tube is maintained for 48–72 h and is removed once the daily output is low. Serum amylase levels to identify early pancreatitis are typically checked on postoperative days 1 and 3. A diet of liquids is begun once the nasogastric tube has been removed. The closed suction drain is then checked for bile and amylase 24 h after initiation of the diet. The drain is removed if the amylase and bilirubin level is normal. Further investigation with Computed Tomography may be required to rule out a pancreatic fluid collection or phlegmon if the closed suction drain amylase or bilirubin levels remain high.

With pancreatitis resolved (or avoided) and the nasogastric tube removed, patients can be rapidly advanced from a fluid to a regular diet.

This typically happens by postoperative day 4 with many patients ready for discharge by postoperative day 6 and an average hospital stay ranging from 5 to 10 days. These patients require long-term follow-up and repeat liver function tests as the chronic inflammation generated by transduodenal sphincteroplasty has been associated with a 6 % incidence of bile duct carcinoma [10]. In addition, some clinicians will provide a recurring prescription for antibiotics that should be initiated with any significant fever, abdominal pain or jaundice to aggressively treat presumed cholangitis until the patient can be evaluated.

Choledochoduodenostomy

Indications

Choledochoduodenostomy should only be performed in patients with dilated common bile ducts (>2 cm). Biliary dilation is an indication of prolonged obstruction with resultant biliary stasis that can create primary stones within the duct. This is the major indication for choledochoduodenostomy. In addition, numerous bile duct stones (that cannot be managed endoscopically), intrahepatic stones or the existence of a long, distal common bile duct stricture may also require cholodeochoduodenostomy. A choledocho- or hepatico-duodenostomy has also been described as part of liver transplantation or malignant bypass but those considerations are beyond the scope of this chapter. Contraindications to choledochoduodenostomy include a common bile duct diameter less than 15 mm, a history of gastric antrectomy and/or resultant scarring from a previous inflammatory process (peptic ulcer disease, perforation treated by Graham patch, etc.). Avoidance of the scarred portion of the proximal duodenum and distal common bile duct can be done via hepaticojejunostomy which is discussed below.

Surgical Technique

The surgeon begins with a right subcostal or upper midline incision and removes the gallbladder if present. An extended Kocher maneuver is performed and the peritoneum overlying the common bile duct incised. Exposure of the common bile duct in the supraduodenal location is accomplished and the duct size confirmed to be 2 cm or greater. An incision is then made in the common bile duct just cephalad to the intrapancreatic portion and extended 2.0–2.5 cm longitudinally and cephalad, often extending onto the common hepatic duct (Fig. 12.4a). The common duct can then be explored as needed ensuring clearance of and adequate drainage from the hepatic ducts. A longitudinal incision centered on the choledochotomy on the superior aspect of the duodenum is then completed. The duodenotomy should be slightly smaller than the choledochotomy as the elasticity of the duodenum will create unnecessary technical difficulty if made too large.

Stay sutures are placed at the ends of the duodenotomy and through the midportion of the choledochotomy (Fig. 12.4b). A third stay suture is then placed at the mid-point of the duodenotomy and through the most caudal portion of the choledochotomy. A posterior row of 4-0 or 5-0 absorbable sutures are placed with the knots tied intraluminally (Fig. 12.4c). The anterior row can then be completed with the knots external (Fig. 12.4d). The goal stoma size is 2.5 cm. A second layer of suture is unnecessary and may narrow the anastomosis creating early stenosis or obstruction. A closed suction drain is then left posterior to the choledochoduodenostomy.

Complications and Postoperative Care

If a large stoma (2.5 cm) is successfully created then the most common late complications, stenosis (1–2 %) or cholangitis (6–11 %), are rare [11, 12]. The risk of perioperative complication such as an anastomotic leak or significant bleeding is low. Suspected leaks are diagnosed with altered physical exam findings, bilious drain output, and postoperative imaging. Well-controlled leaks can be managed expectantly with bowel rest. Large or uncontrolled leaks require additional radiographic or surgical drainage and may require biliary and/or intestinal diversion.

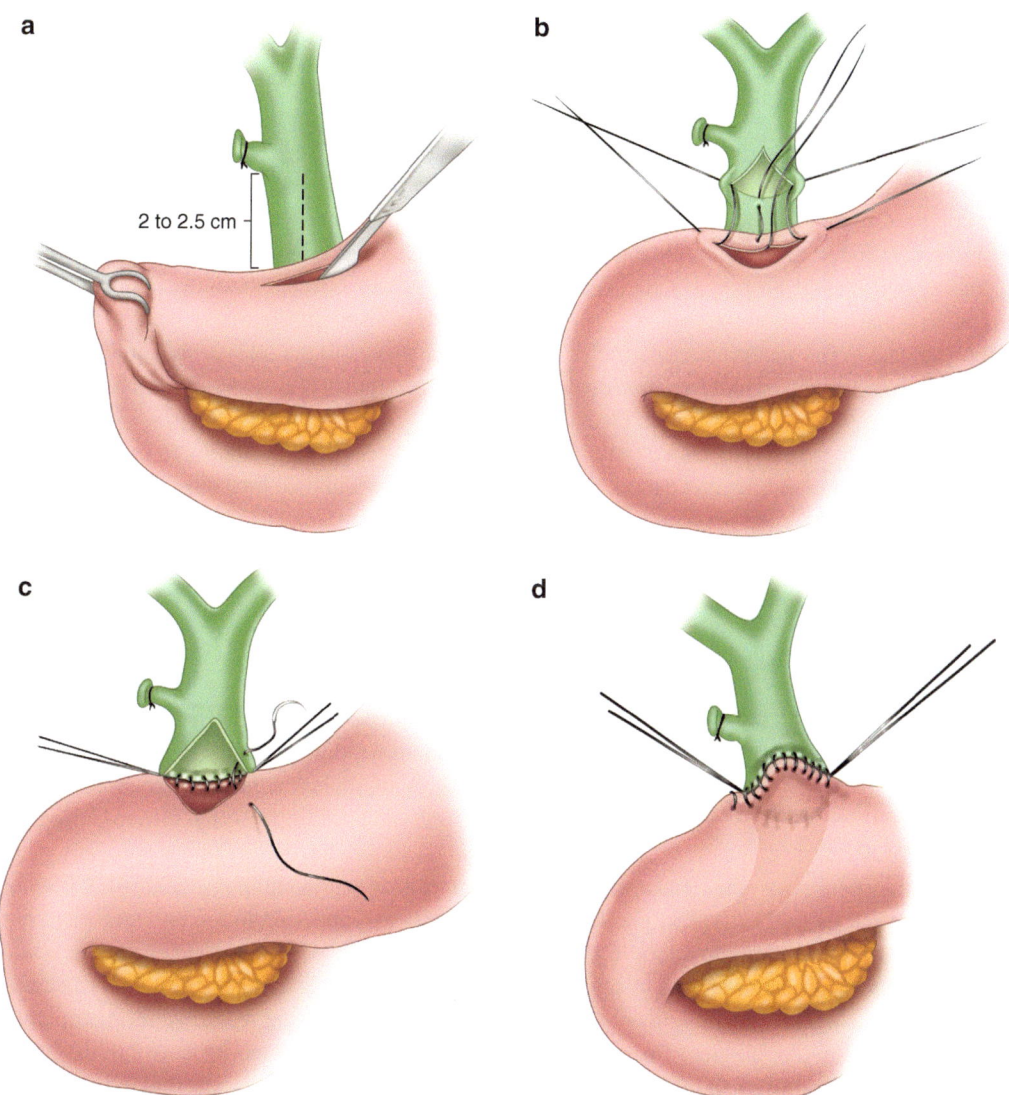

Fig. 12.4 Choledochoduodenostomy. (**a**) Longitudinal incision in the supraduodenal common bile duct extending 2–2.5 cm to match a 1.5–2.0 cm longitudinal incision on the duodenum. (**b**) Stay sutures are placed at apices for anastomosis. (**c**) Completion of the posterior suture line. (**d**) Completion of anterior suture line with goal lumen of 2.0 cm

Significant postoperative bleeding is rare and is treated with transfusion, radiographic embolization and re-exploration as a last resort. Lastly, "sump" syndrome whereby debris collects in the segment of common bile duct distal to the anastomosis has been described and can result in obstruction, cholangitis and pancreatitis. The incidence is less than 1 %. If sump syndrome is encountered, clearance of the distal duct can often be done endoscopically [13]. Both laparoscopic and endoscopic techniques for choledochoduodenostomy have been described in small series but are not widely practiced [14, 15].

In the immediate postoperative period, a nasogastric tube is maintained for 48–72 h and removed once the output is low. A fluid diet can then be started and the closed suction drain sent for a bilirubi level if the output is concerning. The drain is removed once the output is less than 40 cm³/day. Patients who tolerate liquids can be rapidly advanced to a regular diet, transitioned to oral pain medications and can often be discharged as early as postoperative day 4. The average hospital stay ranges from 3 to 8 days.

Long term follow-up including yearly liver function tests is recommended after choledocho-duodenostomy. Many clinicians also provide a recurring prescription for antibiotics to aggressively treat episodes of cholangitis and instruct patients to start the medication for symptoms of fever, abdominal pain and/or jaundice until they can be evaluated. The increased exposure of the bile duct mucosa to bacteria and intestinal contents following bypass of the sphincter of Oddi puts these patients at increased for cholangitis which has been associated with bile duct cancer. In fact, at greater than 10 years post-procedure, Adriano et al. reported a 7.9 % incidence of bile duct cancer in patients following choledochoduodenostomy which was associated with the incidence and severity of postoperative cholangitis [10].

Hepaticojejunostomy

Indications

Hepaticojejunostomy for the management of recurrent bile duct stones is typically performed in patients who have contraindications to choledochoduodneostomy; most often due to prior gastric or duodenal surgery. Most commonly, peptic ulcer disease (and its surgical management) results in severe scarring of the first and second portion of the duodenum preventing safe access to the duodenum and common bile duct. Thus, a more proximal connection from the biliary tree at the hepatic duct level can be made to a Roux limb of jejunum. The indications for hepaticojejunostomy in this context are otherwise the same as for choledochoduodenostomy: a severely dilated bile duct (>2 cm) in patients with recurrent stones after cholecystectomy, primary duct stones, numerous bile duct stones (precluding endoscopic management), intrahepatic duct stones, or a long distal common bile duct stricture.

Roux-en-Y hepaticojejunostomy has the added benefit of a lower rate of cholangitis because the bile duct is not exposed to enteric reflux and less prone to bacterial backflow. This is thought to impart a reduced risk of bile duct malignancy with the incidence of cancer 1.9 % after Roux-en-Y hepaticojejunostomy versus 5.8 % and 7.6 % in patients following transduodenal sphincteroplasty and choledochoduodenostomy, respectively [10]. In patients who are expected to need frequent biliary access (e.g., known biliary stricture, hepatolithiasis), the Roux limb can be tunneled subcutaneously and outlined with a radiopaque marker similar to the intentional jejuno-cutaneous fistula for endoscopic access as first described by Hutson in 1984 [16]. This "Hutson" loop provides long-term access for radiology to perform hepatobiliary interventions including biopsy, stenting, and stone extraction [17].

Surgical Technique

A right subcostal incision or upper midline is followed by cholecystectomy (if not already done) and identification of the left and right hepatic ducts. If significant adhesions are present, initial dissection can begin along the inferior edge of the liver and continue directly on the parenchyma in a posterior direction along segment 4B. Continued dissection should lead to the undisturbed area of the fibrous liver plate. The left hepatic duct can be identified at the inferior edge of this dissection. Identification may be aided by the preoperative placement of percutaneous stents into the hepatic ducts in patients who are expected to have significant adhesions.

Next, careful dissection of the hepatic duct confluence will often identify the right hepatic duct and define a section of common hepatic duct that may be appropriate for the anastomosis. Once the duct(s) have been isolated, a 2 cm (optimal) segment is selected and cleared. Attention can then be turned to the formation of the Roux limb. The jejunum is divided approximately 25 cm distal to the ligament of Treitz. The stapled end must have a good blood supply and is brought up through the transverse mesocolon to lie, without tension, in the right upper quadrant. An antecolic limb can be used if extensive inflammation and scar make access to the lesser sac difficult.

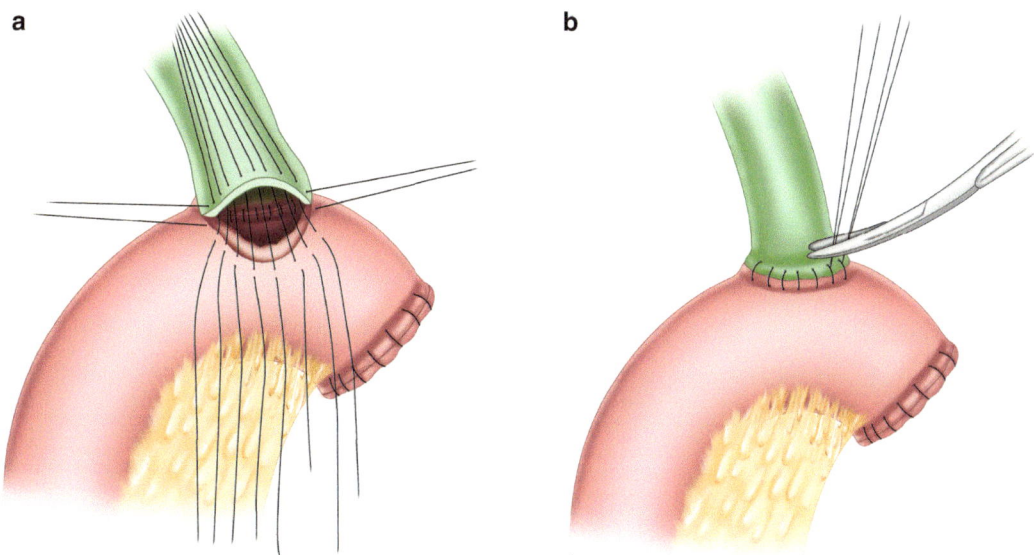

Fig. 12.5 Hepaticojejunostomy. (**a**) An end-to-side bile duct-to-jejunum anastomosis is created. (**b**) Completion of the anastomosis with goal lumen 2.0 cm

This limb should be approximately 40–60 cm in length to limit pancreatic and bacterial enteric reflux. A standard, stapled side-to-side jejunojejunostomy can then be created.

The biliary anastomosis can then be fashioned in an end-to-side anastomosis manner with absorbable, monofilament 3-0 to 5-0 suture (Fig. 12.5). The goal stoma size is 2–2.5 cm. If the left and right hepatic ducts require separate anastomoses, a "cloacal" connection can be made and sewn to single enterotomy (Fig. 12.6). Biliary stents are rarely used as ductal dilation is prominent and the risk of postoperative stricture low. If stenting is desired due to significant inflammation or small caliber ducts then utilization of previously placed percutaneous biliary stents can be done by simply trimming the stent length to extend 1–2 cm into the bowel lumen and completing the anastomosis around the stent. In patients without preoperative biliary drainage, a T-tube can be placed to allow for percutaneous access and internal drainage or an appropriately sized pediatric feeding tube can be shortened and secured with an absorbable suture so that it may pass spontaneously with suture dissolution.

A closed suction drain should be left posterior to the hepaticojejunostomy in all cases.

If continued need for biliary access is expected, then a slightly longer jejunal limb can be brought to the right upper quadrant and tunneled through the transversalis fascia to lie in a subfascial plane for future radiographic access. Radiopaque markers are placed at the access site of the Hutson loop to facilitate access by Radiology.

Complications and Postoperative Care

Complications following hepaticojejunostomy have decreased over time with more recent studies reporting a mortality <2 %, wound infections <10 %, with cholangitis (<3 %), intra-abdominal abscess (3 %) and leak (<5 %) rarely occurring [18, 19]. Cholangitis warrants special mention as it can be quite severe and is associated with an increased risk for malignancy. As such, some clinicians provide patients with a continuous prescription for antibiotics that is filled whenever patients develop concerning fevers, right upper

Fig. 12.6 Double-barrel
hepaticojejunostomy.
Separate right and left
hepatic ducts can be
combined to create a
single anastomosis
utilizing the inferior
duct for the posterior
row and the superior for
the anterior row

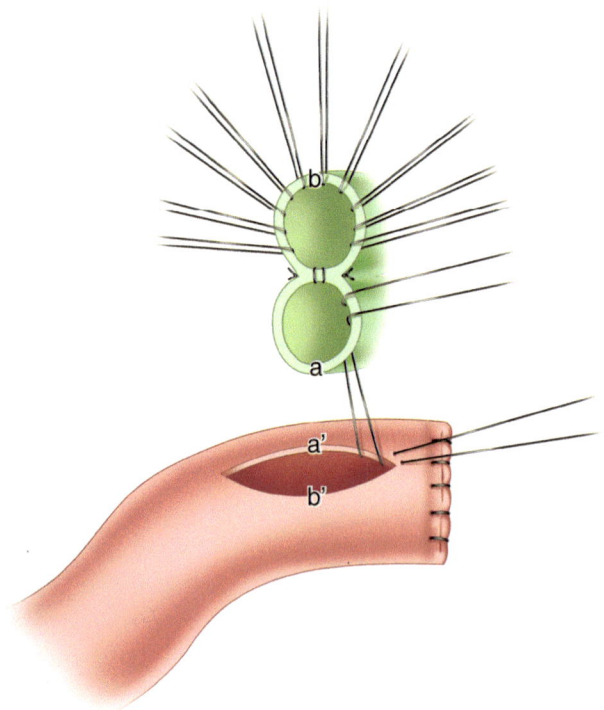

quadrant pain and/or jaundice. Anastomotic leaks can be managed expectantly if they are controlled via the surgical drain; upper gastrointestinal imaging or computed tomography with oral contrast can help clarify this. Additional radiographic or operative drainage in combination with biliary diversion may be required for large leaks.

In the immediate postoperative period, a nasogastric tube is maintained for 24–48 h and removed when the output is low. Liquids can then be started and advanced as tolerated to a regular diet. The closed suction drain is monitored after initiation of the diet and, if it appears bilious, can be sent for a bilirubin level. Low output bile leaks can be managed with continued observation while patients with high output leaks (output >200 cm^3/day) should undergo workup and management as described above. If biliary stents are utilized then they are left in for approximately 6 weeks before removal.

As the diet is advanced the patient is transitioned to oral medications and is typically ready for discharge between postoperative day 4 and 8. Long term follow-up is indicated after discharge as the risk

of biliary malignancy is increased in this patient population likely secondary to the increased inflammation brought on by the altered anatomy [10].

References

1. Oak JH, Paik CN, Chung WC, Lee KM, Yang JM. Risk factors for recurrence of symptomatic common bile duct stones after cholecystectomy. Gastroenterol Res Pract. 2012;2012:417821.
2. Cheon YK, Lehman GA. Identification of risk factors for stone recurrence after endoscopic treatment of bile duct stones. Eur J Gastroenterol Hepatol. 2006;18(5):461–4.
3. Keizman D, Shalom MI, Konikoff FM. An angulated common bile duct predisposes to recurrent symptomatic bile duct stones after endoscopic stone extraction. Surg Endosc. 2006;20(10):1594–9.
4. Grover BT, Kothari SN. Biliary issues in the bariatric population. Surg Clin North Am. 2014;94(2):413–25. doi:10.1016/j.suc.2014.01.003.
5. Jan YY, Chen MF, Wang CS, Jeng LB, Hwang TL, Chen SC. Surgical treatment of hepatolithiasis: long-term results. Surgery. 1996;120(3):509–14.
6. Miccini M, Amore Bonapasta S, Gregori M, Bononi M, Fornasari V, Tocchi A. Indications and results for transduodenal sphincteroplasty in the era of endoscopic sphincterotomy. Am J Surg. 2010;200(2):247–51. doi:10.1016/j.amjsurg.2009.08.048.

7. Morgan KA, Romagnuolo J, Adams DB. Transduodenal sphincteroplasty in the management of sphincter of oddi dysfunction and pancreas divisum in the modern era. J Am Coll Surg. 2008;206(5):908–14. doi:10.1016/j.jamcollsurg.2007.12.032. discussion 914–7.

8. Kune GA. Surgical anatomy of common bile duct. Arch Surg. 1964;89:995–1004.

9. Mirjalili SA, Stringer MD. The arterial supply of the major duodenal papilla and its relevance to endoscopic sphincterotomy. Endoscopy. 2011;43(4):307–11. doi:10.1055/s-0030-1256229.

10. Tocchi A, Mazzoni G, Liotta G, Lepre L, Cassini D, Miccini M. Late development of bile duct cancer in patients who had biliary-enteric drainage for benign disease: a follow-up study of more than 1,000 patients. Ann Surg. 2001;234(2):210–4.

11. Luu C, Lee B, Stabile BE. Choledochoduodenostomy as the biliary-enteric bypass of choice for benign and malignant distal common bile duct strictures. Am Surg. 2013;79(10):1054–7.

12. Panis Y, Fagniez PL, Brisset D, Lacaine F, Levard H, Hay JM. Long term results of choledochoduodenostomy versus choledochojejunostomy for choledocholithiasis. The French Association for Surgical Research. Surg Gynecol Obstet. 1993;177(1):33–7.

13. Zeuge U, Fehr M, Meyenberger C, Sulz MC. Mind the sump! - diagnostic challenge of a rare complication of choledochoduodenostomy. Case Rep Gastroenterol. 2014;8(3):358–63. doi:10.1159/000369298.

14. Khajanchee YS, Cassera MA, Hammill CW, Swanström LL, Hansen PD. Outcomes following laparoscopic choledochoduodenostomy in the management of benign biliary obstruction. J Gastrointest Surg. 2012;16(4):801–5. doi:10.1007/s11605-011-1768-3.

15. Dhir V, Itoi T, Khashab MA, Park DH, Yuen Bun Teoh A, Attam R, Messallam A, Varadarajulu S, Maydeo A. Multicenter comparative evaluation of endoscopic placement of expandable metal stents for malignant distal common bile duct obstruction by ERCP or EUS-guided approach. Gastrointest Endosc. 2015;81:913. doi:10.1016/j.gie.2014.09.054. pii: S0016-5107(14)02274-3.

16. Hutson DG, Russell E, Schiff E, Levi JJ, Jeffers L, Zeppa R. Balloon dilatation of biliary strictures through a choledochojejuno-cutaneous fistula. Ann Surg. 1984;199(6):637–47.

17. Amitha Vikrama KS, Keshava SN, Surendrababu NR, Moses V, Joseph P, Vyas F, Sitaram VJ. Jejunal access loop cholangiogram and intervention using image guided access. Med Imaging Radiat Oncol. 2010;54(1):5–8. doi:10.1111/j.1754-9485.2010.02130.x.

18. Sicklick JK, Camp MS, Lillemoe KD, Melton GB, Yeo CJ, Campbell KA, Talamini MA, Pitt HA, Coleman J, Sauter PA, Cameron JL. Surgical management of bile duct injuries sustained during laparoscopic cholecystectomy: perioperative results in 200 patients. Ann Surg. 2005;241(5):786–92. discussion 793–5.

19. Hirano S, Tanaka E, Tsuchikawa T, Matsumoto J, Shichinohe T, Kato KJ. Techniques of biliary reconstruction following bile duct resection (with video). J Hepatobiliary Pancreat Sci. 2012;19(3):203–9. doi:10.1007/s00534-011-0475-5.

Management of Medical Complications of Gallstone Disease

Victorio Pidlaoan and Somashekar G. Krishna

Introduction

The biliary tree is a low-pressure pathway for excretion of hydrophobic products. Due to this tenuous relationship, bile is vulnerable to precipitation. Once formed, bile crystals or stones rarely dissolve spontaneously. Risk factors for the development of gallstones include female gender, pregnancy, multiparity, chronic hemolytic conditions, obesity and total parenteral nutrition. Gallstone disease manifests by two principal ways, either by obstruction or erosion. Obstruction can be transient or complete. Obstructive gallstone disease can present as choledocholithiasis, biliary pain, acute gallstone pancreatitis, or ascending cholangitis. Acute pancreatitis is the most common gastrointestinal cause of hospital admission and is a cause of significant morbidity and mortality. Severe acute pancreatitis and ascending cholangitis in the presence of an obstructing gallstone are emergent indications for biliary decompression with endoscopic retrograde cholangiopancreatography (ERCP). Rarely gallstones may also erode into adjacent structures causing fistulas. These may manifest as biliary obstruction (Mirrizi's syndrome), biliary enteric fistula which may manifest as small bowel obstruction (gallstone ileus), or fistulization with other interfacing organ systems including integument, vasculature, thorax, or genitourinrary system. Patients with gallstone disease often present with familiar signs and symptoms associated with intra-abdominal disease processes. Hence it is important to deliberate on good clinical practice and elucidate an appropriate differential diagnoses.

Acute Pancreatitis

The Clinical Problem

Acute pancreatitis is the most common gastrointestinal disease leading to inpatient admission [1]. Severe epigastric abdominal pain which may be associated with nausea and vomiting along with at least a threefold elevation in the serum lipase is the characteristic clinical presentation of acute pancreatitis [2]. An abdominal ultrasound is performed to identify gallstones or choledocholithiasis. The diagnosis may be confirmed through cross-sectional imaging but this is usually not necessary and may lead to additional costs. The diagnosis is obtained by ≥2 of these

V. Pidlaoan, M.D. • S.G. Krishna, M.D., M.P.H. (✉)
Division of Gastroenterology, Hepatology and Nutrition, Department of Internal Medicine, The Ohio State University Wexner Medical Center, 2nd Floor Doan Office Tower, 395 W. 12th Avenue, Columbus, OH 43210-1228, USA
e-mail: Victorio.Pidlaoan@osumc.edu; Somashekar. Krishna@osumc.edu

© Springer International Publishing Switzerland 2016
J.W. Hazey et al. (eds.), *Multidisciplinary Management of Common Bile Duct Stones*,
DOI 10.1007/978-3-319-22765-8_13

three clinical findings (abdominal pain, lipase/amylase >3× the upper limit of normal, and imaging characteristics) [3]. Gallstone disease is the most common cause of acute pancreatitis in the western hemisphere and occurs through obstruction of the biliary tree leading to injury of the pancreatic acinar cells, necrosis, and autodigestion [4].

In patients presenting with acute pancreatitis and risk factors for gallstone formation, presence of intermittent epigastric pain suggestive of biliary colic should raise the suspicion of gallstones as a causative agent. This symptom could sometimes be a vague abdominal discomfort. The post-prandial nature of the abdominal pain, when present, contributes to the diagnosis. A history of prior cholecystectomy does not exclude the diagnosis of gallstone pancreatitis because retained stones in the biliary tree may be asymptomatic for years prior to eventual stone migration and obstruction [5]. Physical examination findings typically include epigastric pain associated with components of the systemic inflammatory response syndrome (fever, tachycardia, tachypnea). Patients with mild pancreatitis may not appear acutely ill and present with epigastric pain alone. Increasing severity of pancreatitis is associated with worsening abdominal distention and marked tenderness in the epigastrium. Periumbilical ecchymosis (Cullen's sign) and flank ecchymosis (Grey Turners sign) are rare but when present may suggest extravasation of hemorrhagic pancreatic exudate into those areas, is a poor prognostic sign. The serum amylase and lipase are both equally sensitive but elevations in amylase can occur in non-pancreatic conditions [4]. In comparison, serum amylase tends to be more elevated than serum lipase in gallstone or microlithiasis associated pancreatitis [6]. Furthermore, a more than threefold elevation of alanine aminotransferase (ALT) can contribute to the specificity of gallstone pancreatitis [7]. The degree of elevation in the amylase and lipase do not have any prognostic significance and monitoring the same is not recommended [8].

Approach to Management

Assessment of Severity

The management of pancreatitis begins with an initial assessment of severity. There are several classification systems. While the traditional Ranson criteria are still used widely, a common criticism is the need to wait 48 h before finalizing the same [9]. Other classification systems include Acute Physiology and Chronic Health Evaluation (APACHE) II and Bedside index of severity in acute pancreatitis (BISAP) scoring systems [10]. The BISAP score, being equally sensitive, is simpler although being less involved than the APACHE II system [11]. The criteria for classifying severity using these different systems are detailed in Table 13.1. Serial bedside assessment of the patient is important to assess the patient's initial response to resuscitation. This will enable the clinician to make changes to the strategy of volume management, pain control, and to monitor for evidence of end organ dysfunction.

The Atlanta classification attempts to classify acute pancreatitis into two distinct morphologies based on radiologic appearance [3]. Interstitial edematous pancreatitis shows a relatively homogenous enhancement with mild peripancreatic fat stranding on CT. This is the most common subtype and patient's symptoms typically subside within a week [15]. Necrotizing pancreatitis is less common occurring in 5–15 % of patients. Cross-sectional imaging reveals necrosis of the pancreatic parenchyma, peripancreatic tissue, or both [3]. Pancreatic necrosis develops over several days hence early cross-sectional imaging may underestimate the eventual extent of necrosis [16, 17]. Patients with pancreatic necrosis have increased morbidity and need for intervention compared to interstitial edematous pancreatitis [18]. Areas of pancreatic and peripancreatic necrosis may become infected or remain sterile. There is no correlation between the extent of necrosis and risk of infection [19]. Infected pancreatic necrosis is rare during the first week hence if the concern for infection is high, other etiologies for acute

Table 13.1 Scoring tools in acute pancreatitis, component variables, and prognostic value of scores

Severity scoring tools in acute pancreatitis	Component variables		Prognostic value of scores
Ranson's criteria [9]	*At admission*		≤2=0 % mortality
	Age>55		>3=14.9 % mortality [12]
	White blood cell count>16,000/mm³		
	Serum glucose>200 mg/dL		
	Lactate dehydrogenase>350 U/L		
	AST>250 U/L		
	At 48 h		
	Hematocrit (decrease by ≥10 %)		
	BUN (increase by ≥5 mg/dL despite fluids)		
	Serum calcium<8 mg/dL		
	pO₂<60 mmHg		
	Base deficit>4 meq/L		
	Fluid sequestration>6 L		
Acute physiology and chronic health examination (APACHE) II [13]	Rectal temperature		<7=0 % mortality
	Mean arterial pressure		>7=10.6 % mortality [12]
	Heart rate		
	Alveolar–arterial gradient/PO₂		
	pH or serum HCO₃		
	Serum sodium		
	Serum potassium		
	Serum creatinine		
	Hematocrit		
	White blood cell count		
	Age		
	Glasgow Coma Scale		
	Chronic disease[a]		
Bedside index of severity in acute pancreatitis (BISAP) [11]	BUN>25		≤2=mortality 1.9 %
	Impaired mental status		>3=mortality 15.4 % [12]
	Systemic inflammatory response syndrome (SIRS)		
	Age >60 years		
	Presence of a pleural effusion		
CT severity index (CTSI) [14]	Findings		<2=mortality 0 %
	Normal pancreas	0	>3=mortality 8.5 % [12]
	Focal or diffuse enlargement, contour may show irregularity	1	
	Peripancreatic inflammation	2	
	Intrapancreatic and extrapancreatic fluid collections	3	
	Two or more large collections of gas in the pancreas or retroperitoneum	4	
	Percent necrosis		
	0	0	
	<33	2	
	33–50	4	
	≥50	6	

[a]Cirrhosis, past upper gastrointestinal bleeding due to portal hypertension, prior hepatic failure, prior hepatic encephalopathy, class IV heart failure, chronic restrictive, obstructive, or vascular lung disease causing exercise intolerance, hypoxemia or hypercapnia, secondary polycythemia, severe pulmonary hypertension, ventilator dependence, chronic hemodialysis, immunosuppression for chemotherapy, radiation therapy, high-dose steroids, or immunodeficiency

infection should be considered. If suspected, the diagnosis of infected pancreatic necrosis is important due to the need for treatment including consideration for debridement [20]. The presence of gas in the necrotic areas on cross-sectional imaging or a positive gram stain or culture of fluid obtained via fine needle aspiration confirms the existence of infection [21].

While the vast majority of patients will improve during their hospital stay, some patients will have recurrence of abdominal pain, worsening organ failure or develop multiple laboratory abnormalities. In these scenarios, cross-sectional imaging may be useful in evaluating for local complications that may be contributing to the clinical picture. The Atlanta classification defines four types of local complications which include *acute peripancreatic fluid collections, pancreatic pseudocysts, acute necrotic collections, and walled-off necrosis. Acute peripancreatic fluid collections* are associated with interstitial edematous pancreatitis. These appear as homogenous fluid collections confined to normal peripancreatic planes and are by definition, adjacent to the pancreas. These are likely to resolve without intervention [22]. *Pancreatic pseudocysts* are well-encapsulated fluid collections outside the pancreas and occur greater than 4 weeks after an episode of acute pancreatitis. These are thought to arise from disruption of the pancreatic duct and its branches causing leakage of pancreatic secretions into a localized fluid collection. Aspiration typically reveals an elevated amylase. Acute necrotic collections contain variable amounts of fluid and necrotic tissue. By definition these occur within 4 weeks of an episode of acute pancreatitis. On cross-sectional imaging these appear as heterogeneous areas without a definable wall. These can be seen within the pancreas or in the surrounding tissues. Walled off necrosis refers to an encapsulated collection of pancreatic or peripancreatic necrosis. This usually occurs greater than 4 weeks after an episode of necrotizing pancreatitis. On cross-sectional imaging these appear as heterogeneous areas with a well-defined wall [3]. Systemic complications are exacerbations of preexisting comorbidities such as coronary artery disease or emphysema in the setting of acute pancreatitis not due to acute pancreatitis itself.

Similar to sepsis, the existence and degree of organ failure is what defines the severity of pancreatitis. The Atlanta classification defines three grades of severity based on presence of organ failure, local and systemic complications. Mild acute pancreatitis is defined by the absence of organ failure and lack of local or systemic complications. Mortality is rare and cross-sectional imaging is often not needed [15]. Moderately severe acute pancreatitis is characterized by transient organ failure (resolves within 48 h) and/or the presence of local or systemic complications without the presence of organ failure. Such a patient may be one with acute pancreatitis presenting with acute renal failure which resolves with aggressive fluid repletion or a patient with chronic obstructive pulmonary disease presenting with acute pancreatitis complicated by hypoxia. Patients with moderately severe acute pancreatitis may improve without intervention or may need prolonged nasojejunal feeding due to poor per oral tolerance. Patients with moderately severe acute pancreatitis still have a high morbidity but a low overall mortality [23]. Severe acute pancreatitis is characterized by persistent organ failure. The presence of the systemic inflammatory response syndrome (SIRS) predisposes to development of organ failure. Patients with persistent organ failure typically have associated local complications and are at an increased risk of death with mortality approaching 36–50 % [24, 25]. Infected necrosis in the setting of persistent organ failure is associated with a high mortality [20, 26].

Supportive Care

Initial supportive care should include fluid resuscitation, administration of supplemental oxygen, and correction of electrolyte abnormalities. Nasogastric decompression may be needed should the patient develop an ileus. The presence of shock, delirium, and evidence of respiratory failure are situations that may warrant triage to an ICU environment.

Initiating appropriate therapy is crucial within the first 24 h after presentation. Injury to the pancreas through multiple avenues including gall-stone disease causes third spacing in the capillary-rich pancreatic microcirculation. Decreased blood flow via increasing capillary permeability, vasospasm, and the formation of microthrombi contribute to the development of necrotizing pancreatitis. Fluid resuscitation is performed to prevent further ischemic injury which may eventually lead to pancreatic necrosis [27]. During severe acute pancreatitis vast amounts of fluid may third space in the injured pancreatic bed that may lead to decreased cardiac preload and may lead to circulatory shock and subsequent organ failure.

Aggressive volume repletion is felt to be the mainstay of therapy and is targeted to the under-lying physiology that leads to injury and necro-sis. The development of pancreatic necrosis is associated with organ failure and increased mor-tality [18]. Previous studies have demonstrated that the median time from admission to ICU transfer is 1 day, and hence there may be a so called "therapeutic window" in which measures may be performed to prevent further clinical deterioration [28]. The concept of hemoconcen-tration through volume depletion, marked by an increased hematocrit or serum BUN has been a subject of investigation as a way to prognosticate an individual patient's clinical course. A case control study of patients with pancreatitis dem-onstrated that an admission hematocrit > 47 and/or failure of the admission hematocrit to decrease at 24 h was the best binary risk factor for the development of pancreatic necrosis [29]. A sub-sequent retrospective study of patients with acute pancreatitis determined that an admission hema-tocrit greater than or equal to 44 and/or a failure of the same to decrease within 24 h was a signifi-cant predictor of both pancreatic necrosis and organ failure [30]. However, a second retrospec-tive analysis failed to demonstrate that a hemato-crit of >43 by itself was a sensitive or specific marker for pancreatic necrosis. Whether fluid infusion can prevent pancreatic necrosis is a sub-ject of debate but some studies have shown that drop in hematocrit within 24 h of admission has been shown to be a strong negative predictor for necrosis [31]. The serum BUN is another marker

of hemoconcentration and is a part of several scoring systems for acute pancreatitis [9, 11]. An observational cohort study of patients admitted with acute pancreatitis demonstrated that the serum BUN was significantly higher among non-survivors than survivors. There was a statistically significant trend towards increased mortality for every 5 mg/dL increase in serum BUN for the first 24 h [32]. This observation was validated by the same group using two additional large data sets demonstrating that a BUN > 20 mg/dL or any rise in the BUN within the first 24 h was associ-ated with a fourfold increase in mortality [33].

Many patients with acute pancreatitis require aggressive fluid resuscitation to prevent circula-tory collapse; however, comorbid renal and car-diovascular disease may predispose to volume overload and respiratory insufficiency. To pre-vent necrosis, patients should be given enough fluid to maintain perfusion of the injured pan-creas but only enough to avoid circulatory over-load. A retrospective study found that patients receiving <3.1 L in the first 24 h had no increase in adverse outcomes compared to patients receiv-ing >4.1 L. However, patients who received >4.1 L were found to have an increased rate of respiratory insufficiency, renal insufficiency and local complications. The association persisted despite adjusting for potential confounders such as age, Charlson comorbidity score, body mass index, and the presence of SIRS [34]. A small randomized trial evaluated rapid (10–15 mL/kg/h) versus controlled fluid expansion (5–10 mL/kg/h) in patients presenting with severe acute pancreatitis. The study found that the rate of mechanical ventilation, abdominal compartment syndrome, sepsis were significantly lower in patients receiving controlled fluid expansion. Mortality was also lower in the patients receiving the lower infusion rate [35]. A second trial by the same group demonstrated that patients random-ized to slow hemodilution (goal hematocrit > 35 in 48 h) as compared to rapid (goal hematocrit < 35 within 48 h) had decreased incidence and greater time to the development of sepsis. There was also an increased survival rate in patients randomized to slow hemodilution [36]. Based on the available evidence the International Association of

Pancreatology/American Pancreatic Association (IAP/APA) acute pancreatitis guidelines recommend an initial infusion rate of 5–10 mL/kg/h until a goal heart rate < 120/min, mean arterial pressure of between 65 and 85 mmHg or a urine output of >0.5–1 mL/kg/h. Other physiologic and biochemical targets of a hematocrit of 35–44 %, stroke volume variation and intrathoracic blood volume may also be used [37]. In regard to the type of fluid, lactated Ringer's solution is the preferred choice. This has been shown to decrease the rate of SIRS and serum levels of C-reactive protein after 24 h in a prospective multicenter randomized trial [38].

Abdominal ultrasonography is the preferred initial imaging study because gallstones are the most common etiology of acute pancreatitis. Right upper quadrant abdominal ultrasound gives us a quick assessment for the presence of gallstones and biliary ductal dilation that may suggest the presence of ongoing biliary obstruction. Cross-sectional imaging is recommended when the diagnosis is not certain and only after initial resuscitation due to concerns for contrast induced nephropathy in the setting of profound third spacing of fluid in acute pancreatitis. Early cross-sectional imaging may also underestimate necrosis since these may be better defined 2–3 days after the initial attack [39]. When the diagnosis of acute pancreatitis is established, confirmatory computed tomography (CT) imaging is often unnecessary since clinical scoring systems perform similarly to radiologic scoring systems. Further early CT to detect necrosis has not been demonstrated to improve clinical outcomes or influence treatment [17].

The presence of biliary obstruction in the setting of cholangitis and/or severe acute pancreatitis warrants urgent decompression with ERCP. Clues to this diagnosis include a rising serum bilirubin, persistently elevated transaminases, and an elevated alkaline phosphatase. The presence of jaundice, fever, and abdominal pain are concerning for cholangitis and may warrant initiation of antibiotic therapy. However, ERCP carries a 1.6–15 % risk of pancreatitis [40–42]. If abdominal ultrasonography is negative but the clinical suspicion for gallstones remains high, the diagnosis could be confirmed by more sensitive imaging modalities such as Endoscopic Ultrasonography (EUS) and Magnetic resonance cholangiopancreatography (MRCP) which could then be followed by ERCP. Endosonography can be safely performed in patients with ferromagnetic implants.

A systemic review showed nutrition, either enteral of parenteral, is associated with lower mortality compared to no nutrition [43]. Several other studies have demonstrated that enteral nutrition is associated with fewer complications than parenteral nutrition, though there was no difference in mortality [44–46]. While enteral nutrition can be initiated within 48 h of admission, there is no evidence supporting nasojejunal over a nasoduodenal tube [47]. In a randomized trial of patients with mild acute pancreatitis, there was no difference in the occurrence of pain or exacerbation of acute pancreatitis between patients who fasted and patients initiated on oral feeding after 48 h of the onset of abdominal pain [48]. Given the evidence, the American Gastroenterology Association guidelines recommend initiation of oral feeding when patients are pain free and no longer vomiting. Starting with a low fat solid diet appears to be as safe as a clear liquid diet. In patients with severe acute pancreatitis, when patients are expected to be unable to tolerate oral intake, enteral nutrition is preferred over parenteral nutrition due to the decreased risk of infection, organ failure, need for surgical intervention and hospital stay [46, 49] Initiation of early nasoenteric feeding within 72 h compared to initiation of an oral diet has not been shown to be superior in reducing infection or death in patients with severe acute pancreatitis [50].

Definitive Management

In addition to supportive care, acute gallstone pancreatitis is unique in that procedures are done to treat the underlying cause and prevent its recurrence. A fundamental assumption is that most gallstones eventually originate in the gallbladder and its functions are essential to gallstone formation [51]. To prevent further episodes of acute pancreatitis, cholecystectomy is recommended in all patients presenting with acute gallstone pancreatitis regardless of the severity of the acute attack. Recurrence of acute pancreatitis in patients with gallstones has been reported in 29–63 % when patients are discharged without having a cholecystectomy [52, 53]. The 2012 IAP Guidelines for the Surgical Management of Acute Pancreatitis recommend cholecystectomy for mild acute gallstone pancreatitis as soon as the patient has recovered and ideally within the same hospitalization. In severe acute gallstone pancreatitis, cholecystectomy should be delayed until there is sufficient resolution of the inflammatory response and clinical recovery [54]. Laparoscopic cholecystectomy has a success rate between 80 and 100 %, with a conversion to open rate of between 0 and 16 %.

Biliary Pain

The Clinical Problem

Biliary pain previously known as biliary colic is the most common presentation of cholelithiasis. Typical symptoms are bloating, belching, nausea, epigastric pain, and fatty food intolerance. Clinical assessment is limited because other conditions may present similarly [55]. The pain is typically steady and dull and lasts greater than 30 min to a maximum of 6 h. A history of recurrent attacks of pain is common. The old term biliary colic implying a colicky pain is a misnomer. The pain is caused by gallstone migration into the cystic duct and gallbladder contraction leading intermittent obstruction. Pressure inside the gallbladder increases which thereby causes distension and pain. Pain is relieved when the gallbladder relaxes causing the stone to fall back into the lumen of the gallbladder. The physical exam is typically benign except for occasional epigastric or right upper quadrant tenderness. Peritonitis is rare. Laboratory studies should be normal in patients with biliary pain and any abnormality in the liver function tests, amylase, lipase or evidence of leukocytosis should raise suspicion for acute cholecystitis, acute gallstone pancreatitis or cholangitis depending on the clinical picture [56].

The diagnosis of biliary pain is supported by the presence of gallstones or sludge in the gallbladder. This diagnosis is often made with imaging. Abdominal ultrasonography can detect 95 % of gallstones and may be repeated if the clinical suspicion remains high. EUS can also be used for patients who have had an initial negative abdominal ultrasound to confirm the presence of stones or sludge.

Approach to Management

For symptomatic biliary pain, the mainstay of treatment is elective laparoscopic cholecystectomy. A study of patients who had one episode of biliary pain had a 47.8 % likelihood of biliary symptoms or complications after 5 years [57]. Other studies have shown recurrences as high as 69 % in patients with a history of biliary pain the previous year [58]. The risk of biliary complications is low however and is estimated to be between 1 and 2 % per year [59].

Cholangitis

The Clinical Problem

Cholangitis or inflammation of the bile ducts should be considered a clinical emergency. Diagnosis can be problematic especially in the early phase when signs pointing towards a biliary source may be absent. Charcot's triad which consists of fever, right upper quadrant pain, and jaundice is often cited by many as the hallmark of cholangitis but the presentation can be variable from mild recurrent episodes of abdominal pain to a rapidly progressive illness resulting in septic shock, coma and death [60]. Reynolds pentad (Charcot's triad plus hypotension and confusion) describes a more severe form of cholangitis causing septic shock. Untreated cases may progress to pyogenic liver abscesses.

The development of cholangitis requires the presence of three factors: Biliary obstruction, bacterial colonization of the bile, and elevated biliary pressures [61]. The most common cause is impacted bile duct stones representing 85 % of cases [60]. Etiologies other than gallstones predisposing to cholangitis include biliary strictures from previous surgical procedures, malignancy, HIV cholangiopathy, primary sclerosing cholangitis, chronic pancreatitis causing scarring of the pancreatic portion of the common bile duct [62], infection of biliary/pancreatic stents, complications from bile duct surgery and procedures such as ERCP, and complications of orthotoptic liver transplant. Patients presenting with cholangitis in the absence of gallstones should be worked up for any of these differential diagnoses to guide therapy.

Similar to other manifestations of gallstone disease, the diagnosis of cholangitis is established with a supporting history, laboratory tests and compatible imaging. A long history of recurrent biliary pain may be present. Fever is almost a universal sign and so is right upper quadrant tenderness. Jaundice is present in many patients but may be difficult to determine in dark skinned individuals. Examination of the sclera and mucous membranes may reveal evidence of jaundice not seen on skin exam alone. Because patients may present with delirium from sepsis, the history and physical exam may not be reliable. Laboratory studies are helpful in identifying the biliary tract as a source of infection. Liver function tests may demonstrate an obstructive pattern with marked elevations in the alkaline phosphatase, bilirubin, and serum transaminases. The most sensitive test is the gamma-glutamyl transferase (GGT) which is elevated in 92 % of cases, while the AST may only be elevated in 51 % of patients [63]. The bilirubin is often >2 mg/dL in 80 % of patients. A complete blood count may demonstrate a leukocytosis or a marked left shift [4]. Abdominal ultrasonography for bile duct stones has a lower sensitivity (50–67 %) as opposed to greater than 95 % for gallstones in the gallbladder [64]. The finding of biliary ductal dilation on ultrasonography however may suggest the presence of an obstructing stone in only 75 % of cases [65]. Computed tomography may be helpful to exclude other known complications of gallstones

Table 13.2 2013 Tokyo diagnostic criteria for acute cholangitis

A. Systemic inflammation	B. Cholestasis	C. Imaging
A1. Fever and/or rigors	B1. Jaundice	C1. Biliary dilation
A2. Labs: evidence of inflammatory response[a]	B2. Labs: abnormal liver function tests (LFTs)[b]	C2. Evidence of etiology on imaging (stricture, stone, etc.)
Thresholds Body Temp >38 °C	Thresholds B1. Jaundice Total bilirubin >2 mg/dL B2. AST, ALT, GGT, alkaline phosphatase >1.5 times upper limit of normal	

[a]Abnormal white blood cell counts, increase of serum C-reactive protein levels, and other changes indicating inflammation
[b]Increased serum alkaline phosphatase, GGT, AST, and ALT levels

such as acute pancreatitis or liver abscess but may miss radiolucent stones.

Given the low sensitivity of Charcot's triad, the Tokyo guidelines (Table 13.2) defines three morbidities which represent the manifestations of cholangitis associated with the occurrence of cholangiovenous and cholangiolymphatic reflux due to elevated pressure in the biliary tracts caused by obstruction. A suspected diagnosis is one item in column A plus either any in B or C. A definitive diagnosis is made when a patient has one item in all columns (A, B and C). A multicenter analysis demonstrated a sensitivity of 91.8 % and a specificity of 77.7 % for the Tokyo criteria for the diagnosis of cholangitis. The occurrence of Charcot's triad remains the most specific clinical criteria for the diagnosis of cholangitis with a specificity of 95.9 % [66].

Approach to Management

The initial management of cholangitis starts with making the diagnosis and stabilizing the patient's clinical condition. Fluid resuscitation

Table 13.3 Recommended antibiotic regimens for patients with biliary infections

Infection and risk factors	Recommended antibiotic regimens
Community acquired acute cholecystitis of mild to moderate severity	Cefazolin, cefuroxime, or ceftriaxone
Community acquired acute cholecystitis of severe physiologic disturbance, advanced age or immunocompromised state	Imipenem–cilastatin, meropenem, doripenem, piperacillin–tazobactam, ciprofloxacin, levofloxacin, or cefepime in combination with Metronidazole
Acute cholangitis following bilioenteric anastomosis	Imipenem–cilastatin, meropenem, doripenem, piperacillin–tazobactam, ciprofloxacin, levofloxacin, or cefepime in combination with Metronidazole
Healthcare associated biliary infection of any severity	Imipenem–cilastatin, meropenem, doripenem, piperacillin–tazobactam, ciprofloxacin, levofloxacin, or cefepime with Vancomycin added to each regimen

with vasopressor support may be needed in patients with shock. Antibiotics should be tailored to the most likely pathogen given the patients clinical history. Previously gram negative aerobes such as *E. coli* and *Klebsiella* and enterococci were the most common pathogens in patients with cholangitis. In more recent years polymicrobial infections have become more common. Bacteremia occurs in 21–70 % of patients and results from reflux of infected bile into the lymphatic circulation [67, 68].

The Infectious Disease Society of America (IDSA) published guidelines for empiric antibiotic regimens for patients with biliary infections that include both acute cholecystitis and cholangitis (Table 13.3). Antibiotic regimens can be chosen based on the patient's risk of healthcare associated pathogens. Patients with community acquired infections do not require coverage for enterococci because the pathogenicity of these has not been demonstrated. Anaerobic coverage is not required unless a biliary enteric anastomosis is present [69].

After stabilization and control of sepsis, biliary decompression is a necessary step in the treatment of cholangitis. There are several methods employed for biliary decompression and will depend on the location of the obstruction, anatomy of the patient, available expertise, and comorbid conditions.

Endoscopic sphincterotomy and stone extraction accomplished through ERCP is successful in more than 90 % of cases, with an overall complication rate of approximately 5 % and a mortality rate of less than 1 % in expert hands [70]. When compared to surgical decompression, ERCP was shown to have fewer complications, similar rates of biliary decompression and lower mortality in patients presenting with severe cholangitis [71]. A non-randomized trial comparing all decompressive modalities (ERCP, percutaneous transhepatic cholangiography (PTC) and surgery) demonstrated improved outcomes with ERCP compared to either procedure in patients presenting with acute cholangitis [72].

Using a duodenoscope, the ampulla of Vater is cannulated and then a wire is passed into the common bile duct (CBD) under fluoroscopic guidance. The level of obstruction is visualized by injecting contrast to opacify the bile ducts. The stone can then be extracted with a balloon. If there is a stricture within the ducts or the stone is too large to extract, a stent can be inserted into the bile duct to maintain patency. Sphincterotomy, which is almost always performed, is relatively contraindicated in the presence of coagulopathy and sepsis [61]. Although ERCP is the preferred procedure for biliary decompression, failure of ERCP may occur especially in patients with a history of a Roux-en-y gastric bypass and difficult cannulation of the ampulla of Vater. When ERCP fails or if the patient is deemed to be too unstable, PTC may be attempted to quickly decompress the biliary tree. Known complications of PTC are intraperitoneal hemorrhage, biliary peritonitis, catheter dislodgement, hemobilia, hemoperitoneum, and choleperitoneum. PTC may be the preferred modality in cases of proximal biliary obstruction. Surgery is only attempted when the all noninvasive procedures have failed.

Uncommon Manifestations of Gallstones

The Clinical Problem

Mirrizi's syndrome is a rare cause of extrinsic biliary obstruction caused by gallstones. This was described by Mirizzi in 1948 [73]. This clinical entity is rare in developed countries because the diagnosis of gallstone associated disease is made at an earlier stage. Patients typically present in the fifth to seventh decade of life and may endorse a long history of gallstone disease.

The syndrome itself is caused by either a large stone or multiple stones impacted in the neck of the gallbladder or cystic duct. The large stone burden may either cause obstruction through extrinsic compression of the common bile duct or cause a fistula between the gallbladder and common bile duct leading to direct obstruction. Following anatomic alignment of the cystic duct parallel to the common bile duct and impaction of a stone in the cystic duct or neck of the gall bladder, there is obstruction of the common hepatic duct from the stone or from the inflammatory response. Eventually, intermittent or constant jaundice manifests occasionally causing cholangitis and with long standing obstruction, secondary biliary cirrhosis [74].

There are five types classified by the manner of obstruction and the occurrence of a biliary enteric fistula. Type 1 is caused by extrinsic compression of the common bile duct (without erosion) by an impacted gallstone. Type 2 is caused by cholecystobiliary fistula secondary to an eroded gallstone involving one third of the circumference of the common bile duct. Type 3 is caused by a cholecystobiliary fistula involving two thirds of the circumference of the common bile duct. Type 4 is caused by cholecystobiliary fistula comprising the whole circumference of the common bile duct. Type 5 is any of the previous types with an associated cholecystoenteric fistula [75].

Diagnosis and Management

Patients typically present with symptoms suggestive of acute cholecystitis or choledocholithiasis. Episodic right upper quadrant pain, jaundice, or elevated liver function tests may be elicited from the history and initial laboratory workup. Occasionally they may present more acutely with clinical findings consistent with acute cholangitis or pancreatitis. Because of the complex nature of the obstruction, imaging is essential to make the correct diagnosis. For most patients ultrasonography is the first step followed by CT and/or MRI. Diagnosis via ultrasonography is limited given its lack of unique features [76]. Combined CT and MRCP has a sensitivity of 95 % and specificity of 93.5 %. CT alone had a very low sensitivity of 42 % but a very high specificity (98 %) [77]. ERCP remains the gold standard imaging modality with nearly 100 % sensitivity in one case series [78]. During ERCP, stenting can be also performed to temporarily decompress the bile duct. Definitive therapy is accomplished by surgical intervention.

Biliary Enteric Fistula

The Clinical Problem

Chronic untreated gallstone disease may occasionally cause fistula formation between the biliary tract and adjacent bowel. Patients who develop these are typically between 60 and 80 years of age and the majority are women. Gallstones from prior attacks cause inflammation leading to adhesion with the adjacent bowel wall. With subsequent pressure and ischemia, gallstones erode into the bowel resulting in fistula formation. Cholecystoduodenal fistulas are the most common followed by cholecystocolonic fistulas. Less common biliary enteric fistulas include cholecystogastric, cholecystocholedochal, choledochoduodenal, cholecystojejunal, and hepaticobronchial fistulas. Biliary enteric fistulas are not a phenomenon caused by gallstones alone but can be seen in inflammatory bowel disease, duodenal ulcers eroding into the gallbladder, or gallbladder carcinoma [79, 80].

Cholecystoduodenal fistulas account for 75–80 % of biliary enteric fistulas. Most are clinically silent or have vague symptoms. Occasionally they may present with more dramatic clinical presentations. A gallstone ileus refers to a mechanical small bowel obstruction caused by large gallstones, typically greater than 2–2.5 cm. The site of obstruction is typically at the terminal ileum that is the narrowest portion of the small bowel, but may occur at other sites. It accounts for 1–3 % of all small bowel obstructions but accounts for up to 25 % of cases in patients greater than age 65 [79]. Very early studies have demonstrated a high mortality up to 40 % but more recent studies have shown improved survival [81, 82]. The diagnosis is difficult to make preoperatively due to lack of specific symptoms [79, 82]. In 1941 the classic triad of pneumobilia, partial or complete small bowel obstruction and an aberrant gallstone in the GI tract known Rigler's triad was coined to be diagnostic of gallstone ileus. However, the presence of all three findings is only reported in 17–35 % of cases. Further there may be other causes of pneumobilia related to prior sphincterotomy or a surgically placed bilioenteric anastomosis hence the finding of pneumobilia in the setting of a small bowel obstruction may not be pathognomonic. The diagnosis of gallstone ileus can be aided with imaging. Multidetector CT has been demonstrated to be effective in obtaining the diagnosis rapidly. In a series of 40 patients with gallstone ileus obstruction was identified in 32/40 patients, pneumobilia in 35/40 and the site of obstruction in 35/40 patients. The biliary enteric fistula was only visualized in five patients [83].

Treatment begins with attaining hemodynamic stability. Relief of obstruction is the primary objective and can be performed through a simple enterotomy. The decision to close the biliary enteric fistula remains controversial [81].

Bouveret's syndrome is a rare form of gastric outlet obstruction due to a large gallstone migrating through a cholecystoduodenal fistula lodging at the proximal duodenum, post-bulbar duodenum, pylorus, or prepyloric area. Patients typically present with nausea, vomiting, and abdominal pain. The most common findings on abdominal imaging are pneumobilia and a calcified mass in the right upper quadrant. Endoscopy most often reveals an obstructing stone in the majority of cases [84]. The condition is often managed surgically with a laparoscopic or open enterolithotomy to relieve the obstruction. CT may be helpful in delineating the extent and location of the biliary enteric fistula [81].

Cholecystocolic fistulas are the second most common biliary enteric fistula. Obstruction though rare may occur at the sigmoid colon and is often associated with a colonic stricture [81].

Biliary Vascular Fistulas

Biliary vascular fistulas manifests often as bleeding into the biliary tree or hemobilia. In this situation blood preferentially flows from the high-pressure vascular structures into the low pressure biliary system. These anomalous connections may originate from the liver, gallbladder, pancreas (hemosuccus pancreaticus), or bile ducts. Bleeding can be severe if the source is arterial or a venous source in the setting of portal hypertension. Accidental trauma or iatrogenic injury from various percutaneous and endoscopic interventions to the liver, gall bladder, and biliary tree are the most common causes of hemobilia [81, 85]. Biliary vascular fistulas from gallstone erosion account for approximately 10 % of cases of hemobilia [61]. Biliary tract hemorrhage is described in the literature to present as a triad of upper GI bleeding, biliary pain and jaundice although it is rare that all features are seen in an individual patient [81, 86]. Rupture of a pseudoaneurysm from gallstone erosion may result in massive hemobilia or intraperitoneal bleeding which may prove fatal. Upper endoscopy is the initial examination of choice to exclude more common sources of bleeding. Blood seen exiting the ampulla of Vater is highly suggestive of a biliary source. Abdominal ultrasonography, CT or MRI may demonstrate blood in the biliary tree. Selective hepatic angiography is the most specific method of identifying the site of bleeding and provides the opportunity for embolization [86]. In addition gallstone related hemobilia is treated with cholecystectomy and removal of the bile duct stones [81].

Bilehemia refers to direct flow of bile into the blood stream through a biliary vascular fistula. Bile flows preferentially from an obstructed biliary system to a lower pressure portal vein, hepatic vein or inferior vena cava that may manifest as sepsis or pulmonary embolism [87]. The most common causes include rupture of the liver from trauma, iatrogenic injury from percutaneous drainage, liver biopsies, endoscopic stent placement or transjugular intrahepatic portosystemic shunts or erosion of gallstones into venous structures [88, 89]. Patients present with a triad of progressive jaundice, marked direct hyperbilirubinemia in the absence of transaminase elevations. ERCP or percutaneous transhepatic cholangiography are the best methods to visualize the fistula. Angiography is not diagnostic. Relief of biliary obstruction may result in spontaneous fistula closure. Occlusion of the fistula with stents, angiographic coils, or balloon tamponade has been successful [90, 91].

Biliary Thoracic Fistula

A biliary thoracic fistula is an abnormal communication between the biliary tract and thoracic cavity. The fistula may communicate between the pleural space or bronchial tree. Trauma, iatrogenic causes, malignancy, and biliary obstruction are the most common causes in developed countries [92]. In the developing world, amoebic liver abscesses are a common cause. Patients present with right upper quadrant pain and pleuritic chest pain. In patients with bronchobiliary fistulas, patients may complain of a bitter productive cough suggestive of biliptysis. Imaging may demonstrate a right sided pleural effusion [93, 94]. Signs of infection may be seen in half the patients. Treatment usually starts with drainage of abscess or pleural effusion either with a chest tube or percutaneous drain. If the fistula persists, endoscopic sphincterotomy is performed to preferentially drain the bile towards the duodenum. Surgery is only attempted if the fistula persists [95, 96].

References

1. Peery AF, Dellon ES, Lund J, Crockett SD, McGowan CE, Bulsiewicz WJ, et al. Burden of gastrointestinal disease in the United States: 2012 update. Gastroenterology. 2012;143:1179–87. e1–3.
2. Bradley III EL. A clinically based classification system for acute pancreatitis. Summary of the International Symposium on Acute Pancreatitis, Atlanta, GA, September 11 through 13, 1992. Arch Surg. 1993;128:586–90.
3. Banks PA, Bollen TL, Dervenis C, Gooszen HG, Johnson CD, Sarr MG, et al. Classification of acute pancreatitis—2012: revision of the Atlanta classification and definitions by international consensus. Gut. 2013;62:102–11.
4. Feldman M, Friedman LS, Sleisenger MH. Sleisenger & Fordtran's gastrointestinal and liver disease: pathophysiology, diagnosis, management. 7th ed. Philadelphia, PA: Saunders; 2002.
5. Kaw M, Al-Antably Y, Kaw P. Management of gallstone pancreatitis: cholecystectomy or ERCP and endoscopic sphincterotomy. Gastrointest Endosc. 2002;56:61–5.
6. Gumaste VV, Dave PB, Weissman D, Messer J. Lipase/amylase ratio. A new index that distinguishes acute episodes of alcoholic from nonalcoholic acute pancreatitis. Gastroenterology. 1991; 101:1361–6.
7. Gwozdz GP, Steinberg WM, Werner M, Henry JP, Pauley C. Comparative evaluation of the diagnosis of acute pancreatitis based on serum and urine enzyme assays. Clin Chim Acta. 1990;187:243–54.
8. Yadav D, Agarwal N, Pitchumoni CS. A critical evaluation of laboratory tests in acute pancreatitis. Am J Gastroenterol. 2002;97:1309–18.
9. Ranson JH, Rifkind KM, Roses DF, Fink SD, Eng K, Localio SA. Objective early identification of severe acute pancreatitis. Am J Gastroenterol. 1974;61: 443–51.
10. LeGall JR, Loirat P, Alperovitch A. APACHE II—a severity of disease classification system. Crit Care Med. 1986;14:754–5.
11. Wu BU, Johannes RS, Sun X, Tabak Y, Conwell DL, Banks PA. The early prediction of mortality in acute pancreatitis: a large population-based study. Gut. 2008;57:1698–703.
12. Khanna AK, Meher S, Prakash S, Tiwary SK, Singh U, Srivastava A, et al. Comparison of Ranson, Glasgow, MOSS, SIRS, BISAP, APACHE-II, CTSI Scores, IL-6, CRP, and Procalcitonin in predicting severity, organ failure, pancreatic necrosis, and mortality in acute pancreatitis. HPB Surg. 2013;2013: 367581.
13. Knaus WA, Draper EA, Wagner DP, Zimmerman JE. APACHE II: a severity of disease classification system. Crit Care Med. 1985;13:818–29.
14. Balthazar EJ, Ranson JH, Naidich DP, Megibow AJ, Caccavale R, Cooper MM. Acute pancreatitis: prognostic value of CT. Radiology. 1985;156:767–72.
15. Singh VK, Bollen TL, Wu BU, Repas K, Maurer R, Yu S, et al. An assessment of the severity of interstitial pancreatitis. Clin Gastroenterol Hepatol. 2011;9:1098–103.
16. Spanier BW, Nio Y, van der Hulst RW, Tuynman HA, Dijkgraaf MG, Bruno MJ. Practice and yield of early CT scan in acute pancreatitis: a Dutch Observational Multicenter Study. Pancreatology. 2010;10:222–8.

17. Bollen TL, Singh VK, Maurer R, Repas K, van Es HW, Banks PA, et al. A comparative evaluation of radiologic and clinical scoring systems in the early prediction of severity in acute pancreatitis. Am J Gastroenterol. 2012;107:612–9.

18. Sakorafas GH, Tsiotos GG, Sarr MG. Extrapancreatic necrotizing pancreatitis with viable pancreas: a previously under-appreciated entity. J Am Coll Surg. 1999;188:643–8.

19. Besselink MG, van Santvoort HC, Boermeester MA, Nieuwenhuijs VB, van Goor H, Dejong CH, et al. Timing and impact of infections in acute pancreatitis. Br J Surg. 2009;96:267–73.

20. van Santvoort HC, Bakker OJ, Bollen TL, Besselink MG, Ahmed Ali U, Schrijver AM, et al. A conservative and minimally invasive approach to necrotizing pancreatitis improves outcome. Gastroenterology. 2011;141:1254–63.

21. Banks PA, Gerzof SG, Langevin RE, Silverman SG, Sica GT, Hughes MD. CT-guided aspiration of suspected pancreatic infection: bacteriology and clinical outcome. Int J Pancreatol. 1995;18:265–70.

22. Lenhart DK, Balthazar EJ. MDCT of acute mild (non-necrotizing) pancreatitis: abdominal complications and fate of fluid collections. AJR Am J Roentgenol. 2008;190:643–9.

23. Vege SS, Gardner TB, Chari ST, Munukuti P, Pearson RK, Clain JE, et al. Low mortality and high morbidity in severe acute pancreatitis without organ failure: a case for revising the Atlanta classification to include "moderately severe acute pancreatitis". Am J Gastroenterol. 2009;104:710–5.

24. Johnson CD, Abu-Hilal M. Persistent organ failure during the first week as a marker of fatal outcome in acute pancreatitis. Gut. 2004;53:1340–4.

25. Mofidi R, Duff MD, Wigmore SJ, Madhavan KK, Garden OJ, Parks RW. Association between early systemic inflammatory response, severity of multiorgan dysfunction and death in acute pancreatitis. Br J Surg. 2006;93:738–44.

26. Beger HG, Bittner R, Block S, Buchler M. Bacterial contamination of pancreatic necrosis. A prospective clinical study. Gastroenterology. 1986;91:433–8.

27. Gardner TB, Vege SS, Pearson RK, Chari ST. Fluid resuscitation in acute pancreatitis. Clin Gastroenterol Hepatol. 2008;6:1070–6.

28. Harrison DA, D'Amico G, Singer M. The Pancreatitis Outcome Prediction (POP) Score: a new prognostic index for patients with severe acute pancreatitis. Crit Care Med. 2007;35:1703–8.

29. Baillargeon JD, Orav J, Ramagopal V, Tenner SM, Banks PA. Hemoconcentration as an early risk factor for necrotizing pancreatitis. Am J Gastroenterol. 1998;93:2130–4.

30. Brown A, Orav J, Banks PA. Hemoconcentration is an early marker for organ failure and necrotizing pancreatitis. Pancreas. 2000;20:367–72.

31. Gardner TB, Olenec CA, Chertoff JD, Mackenzie TA, Robertson DJ. Hemoconcentration and pancreatic necrosis: further defining the relationship. Pancreas. 2006;33:169–73.

32. Wu BU, Johannes RS, Sun X, Conwell DL, Banks PA. Early changes in blood urea nitrogen predict mortality in acute pancreatitis. Gastroenterology. 2009;137:129–35.

33. Wu BU, Bakker OJ, Papachristou GI, Besselink MG, Repas K, van Santvoort HC, et al. Blood urea nitrogen in the early assessment of acute pancreatitis: an international validation study. Arch Intern Med. 2011;171:669–76.

34. de-Madaria E, Soler-Sala G, Sanchez-Paya J, Lopez-Font I, Martinez J, Gomez-Escolar L, et al. Influence of fluid therapy on the prognosis of acute pancreatitis: a prospective cohort study. Am J Gastroenterol. 2011;106:1843–50.

35. Mao EQ, Tang YQ, Fei J, Qin S, Wu J, Li L, et al. Fluid therapy for severe acute pancreatitis in acute response stage. Chin Med J (Engl). 2009;122:169–73.

36. Mao EQ, Fei J, Peng YB, Huang J, Tang YQ, Zhang SD. Rapid hemodilution is associated with increased sepsis and mortality among patients with severe acute pancreatitis. Chin Med J (Engl). 2010;123:1639–44.

37. IAP/APA evidence-based guidelines for the management of acute pancreatitis. Pancreatology. 2013;13:e1–15.

38. Wu BU, Hwang JQ, Gardner TH, Repas K, Delee R, Yu S, et al. Lactated Ringer's solution reduces systemic inflammation compared with saline in patients with acute pancreatitis. Clin Gastroenterol Hepatol. 2011;9:710–7. e1.

39. Wu BU, Conwell DL. Acute pancreatitis part I: approach to early management. Clin Gastroenterol Hepatol. 2010;8:410–6. quiz e56–8.

40. Masci E, Toti G, Mariani A, Curioni S, Lomazzi A, Dinelli M, et al. Complications of diagnostic and therapeutic ERCP: a prospective multicenter study. Am J Gastroenterol. 2001;96:417–23.

41. Loperfido S, Angelini G, Benedetti G, Chilovi F, Costan F, De Berardinis F, et al. Major early complications from diagnostic and therapeutic ERCP: a prospective multicenter study. Gastrointest Endosc. 1998;48:1–10.

42. Cotton PB, Garrow DA, Gallagher J, Romagnuolo J. Risk factors for complications after ERCP: a multivariate analysis of 11,497 procedures over 12 years. Gastrointest Endosc. 2009;70:80–8.

43. Petrov MS, Pylypchuk RD, Emelyanov NV. Systematic review: nutritional support in acute pancreatitis. Aliment Pharmacol Ther. 2008;28:704–12.

44. Petrov MS, Kukosh MV, Emelyanov NV. A randomized controlled trial of enteral versus parenteral feeding in patients with predicted severe acute pancreatitis shows a significant reduction in mortality and in infected pancreatic complications with total enteral nutrition. Dig Surg. 2006;23:336–44. discussion 44–5.

45. Casas M, Mora J, Fort E, Aracil C, Busquets D, Galter S, et al. Total enteral nutrition vs. total parenteral

nutrition in patients with severe acute pancreatitis. Rev Esp Enferm Dig. 2007;99:264–9.

46. Yi F, Ge L, Zhao J, Lei Y, Zhou F, Chen Z, et al. Meta-analysis: total parenteral nutrition versus total enteral nutrition in predicted severe acute pancreatitis. Intern Med. 2012;51:523–30.

47. Petrov MS, McIlroy K, Grayson L, Phillips AR, Windsor JA. Early nasogastric tube feeding versus nil per os in mild to moderate acute pancreatitis: a randomized controlled trial. Clin Nutr. 2013;32:697–703.

48. Eckerwall GE, Tingstedt BB, Bergenzaun PE, Andersson RG. Immediate oral feeding in patients with mild acute pancreatitis is safe and may accelerate recovery—a randomized clinical study. Clin Nutr. 2007;26:758–63.

49. Gupta R, Patel K, Calder PC, Yaqoob P, Primrose JN, Johnson CD. A randomised clinical trial to assess the effect of total enteral and total parenteral nutritional support on metabolic, inflammatory and oxidative markers in patients with predicted severe acute pancreatitis (APACHE II > or =6). Pancreatology. 2003;3:406–13.

50. Bakker OJ, van Brunschot S, van Santvoort HC, Besselink MG, Bollen TL, Boermeester MA, et al. Early versus on-demand nasoenteric tube feeding in acute pancreatitis. N Engl J Med. 2014;371:1983–93.

51. O'Connell K, Brasel K. Bile metabolism and lithogenesis. Surg Clin North Am. 2014;94:361–75.

52. Frei GJ, Frei VT, Thirlby RC, McClelland RN. Biliary pancreatitis: clinical presentation and surgical management. Am J Surg. 1986;151:170–5.

53. Ranson JH. The timing of biliary surgery in acute pancreatitis. Ann Surg. 1979;189:654–63.

54. Uhl W, Warshaw A, Imrie C, Bassi C, McKay CJ, Lankisch PG, et al. IAP guidelines for the surgical management of acute pancreatitis. Pancreatology. 2002;2:565–73.

55. Diehl AK, Sugarek NJ, Todd KH. Clinical evaluation for gallstone disease: usefulness of symptoms and signs in diagnosis. Am J Med. 1990;89:29–33.

56. Cafasso DE, Smith RR. Symptomatic cholelithiasis and functional disorders of the biliary tract. Surg Clin North Am. 2014;94:233–56.

57. Del Favero G, Caroli A, Meggiato T, Volpi A, Scalon P, Puglisi A, et al. Natural history of gallstones in non-insulin-dependent diabetes mellitus. A prospective 5-year follow-up. Dig Dis Sci. 1994;39:1704–7.

58. Thistle JL, Cleary PA, Lachin JM, Tyor MP, Hersh T. The natural history of cholelithiasis: the National Cooperative Gallstone Study. Ann Intern Med. 1984;101:171–5.

59. Newman HF, Northup JD, Rosenblum M, Abrams H. Complications of cholelithiasis. Am J Gastroenterol. 1968;50:476–96.

60. Lipsett PA, Pitt HA. Acute cholangitis. Surg Clin North Am. 1990;70:1297–312.

61. Jarnagin WR, Blumgart LH. Blumgart's surgery of the liver, biliary tract, and pancreas. 5th ed. Philadelphia, PA: Elsevier Saunders; 2012.

62. Abdallah AA, Krige JE, Bornman PC. Biliary tract obstruction in chronic pancreatitis. HPB (Oxford). 2007;9:421–8.

63. Pereira-Lima JC, Jakobs R, Busnello JV, Benz C, Blaya C, Riemann JF. The role of serum liver enzymes in the diagnosis of choledocholithiasis. Hepatogastroenterology. 2000;47:1522–5.

64. Chau EM, Leong LL, Chan FL. Recurrent pyogenic cholangitis: ultrasound evaluation compared with endoscopic retrograde cholangiopancreatography. Clin Radiol. 1987;38:79–85.

65. Yusoff IF, Barkun JS, Barkun AN. Diagnosis and management of cholecystitis and cholangitis. Gastroenterol Clin North Am. 2003;32:1145–68.

66. Mayumi T, Someya K, Ootubo H, Takama T, Kido T, Kamezaki F, et al. Progression of Tokyo Guidelines and Japanese Guidelines for management of acute cholangitis and cholecystitis. J UOEH. 2013;35:249–57.

67. Cotton PB, Lehman G, Vennes J, Geenen JE, Russell RC, Meyers WC, et al. Endoscopic sphincterotomy complications and their management: an attempt at consensus. Gastrointest Endosc. 1991;37:383–93.

68. Csendes A, Mitru N, Maluenda F, Diaz JC, Burdiles P, Csendes P, et al. Counts of bacteria and pyocites of choledochal bile in controls and in patients with gallstones or common bile duct stones with or without acute cholangitis. Hepatogastroenterology. 1996;43:800–6.

69. Solomkin JS, Mazuski JE, Bradley JS, Rodvold KA, Goldstein EJ, Baron EJ, et al. Diagnosis and management of complicated intra-abdominal infection in adults and children: guidelines by the Surgical Infection Society and the Infectious Diseases Society of America. Surg Infect (Larchmt). 2010;11:79–109.

70. Carr-Locke DL. Therapeutic role of ERCP in the management of suspected common bile duct stones. Gastrointest Endosc. 2002;56:S170–4.

71. Lai EC, Mok FP, Tan ES, Lo CM, Fan ST, You KT, et al. Endoscopic biliary drainage for severe acute cholangitis. N Engl J Med. 1992;326:1582–6.

72. Sugiyama M, Atomi Y. Treatment of acute cholangitis due to choledocholithiasis in elderly and younger patients. Arch Surg. 1997;132:1129–33.

73. Mirizzi PL. Rev Asoc Med Argent. 1948;62:529–33. Sindrome del conducto hepatico

74. Johnson LW, Sehon JK, Lee WC, Zibari GB, McDonald JC. Mirizzi's syndrome: experience from a multi-institutional review. Am Surg. 2001;67:11–4.

75. Beltran MA, Csendes A, Cruces KS. The relationship of Mirizzi syndrome and cholecystoenteric fistula: validation of a modified classification. World J Surg. 2008;32:2237–43.

76. Becker CD, Hassler H, Terrier F. Preoperative diagnosis of the Mirizzi syndrome: limitations of sonography and computed tomography. AJR Am J Roentgenol. 1984;143:591–6.

77. Yun EJ, Choi CS, Yoon DY, Seo YL, Chang SK, Kim JS, et al. Combination of magnetic resonance cholangiopancreatography and computed tomography for

preoperative diagnosis of the Mirizzi syndrome. J Comput Assist Tomogr. 2009;33:636–40.

78. Yeh CN, Jan YY, Chen MF. Laparoscopic treatment for Mirizzi syndrome. Surg Endosc. 2003;17:1573–8.

79. Reisner RM, Cohen JR. Gallstone ileus: a review of 1001 reported cases. Am Surg. 1994;60:441–6.

80. Clavien PA, Richon J, Burgan S, Rohner A. Gallstone ileus. Br J Surg. 1990;77:737–42.

81. Luu MB, Deziel DJ. Unusual complications of gallstones. Surg Clin North Am. 2014;94:377–94.

82. Lobo DN, Jobling JC, Balfour TW. Gallstone ileus: diagnostic pitfalls and therapeutic successes. J Clin Gastroenterol. 2000;30:72–6.

83. Lassandro F, Romano S, Ragozzino A, Rossi G, Valente T, Ferrara I, et al. Role of helical CT in diagnosis of gallstone ileus and related conditions. AJR Am J Roentgenol. 2005;185:1159–65.

84. Cappell MS, Davis M. Characterization of Bouveret's syndrome: a comprehensive review of 128 cases. Am J Gastroenterol. 2006;101:2139–46.

85. Sandblom P, Mirkovitch V. Hemobilia: some salient features and their causes. Surg Clin North Am. 1977;57:397–408.

86. Munoz C, Fernandez M, Brahm J. Traumatic hemobilia: a case report and literature review. Gastroenterol Hepatol. 2008;31:79–81.

87. Sandblom P, Jakobsson B, Lindgren H, Lunderquist A. Fatal bilhemia. Surgery. 2000;127:354–7.

88. Mallery S, Freeman ML, Peine CJ, Miller RP, Stanchfield WR. Biliary-shunt fistula following transjugular intrahepatic portosystemic shunt placement. Gastroenterology. 1996;111:1353–7.

89. Siddiqui J, Jaffe PE, Aziz K, Forouhar F, Sheppard R, Covault J, et al. Fatal air and bile embolism after percutaneous liver biopsy and ERCP. Gastrointest Endosc. 2005;61:153–7.

90. Struyven J, Cremer M, Pirson P, Jeanty P, Jeanmart J. Posttraumatic Bilhemia: diagnosis and catheter therapy. AJR Am J Roentgenol. 1982;138:746–7.

91. Rankin RN, Vellet DA. Portobiliary fistula: occurrence and treatment. Can Assoc Radiol J. 1991; 42:55–9.

92. Liao GQ, Wang H, Zhu GY, Zhu KB, Lv FX, Tai S. Management of acquired bronchobiliary fistula: a systematic literature review of 68 cases published in 30 years. World J Gastroenterol. 2011;17: 3842–9.

93. Cunningham LW, Grobman M, Paz HL, Hanlon CA, Promisloff RA. Cholecystopleural fistula with cholelithiasis presenting as a right pleural effusion. Chest. 1990;97:751–2.

94. Delco F, Domenighetti G, Kauzlaric D, Donati D, Mombelli G. Spontaneous biliothorax (thoracobilia) following cholecystopleural fistula presenting as an acute respiratory insufficiency. Successful removal of gallstones from the pleural space. Chest. 1994;106:961–3.

95. Aydin U, Yazici P, Tekin F, Ozutemiz O, Coker A. Minimally invasive treatment of patients with bronchobiliary fistula: a case series. J Med Case Rep. 2009;3:23.

96. Chong CF, Chong VH, Jalihal A, Mathews L. Bronchobiliary fistula successfully treated surgically. Singapore Med J. 2008;49:e208–11.

Helmi Khadra, Terence Jackson, and Jeffrey Marks

Introduction

Major changes have occurred in the management of common bile duct stones in the past three decades. For many years, open CBD exploration was the gold standard for management of choledocholithiasis. Advent of endoscopy and minimally invasive surgery, with considerably lower morbidity and mortality, has now replaced open surgery as the first choice treatment. Understanding of potential complications is an essential part of treatment planning and postoperative care. The most common complications of laparoscopic and open approaches of common bile duct exploration include retained and recurrent common bile duct of stones, bile leak, bile duct injury, abscess/cholangitis, and pancreatitis. This chapter reviews the potential complications of surgical approaches for choledocholithiasis and discusses the management of major intraoperative, postoperative, and delayed complications related to surgical treatments of common bile duct stones.

H. Khadra, M.D. • T. Jackson, M.D. (✉)
J. Marks, M.D.
Department of Surgery, University Hospitals Case Medical Center, 11100 Euclid Avenue, Cleveland, OH 44106, USA
e-mail: helmikhadra@gmail.com;
Helmi.Khadra@UHhospitals.org;
Terence.Jackson@UHhospitals.org;
Jeffrey.Marks@UHhospitals.org

Technical Overview

The relative risks and complications increase proportionately according to the type of procedure performed and the nature of the pathology or underlying disease process. In general, the more complex the biliary procedure is, the risk of complications inherently increase. This is principally related to the technical difficulty, ability to expose the field, blood supply, risk of tissue injury, hematoma formation, and technical ease of achieving the resection and/or anastomosis. Here is a summarized overview of the surgical techniques involved in management of common bile duct stones and key steps of the procedures with potential for complications.

Laparoscopic Transcystic Common Bile Duct Exploration

The transcystic duct approach is mainly reserved for smaller diameter ducts and small CBD stones. When indicated, the transcystic approach is preferred over choledochotomy, because it is avoids the need for a choledochotomy repair and associated with less postoperative morbidity. Regardless of the approach, proper exposure and dissection to achieve critical view should be obtained for clear visualization of biliary structures and to avoid injuries to nearby structures. Dissection of

© Springer International Publishing Switzerland 2016
J.W. Hazey et al. (eds.), *Multidisciplinary Management of Common Bile Duct Stones*,
DOI 10.1007/978-3-319-22765-8_14

Fig. 14.1 Posterior
rupture of cystic duct by
pushing the catheter in
wrong direction.
(Courtesy of SAGES
Image Library and
Shahram Nazari, MD.)

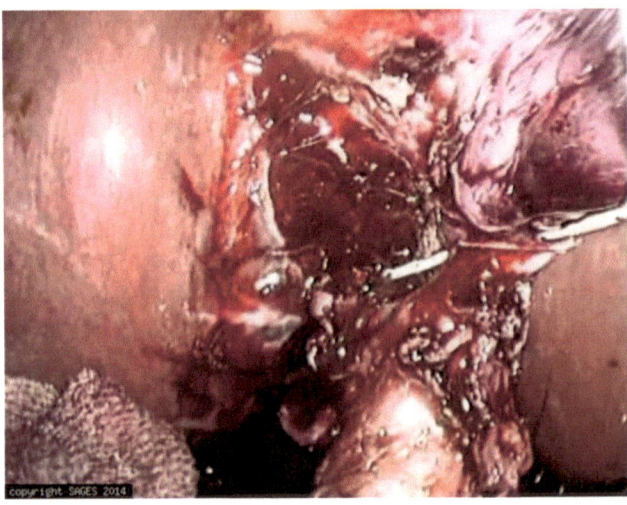

the porta hepatis is done more thoroughly than it
is for routine laparoscopic cholecystectomy since
access to the cystic duct–common duct junction
or the anterior surface of the common duct itself
is frequently required for adequate ductal exploration. When the cystic duct is adequately
exposed, a 2–3 cm incision is made. The duct
may be dilated with either mechanical over-the-
wire graduated dilators or pneumatic dilators if
the duct is not large to properly insert choledo-
choscopes or baskets. This must be done cau-
tiously to avoid injury to the cystic duct–common
duct junction (Fig. 14.1).

Under fluoroscopy, transcystic flushing of the
common bile duct with saline can often flush
small (1–2 mm) stones. Flushing must be performed at low pressures. High pressure can result
in injury to the papilla and also may result in bacterial translocation from the biliary system into
the bloodstream. If flushing is unsuccessful in
clearing the stones, either retrograde retrieval of
stones with a basket/balloon or antegrade removal
using balloon catheters is performed. During retrograde retrieval, care must be taken not to drag
the stones higher into the hepatic ducts. Retrieval
using balloon catheters involves a 4 French
Fogarty balloon catheter inserted through the
cystic duct and into the duodenum where it is
inflated, and withdrawn through the cystic duct.
Papillary dilatation must be performed with care
given the risk for bleeding, ductal trauma, and

pancreatitis. Stones retrieved will be removed via
forceps and withdrawn through the cystic duct.
Excessive or aggressive maneuvers of the catheter can easily perforate the ductal system when
the stone is impacted in the distal duct. Excessive
or aggressive maneuvers of the basket can injure
the ductal system or the papilla of Vater by retrac-
tion. Following retrieval of stones, a completion
cholangiogram is performed to ensure clearance
of the biliary tract and to evaluate for leak or
injury. The cystic duct is then ligated using an
endoloop or clipped. Increased ampullary spasm
secondary to manipulation may result in increased
back pressure and cause cystic stump leaks [1, 2].

Laparoscopic Transcholedochal Common Bile Duct Exploration

After adequate exposure and careful dissection of
the common bile duct is ensured, a choledochotomy should only be performed if there is favorable anatomy and minimal inflammation—A
longitudinal incision approximately 10–15 mm
in length, or as long as the diameter of the largest
stone on the anterior surface of the duct, as distal
on the duct as possible. This helps preserve the
proximal portion of the duct for potential further
procedures. Supraduodenal choledochotomy
may also be performed in cases where stones
cannot be readily removed from above.

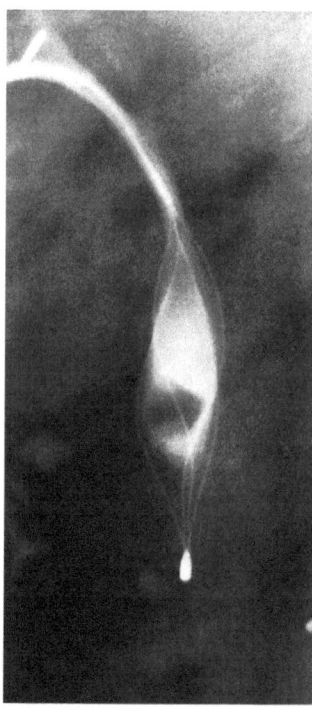

Fig. 14.2 Basket extraction of CBD stone. (From Papalezova and Clary [6].)

Exploration should be as atraumatic as possible. Grasping forceps may damage the duct wall leading to late strictures. Care must be taken to avoid the vascular supply to the duct, at 3 and 9'o clock positions. Devascularization of the duct leads to increased risk for leaks and postoperative strictures. The techniques for stone clearance are generally identical to the trans-cystic approach. During retrograde retrieval, care must be taken to use only superior (proximal) traction on the basket/balloon rather than anterior (Fig. 14.2). There is a risk of lacerating the common bile duct if too much anterior traction is applied. Following stone clearance, management of the choledochotomy can be performed via placement of a T-tube, or primary closure alone. Primary closure of the common bile duct without a T-Tube has been advocated by some authors because of the potential complications associated with T-Tube placement, and no increased incidence of bile leak, peritonitis, or retained bile duct stones [3–5]. Also, higher patient satisfaction with shorter length of stay and operative times has been observed with primary closure. If primary closure of the ductotomy is performed it is recommended to use running or interrupted absorbable sutures as studies have indicated that resorbable sutures may reduce stone formation at the suture site [1, 2]. Following primary closure of the choledochotomy, a closed suction drain should be placed in the subhepatic bed with the catheter tip near the choledochotomy site.

Proponents of the use of T-Tubes state that primary closure is associated with a greater incidence of stenosis and placement of a T-tube can be used for removal of any residual stones should they be seen postoperatively. If a T-tube was placed, adequate time is allowed for tract formation to occur around the T-tube. Generally, 10–14 days is sufficient and the T-tube may be removed following a T-tube cholangiogram.

Open Common Bile Duct Exploration

Although infrequently performed, open common bile duct exploration remains a viable option in situations in which laparoscopy and endoscopy approaches are contraindicated or when these modalities have failed. It offers the advantages of being able to directly manipulate the duct and catheters. It also enables the surgeon to perform a Kocher's maneuver and transduodenal sphincteroplasty when indicated. The profile of complications after open common bile duct exploration is similar to the laparoscopic approach, although with significantly higher complication rates [7].

Choledochoscopy

Choledochoscopy is typically utilized during laparoscopic procedures; however, it can also be utilized with an open approach to allow the removal of stones under direct vision (Fig. 14.3). During transcystic choledochoscopy, a 1.2-mm choledochoscope or ureteroscope is advanced into the common bile duct via the choledochotomy or the cystic duct. The cystic duct sometimes requires dilation prior to inserting the choledochoscopy. This dilation may be performed using a balloon

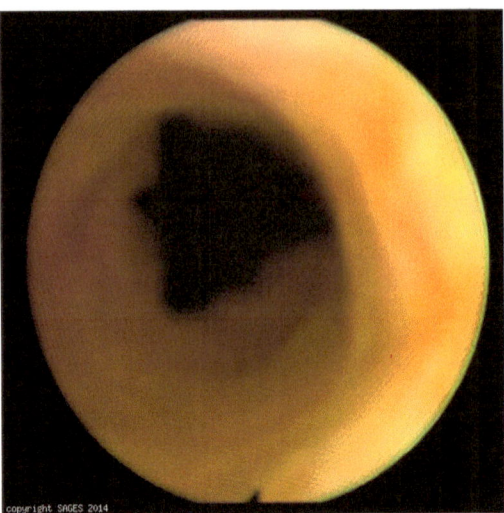

Fig. 14.3 Stone on choledochoscopy. (Courtesy of SAGES Image Library and Shahram Nazari, MD.)

catheter or curved forceps. Dilation must be performed up to 5 mm but not beyond 7 mm to avoid disruption of the cystic duct–CBD junction. This may require an open repair. Care must be taken not to create a false passage while performing a choledochoscopy. Care must also be taken to irrigate with no more than 80 mmHg of irrigation pressure [8, 9]. Creating a false passage or disruption of the CBD using rigid instruments in the CBD must be promptly diagnosed using a post procedure cholangiogram.

T-Tube Placement

When used, the size and length of the T-tube must be appropriate for the individual bile duct. T-tubes can become obstructed if they are too tight fitting. This can be avoided by using smaller bore T-tubes (14 fr) and cutting off the back wall of the T-limb. The length of the T-limbs must be cut to appropriate size. A limb that extends too far proximally into the hepatic ducts may become a cause of obstruction. While closing the choledochotomy around the T-tube, care must be taken to avoid catching the tube in the sutures and the sutures must not be tied around the tube. This will potentially cause tearing of the CBD when

the tube is removed. A subhepatic drain should always be place following T-tube placement with the tip of the drain near the choledochotomy.

Intraoperative Complications

Cystic Duct Stump Leak/Duct of Luschka Leak

A cystic duct stump leak or leaks from small accessory ducts in the cystic plate (ducts of Luschka) are most commonly encountered during dissection and manipulation of these structures following a cholecystectomy [10], or laparoscopic common bile duct exploration [11]. Cystic duct stump or ducts of Luschka injuries may occur due to inaccurate clip placement, perforation proximal to the clip, cystic duct necrosis, or clip dislodgment due to increased intraductal pressure secondary to a retained common bile duct stone. These injuries are rarely discovered intraoperatively. They typically present within the first week postoperatively with signs and symptoms of a biliary leak or biloma consisting of abdominal pain, nausea, and fevers. Jaundice is infrequently seen; however, hyperbilirubinemia in the range of 2–3 mg/dL may occur due to absorption of bile from the peritoneum.

Since these injuries maintain continuity with the rest of the bile ducts, they can often be easily visualized and treated with endoscopic therapy. ERCP has the additional advantage of evaluating the CBD for choledocholithiasis, which may be associated with these biliary leaks [12]. The objective of endoscopic sphincterotomy is to decrease intraductal pressure distal to the bile leak, allowing diversion of bile away from the leaking cystic duct stump or accessory hepatic duct. During this procedure, the placement of an enterobiliary stent will usually cease any further leakage. The stent is typically removed after 4–6 weeks. Since the extrahepatic biliary drainage was not directly compromised, the risk of subsequent stricture is minimal. If endoscopy is not available, percutaneous drainage of bile collections and referral to a specialized center for further management is another option.

Common Bile Duct Injury

Bile duct injuries are a common complication related to laparoscopic or open CBD exploration. Improper identification of the anatomy during dissection may lead to injury to the duct. This may be more likely when there is intense inflammation in the porta hepatis. Familiarizing yourself with a thorough knowledge of the anatomy, including laparoscopically, is your best aid in preventing biliary injuries. During the ductal exploration, aggressive manipulation of instruments can lead to ductal tears or perforations. Baskets are especially prone to puncture the duct, owing to the small size and configuration of the tip. Similarly, electrohydraulic lithotripsy must be used under direct visual control, and applied accurately and with care to avoid injury to the duct wall. The universally accepted techniques for managing serious common bile duct injury are either a choledochoduodenostomy (for distal common bile duct injury) or a Roux-en-Y hepaticojejunostomy. Injury of a small diameter (less than 5 mm) low posterior sectoral bile duct takeoff can be managed with proximal ligation alone, but if the duct diameter is larger, then biliary reconstruction with either the duodenum or a Roux-en-Y of jejunum is indicated.

Bile duct perforation or mucosal tears may result from attempted placement of the choledochoscope into a bile duct that is too small or into a variant biliary duct. If perforation is appreciated at the time of choledochotomy, primary repair may not provide a long-term effective solution and a Roux-en-Y hepaticojejunostomy should be considered. The incidence of biliary stricture after undergoing a biliary exploration is usually small, but when this complication develops it is significant, often requiring further surgery, sometimes including biliary bypass procedures. Stricture results from bile duct trauma, either from chronic choledocholithiasis or iatrogenic from choledochotomy, choledochoscopy, instrumentation or inadvertent laceration, or ligation. This can occur at any level in the biliary tree and may only become evident years after biliary surgery. Damage to the ampulla from chronically impacted CBD stones at the ampulla, edema, mucosal irritation, and scarring can also occur. After the removal of an impacted CBD stone, further instrumentation of the ampulla with the choledochoscope can lead to mucosal tears, which can lead to long-term stricture formation and require further biliary instrumentation for drainage.

The best time to recognize a CBD injury is at the time of surgery. The management of bile duct injuries largely depends on surgeon experience and comfort level with biliary tree reconstruction procedures. These are complex operations, and the best chance for a good, long-term outcome is during the first reconstruction. If the surgeon is uncomfortable or inexperienced, arrangements should be made for immediate transfer to a tertiary hepatobiliary center. Hepatobiliary surgeons prefer to encounter these injuries in an undisturbed field, where the results of repair are clearly better than when having to redo a suboptimal repair [14, 15]. If the primary surgeon recognizes a transection injury, attempting to remove clips and sutures can be challenging and requires additional maneuvers. Leaving the biliary tract obstructed in the acute setting does not typically cause immediate morbidity and may even assist the placement of transhepatic catheters if the CBD dilates proximally. However, the CBD should never be intentionally ligated in hopes that it will dilate and facilitate future identification. Dilation occurs in only 10 % of patients and often leads to necrosis of the ligated bile duct and bile leakage (Fig. 14.4). Bile ducts with active extravasation of bile can have a silastic feeding tube placed in the proximal duct to control the biliary outflow if excessive maneuvers are not needed to suture in the tube, place a balloon catheter, or other means to control the biliary drainage. These supplementary maneuvers may cause further injury to the remnant duct, which potentially shortens the amount of hepatic duct available to the repairing surgeon [16]. Leaving large subhepatic drains is often perfectly adequate to control biliary drainage during the transit to the nearest hepatobiliary tertiary center where definitive repair or drainage can be achieved.

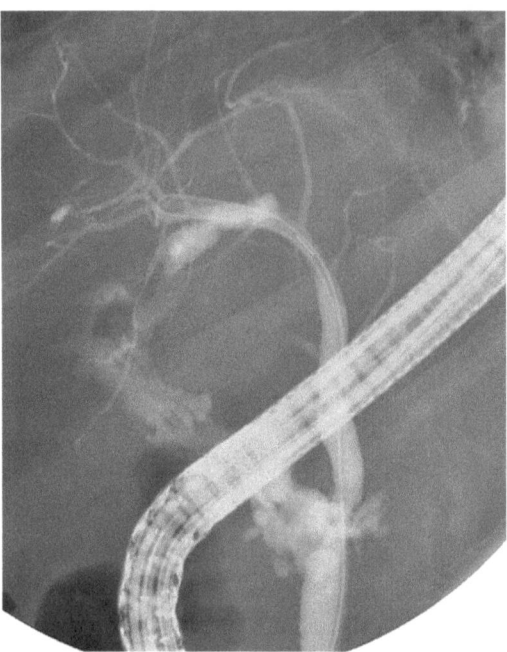

Fig. 14.4 Postsurgical bile leak. (From Baron [13]; with permission.)

Vascular Injury

Evaluation of vascular structures is imperative when performing common bile duct explorations. Studies have suggested that even though the liver may not be affected, vascular injuries resulting in bile duct ischemia and are associated with higher rates of hemobilia, abscess formation, postoperative bile leaks, and anastomotic stricture rates [17, 18]. It is therefore extremely important to evaluate for concomitant vascular injuries with bile duct injuries as the outcome of patients is worse than in patients with an intact blood supply of the bile ducts.

During dissection of the common bile duct, hepatic artery variant anatomy should also be identified. In a small subset of patients, a right hepatic artery can transverse anterior to the bile duct and is in danger of injury or ligation during dissection. Before choledochotomy, it should be verified that the portal vein (PV) lies on the medial-posterior aspect of the common bile duct to avoid catastrophic injury of an aberrant PV during the (anterior) dissection of the common

bile duct. Injury to the portal vein, vena cava, or liver parenchyma is very uncommon, but is a serious complication when it occurs.

Management of vascular injuries in the postoperative period is not as well defined. Controversy exists mainly because delayed vascular repair will not prevent the already existing hepatic necrosis. If a vascular injury is suspected in the immediate postoperative period, a complete abdominal angiography, including portal vein evaluation should be done. Doppler ultrasound of the liver is not recommended as the existence of collateral circulation produces false-positive results [19]. If lobar ischemia is evident, hepatic resection is indicated with a hepaticojejunostomy in the remaining duct. It is important to maintain these patients with broad-spectrum antibiotics to avoid further septic complications due to the translocated intestinal bacteria and decreased hepatic clearing functions after ischemia.

Bowel Injury

Injury to the colon, antrum of the stomach, small bowel, or more commonly, the second portion of the duodenum can occur especially with dissection of dense adhesions from GB wall inflammation. Immediate primary repair, depending on the size and extent of injury, is indicated if this occurs.

Retained Common Bile Duct Stones

Laparoscopic or open CBD exploration leads to a greater than 90 % stone clearance rate. However, they have a 2–6 % incidence of retained or residual stones. Large size (>2 cm) or impaction may be reasons for retained stones after exploration. Management options when a retained stone is diagnosed vary depending on when it was diagnosed. The incidence of retained or recurrent stones after a positive common bile duct exploration is 5–10 %, and approximately 2–3 % of patients develop stones even after correction reoperation [20, 21].

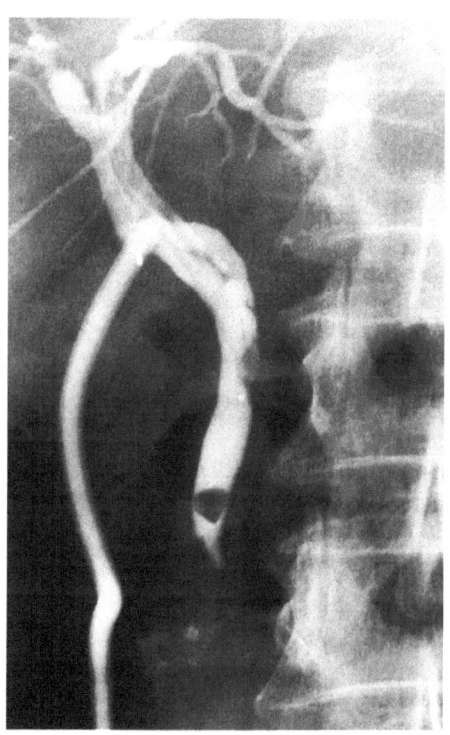

Fig. 14.5 Retained CBD stone. (From Papalezova and Clary [6].)

Intraoperatively Diagnosed Retained Stone

A retained stone is diagnosed intraoperatively by cholangiography (fluoroscopic or ultrasound) (Fig. 14.5). When diagnosed during a laparoscopic procedure, management options include (1) Intraoperative simultaneous ERCP (2) closure of the choledochotomy over a T-tube and postoperative ERCP (3) Conversion to open common bile duct exploration for a possible transduodenal approach or bilio-enteric bypass, if needed. The availability of specialist and experienced staff becomes a major limiting factor when planning for an intraoperative ERCP. When available, it serves as an effective means of treating intraoperatively diagnosed retained stones. However, when endoscopy is not available at the time of diagnosis, closing over a T-tube and planning for a postoperative ERCP or re-exploration via the T-tube is a valid option. The primary function of a T-tube is to ensure adequate drainage of the biliary tract in the case of a retained stone and allows the edema and spasm of the sphincter to subside after exploration. It also provides access to the CBD to help with postoperative cholangiography and stone extraction. It has however been associated with an increased risk of biliary infections, migration of the tube causing obstruction, bile leaks following removal, injury to CBD following removal, and a longer hospital stay [22, 23]. Postoperative ERCP or re-exploration of the common bile duct via T-tube may fail in 3–10 % of patients [24]. This may require a reoperation and depending on the degree of impaction, may require a bilio-enteric bypass procedure. Some stones, if small (>2 mm) in size, may be observed without intervention.

Postoperatively Diagnosed Retained Stone

Five to 12 % of these stones remain asymptomatic. These are diagnosed when patient presents with recurrent symptoms and/or cholangitis. Diagnosis is confirmed by abnormal laboratory studies and imaging, most commonly a transabdominal or endoscopic ultrasound or cholangiography. Management of patients with symptomatic or obstructing retained CBD stones begins much the same way as a patient with newly diagnosed CBD stone; intravenous antibiotics, hydration and bowel rest. Several options are available for stone extraction. If a T-tube has been left in situ during the first exploration, cholangiography and stone extraction may be performed via the T-tube safely and in a cost-effective manner [25]. If the CBD is not already accessed with a T-tube, stone extraction and biliary decompression may be performed endoscopically. Endoscopic retrograde cholangiopancreatography can be diagnostic and therapeutic. Stone extraction and sphincterotomy can be performed with over 90 % clearance. To ensure biliary drainage in cases of CBD stones that cannot be retrieved, biliary stenting can also be performed, as a bridge to further definitive therapy. Biliary decompression may also be achieved using percutaneous transhepatic cholangiography and drain placement. As mentioned previously, ERCP and stone extraction fails in 3–10 % of cases. Laparoscopic re-exploration, either by transcystic approach or by choledochotomy is a safe option with great efficacy and minimal morbidity. Some cases might require conversion to an open procedure secondary to difficult dissection [26].

Recurrrent Common Bile Duct Stones

Review of literature shows that the incidence of recurrent CBD stones after open CBD exploration varies from 7 to 14 % in 40–60 months [27, 28] and is approximately 3–6 % in 30–70 months after laparoscopic CBD exploration [29, 30]. Risk factors for recurrent stones include larges sized CBD stones, peripapillary diverticula and primary CBD stones. Preoperative sphincterotomy, use of a T-tube, primary closure and number of stones have not shown any association with recurrence. Management options for recurrent choledocholithiasis include endoscopic stone extraction, bilioenteric anastomosis or observation depending on clinical presentation and the type of expertise available.

Biliary Reconstruction and Bile Leak

CBD stones are the most common indication for biliary reconstruction. Surgical options for biliary reconstruction include hepaticojejunostomy, choledochojejunostomy, choledochoduodenostomy, cholecystoenterostomy, and choledochocholedochostomy.

A duct to duct anastomosis is relatively easy to perform compared to other biliary enteric anastomosis. It also provides easy access for future endoscopic interventions, if needed. This can also be a difficult procedure to perform if the ducts are small in size. Choledochoduodenostomy is created in the most distal portion of CBD to a kocherized, well mobilized duodenum. Complications related to this anastomosis include sump syndrome, bile leak, stenosis/stricture and surgical site infections. An incidence of 3 % biliary leaks has been reported

[31]. An alternative to choledochoduodenostomy is choledochojejunostomy. This can be performed wither in an end to side or side to side manner with a loop of jejunum or in a Roux-en-Y manner. The roux-en-y configuration has been found to have the lowest complication rate as it protects against intestinal reflux and cholangitis. However, the Roux-en-Y configuration makes this anastomosis inaccessible by endoscopy if any such interventions are required.

A well performed Roux-en-Y hepaticojejunostomy is critical to the long term outcomes of all patients with bile duct injuries in discontinuity with the bowel. The hepaticojejunostomy ideally should be widely patent with a tension free mucosa-to-mucosa anastomosis using well-vascularized bile ducts that drain all aspects of the liver [32]. A choledochodochostomy, choledochoduodenostomy, or hepaticoduodenostomy are not as favored because devascularized ducts are used for the reconstruction and the duodenum tends to move downwards, increasing anastomotic tension, even if a Kocher maneuver is performed well in advance [33]. Performing a side-to-side hepaticojejunostomy anastamosis is favored over a direct duct-to-duct anastomosis due to the associated 50 % failure rate and late stenosis seen in direct duct-to-duct anastomosis [34, 35].

The major complication in performing any biliary bypass procedures is related to postoperative biliary leak and strictures, caused by inadequate identification of healthy bile duct mucosa, an inadequate anastomosis to the jejunum, or leakage from small biliary radicals. These can predominately be managed with the use of a drain placed intraoperatively, by endoscopy and by reoperation.

Strictures

The incidence of biliary stricture after undergoing a biliary exploration is usually small (<1 %) [36]. Benign strictures or stenosis of the bile duct occur most commonly secondary to CBD injury during the primary procedure. Timing of identification of injury and referral, timing of repair, and experience of the repairing surgeon have been cited as factors governing the incidence of biliary strictures [37]. Injury to the duct mucosa from instrumentation or damage to duct wall from grasping forceps can also cause result in delayed stricture formation. Ischemic injury is another important factor leading to delayed strictures of the common bile duct. Blood supply to the CBD comes distally from the gastroduodenal artery via longitudinal vessels in the 3'o clock and 9'o clock position. Proximally it is supplied by branches from the hepatic arteries. Since choledochotomies are performed at the lowest supraduodenal part of the CBD, care must be taken during dissection to avoid manipulation of the vessels. Improper suturing of the choledochotomy site may also result in stenosis or structuring of the CBD. Most of these strictures present within 2 years of the index procedure [37, 38]. Endoscopic retrograde or percutaneous stenting and dilatation are minimally invasive methods of treatment of benign strictures. However, severe bile duct strictures and recurrent strictures may require operative interventions. A biliary-enteric anastomosis (i.e., Roux-en-Y hepaticojejunostomy) is a safe and viable option for management of strictures [39].

Infectious Complications

Surgical Site Infections

Advancement in surgery has meant that open and laparoscopic bile duct surgery is now much safer than before. However, it still comes with significant morbidity. The incidence of surgical site infections after bile duct surgery is approximately 10 % [40]. Current recommendations for antibiotic prophylaxis prior to biliary surgery include a dose of cefazolin preoperatively and redosed as appropriate during a prolonged case. Reports have shown that intraoperative cultures, treatment of bacteriobilia/fungobilia, and a short course of postoperative antibiotic therapy after surgery is associated with decreased surgical site infection [41, 42]. A prospective randomized trial is warranted to investigate this practice.

Hepatic Pyogenic Abscess

Biliary stones are the most common cause of pyogenic liver abscesses [43]. Determination of the pathology of the hepatic abscess is crucial in management planning. Other causes of pyogenic hepatic abscesses include parasites, cholangitis and previous gastric or duodenal surgery. Several factors including size, multiplicity, location, loculation, and patient's operative risk must be taken into account prior to treatment planning. Open surgical drainage, percutaneous drainage and antibiotic therapy alone, are all valid options for the management of a pyogenic liver abscess. Open drainage offers the best chance of clearance of disease and a marked improvement in mortality and low recurrence rates [44, 45]. Percutaneous drainage is an attractive option and offers resolution without the morbidity of open drainage. Antibiotic therapy alone has been recommended in the past for management of hepatic abscesses; however, a relatively poor success rate of antibiotic therapy alone is well documented. Percutaneous drainage along with broad spectrum or culture/sensitivity directed antibiotic therapy is our management method of choice. Following drainage, patients are followed clinically and by imaging to look for response.

Pancreatitis

Choledochoscopy uses a fiber-optic flexible endoscope and saline infusion at low rate through the endoscope to evaluate the CBD. Infusion at high rates and manipulation of the papilla may result in peri-ampullary edema. This could result in transient pancreatitis usually successfully managed conservatively with bowel rest. Preprocedure glucagon helps relax the ampulla and thus decrease the amount of manipulation and instrumentation required. This in turn reduces the incidence of post procedural ampullary edema and pancreatitis. Prophylactic pancreatic stenting has been discussed in the setting of high risk for post-ERCP pancreatitis alone, and is not indicated for in CBD exploration. Post ERCP pancreatitis along with duodenal perforation is a rare but serious entity whose management is addressed in a later section.

Biliary-Enteric Fistula

Choledochoscopy or inaccurate delivery of a rigid instrument may also result in the creation of an iatrogenic fistulous tract between the CBD and nearby structures, most commonly bowel. This may present as recurrent cholangitis, recurrent cholelithiasis, or bile leak and peritonitis, with air in the biliary tree. ERCP helps identify the fistula. Management methods include CBD stenting across the fistula and diversion of bile across the stent. Refractory symptomatic fistulae might require bilio-enteric diversion [46].

Surgical Management of ERCP Complications

ERCP is an important modality in the evaluation and treatment of choledocholithiasis. As described in previous chapters, ERCP involves the advancement of an endoscope into the oropharynx and through the esophagus and stomach and into the second portion of the duodenum. The papilla is then identified and selective cannulation of the bile duct is performed. Contrast is then injected to visualize the ducts or a wire may be advanced to provide access for other interventions such as endoscopic balloon dilation of the biliary sphincter or endoscopic sphincterotomy to extract common bile duct stones.

Complications occur in 5–10 % of patients undergoing ERCP with post ERCP pancreatitis being the most common complication, occurring in about 5–15 % of patients, followed by bleeding (0.3–2 %), biliary infection (1 %), and perforation (<1 %) [47–51]. Surgical management of ERCP-related complications is generally related to duodenal perforations, and however is rarely required for intractable bleeding, or mechanical complications, such as basket impaction or guidewire fracture. Migration of biliary stents may present as obstruction or peritonitis, which may require surgical intervention.

ERCP-Related Hemorrhage

Bleeding related to ERCP occurs almost exclusively in the setting of endoscopic sphincterotomy (ES) and complicates 0.3–1.2 % of procedures [47, 49, 51]. The majority of ES bleeding is self-limiting; however, delayed bleeding can present days to weeks post-procedure. Endoscopic management of post-endoscopic bleeding is effective in well over 90 % of cases using submucosal epinephrine injections, or placement of endoscopic clips [52, 53]. If bleeding fails to cease, the use of electrosurgical coagulation, placement of covered metallic biliary stents, balloon tamponade, or fibrin glue application have also been reported to be effective [53–56]. In the event of failed endoscopic hemostasis, angiography with selective embolization of the GDA is another alternative prior to surgical management [57]. With the continued advances in endoscopic and interventional technique, technology, and experience, surgical intervention is rarely needed and reported.

Unfortunately, when the decision for surgical intervention is indicated there is no standard surgical approach, leaving the decision to the judgment and experience of the surgeon. Anatomically, the ampulla derives its blood supply from the GDA and its branches, making ligation an ideal option for hemostasis; however, this can be accomplished using angiography to selectively embolize the GDA preoperatively. The papilla can be approached via a longitudinal anterior duodenotomy, a supraduodenal gastrotomy, or a posterior distal duodenotomy [58, 59]. Direct control of hemorrhage at the papilla with suture ligation or cauterization has been shown to be effective; however, blind placement of sutures or excessive use of cautery may lead to the formation of delayed strictures or acute pancreatitis [60]. The risk of leak from duodenotomy repair, and fistula development, should also be considered.

ERCP-Related Perforation

The incidence of perforation during ERCP is rare and reported to be less than 1 % [47–49, 51]. Both the severity and the management of ERCP-related perforations vary according to location

Table 14.1 Stapfer classification of ERCP-related perforations

		Mechanism of injury
Type I	Perforation of lateral duodenal wall (remote from papilla)	Direct scope trauma
Type II	Periampullary perforation	Endoscopic sphincterotomy
Type III	Perforation of bile duct	Guidewire or other instrumentation
Type IV	Retroperitoneal free air with no demonstrable perforation	Insufflation of compressed air during ERCP

Adapted from Stapfer et al. [61]

and mechanism. Perforations are classified according to its location, and the management of each type varies significantly. Stapfer et al. proposed the most widely accepted classification system of ERCP related perforations (Table 14.1) [61] which is used in this chapter. The risk of biliopancreatic perforation from duct cannulation with guidewires, baskets or stents is more likely to occur during technically challenging procedures, in patients with choledocholithiasis, biliary stricture or tumor due to increased use of guidewires and instrument manipulation.

Any suspicion of perforation should prompt immediate evaluation. Patients with a suspected perforation should immediately undergo contrasted imaging with fluoroscopy or CT. Findings of large pneumoperitoneum or extravasation of contrast into the peritoneal cavity are clear indications for surgery; however, the presence of retroperitoneal free air does not correlate with the degree of injury or the indication for surgery since up to a third of asymptomatic patients have pneumoretroperitoneum 24 h following ERCP. Similarly, the presence of pneumatosis on CT can occur from submucosal air injection with misdirection of cannulation device, which is also without clinical significance [62–64].

Again, there is no standard surgical approach when intervention is deemed necessary. The surgical approach depends on the surgeon judgement and experience, location and size of the perforation, time to recognition of the injury, and degree of peritoneal or retroperitoneal contamination. Also, additional concomitant procedures, such as cholecystectomy, CBD exploration, or biliary-enteric bypass, are indicated in the event of failed ERCP stone extraction or common bile duct injury.

Surgical Management of Perforations Remote to the Papilla

Type I perforations usually occur at the lateral posterior duodenal wall. Due to the use of side viewing endoscopes, these perforations are usually not recognized at the time of ERCP. All type I perforations require surgical intervention. When recognized early, primary repair of the enterotomy should be done in two layers in a transverse fashion and reinforced with an omental patch along with nasogastric drainage [65]. Closure of larger perforations can be repaired with a jejunal serosal patch and local closed suction drain placement.

When encountered with a delayed perforation, consideration should be taken that the risk of anastomotic leak or dehiscence is high, potentially leading to formation of an enterocutaneous fistula or intraabdominal sepsis. It has been described that duodenal diversion with pyloric exclusion and gastrojejunostomy should be considered in these circumstances [66, 67] with placement of enteral feeding access with a jejunostomy at the time of surgery as well.

Surgical Management of Periampullary Duodenal Perforations

Type II injuries are usually recognized at the time of ERCP. Immediate decompression with nasoenteric, nasobiliary, or internal biliary stents with close observation is usually adequate as the majority of these injuries can be managed conservatively without surgery. However, worsening of clinical presentation after attempting conservative management, or extensive retroperitoneal contrast extravasation are clear indications for surgery; as delayed operative intervention carries

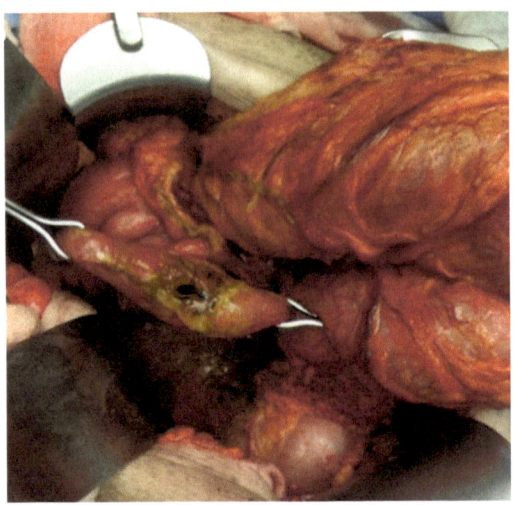

Fig. 14.6 Operative image of type 1 duodenal perforation. (From Warren et al. [70].)

a significantly higher risk of mortality and prolonged hospital course (Fig. 14.6) [68, 69].

Simple retroperitoneal drainage may be treated nonoperatively in stable patients that are diagnosed early with minimal contamination and small injuries. Retroperitoneal duodenal perforations can be repaired through a transduodenal approach by direct repair or sphincteroplasty using absorbable suture. Duodenal drainage, biliary drainage with a T-tube, pyloric exclusion, and gastrojejunostomy have commonly been described as well; however, they are typically reserved for cases with significant contamination. Concurrent CBDE and cholecystectomy should also be performed at the time of surgery if choledocholithiasis was initial indication for the ERCP.

Surgical Management of ERCP Bile Duct Perforations

Type III injuries are usually detected at the time ERCP by visualization of extravasated contrast from the bile duct. The vast majority of these injuries can be managed nonoperatively with percutaneous or endoscopic biliary drainage. In the event of a large injury to the CBD outcomes are significantly better when repair is done by an

experienced hepatobiliary surgeon [14, 15]. If immediate expertise is not available, placement of large bore drains and transfer to a tertiary hepatobiliary center is recommended. Suboptimal repair should not be attempted as hepatobiliary surgeons prefer to encounter these injuries in an undisturbed field, where the results of repair are clearly better than when having to redo a suboptimal repair.

Retroperitoneal Free Air with No Demonstrable Perforation

Type IV injuries is the presence of pneumoretroperitoneum with the absence of perforation. It is thought to be caused by insufflation of compressed air used to maintain visualization during ERCP. The majority of these patients are asymptomatic; however, they can present with pain. Pneumoretroperitoneum is seen on CT imaging in up to 30 % of patients following ERCP with no correlation to the extent or location of the injury or the need for surgery [62–64]. In an otherwise stable patient, no intervention is indicated; however, patients should be monitored to ensure there is no clinical deterioration [61].

Surgical Management of Endoscopic Instrument Complications

There is a scant amount of literature describing surgical techniques for the treatment of instrument complications during ERCP. Basket impaction is an uncommon but recognized complication of ERCP stone extraction. Extraction of a retained basket or wire can be done via duodenotomy or choledochotomy [71, 72]; however, endoscopic maneuvers can be attempted before surgical intervention. Some baskets have a built-in safety mechanism to break upon excess force of closure; however, most baskets require an external crushing sheath such as the Soehendra lithotriptor to either crush the stone or break the basket wire to retrieve the device. Other alternative techniques described include the use of laser, mechanical, and extracorporeal shockwave lithotripsy [73, 74], intracorporeal electrohydraulic lithotriptor, or extending the sphincterotomy using a needle knife. Erosion of a retained guidewire fragment through the bile duct, pancreatic duct or intestine could theoretically lead to abscess, fistula, or pancreatitis; however, none of these potential complications have been reported in the literature (Figs. 14.7 and 14.8).

Biliary stent migration is fairly common, occurring in up to 7 % of cases; with reported complications of bowel obstruction, biliary obstruction with cholangitis, abscess, perforation, or enteroenteric fistula [77]. When distal stent migration is recognized early, it is often retrievable endoscopically. The retrieval techniques included forceps, Dormia basket, snare, Soehendra stent retriever, and balloon. Also spontaneous passage with more distal migrations generally occurs and surgery is rarely needed.

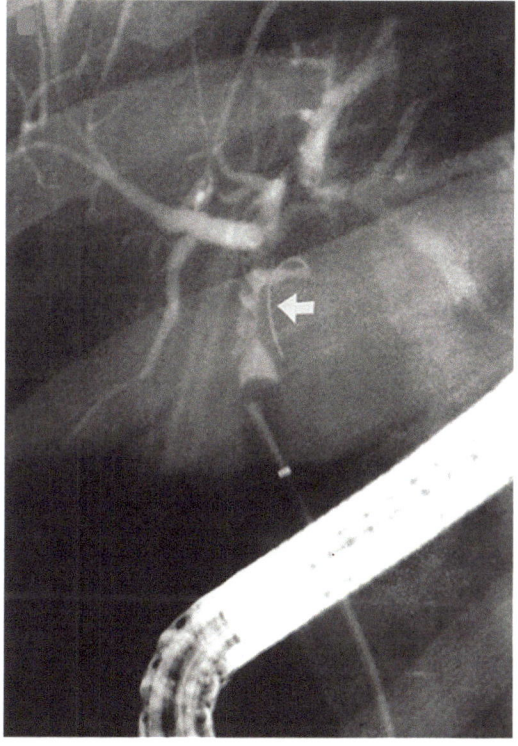

Fig. 14.7 Fractured guidewire. (From Pruitt et al. [75]; with permission.)

Conclusion

Common bile duct exploration is an important tool in a surgeon's arsenal while dealing with choledocholithiasis. This procedure is associated with several, clinically important early and late complications. Patients with complications resulting from this procedure may present to any physician. It is thus crucial for us to understand the mechanics of each complication and learn its appropriate management.

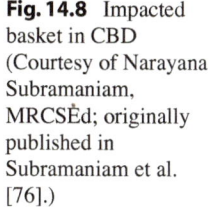

Fig. 14.8 Impacted basket in CBD (Courtesy of Narayana Subramaniam, MRCSEd; originally published in Subramaniam et al. [76].)

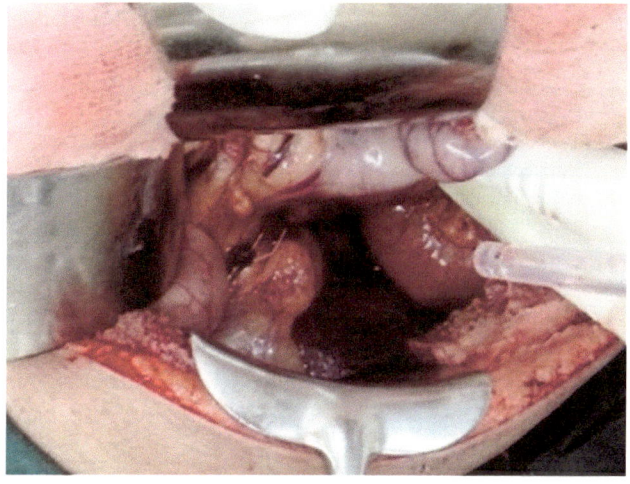

References

1. Petelin JB. Laparoscopic common bile duct exploration. Surg Endosc. 2003;17(11):1705–15.

2. Carroll BJ, Phillips EH, Rosenthal R, Liberman M, Fallas M. Update on transcystic exploration of the bile duct. Surg Laparosc Endosc. 1996;6(6):453–8.

3. Martin IJ, Bailey IS, Rhodes M, O'Rourke N, Nathanson L, Fielding G. Towards T-tube free laparoscopic bile duct exploration: a methodologic evolution during 300 consecutive procedures. Ann Surg. 1998;228(1):29–34.

4. Dorman JP, Franklin ME, Glass JL. Laparoscopic common bile duct exploration by choledochotomy. An effective and efficient method of treatment of choledocholithiasis. Surg Endosc. 1998;12(7):926–8.

5. Decker G, Borie F, Millat B, Berthou JC, Deleuze A, Drouard F, Guillon F, Rodier JG, Fingerhut A. One hundred laparoscopic choledochotomies with primary closure of the common bile duct. Surg Endosc. 2003;17(1):12–8.

6. Papalezova K, Clary B. Blumgart's surgery of the liver, pancreas and biliary tract. Philadelphia, PA: Elsevier; 2012.

7. Grubnik VV, Tkachenko AI, Ilyashenko VV, Vorotyntseva KO. Laparoscopic common bile duct exploration versus open surgery: comparative prospective randomized trial. Surg Endosc. 2012; 26(8):2165–71.

8. Lau WY, Fan ST, Yip WC, Poon GP, Wong KK. Optimal irrigation pressures in operative choledochoscopy. Aust N Z J Surg. 1988;58(1):63–6.

9. Orenstein SB, Marks JM, Hardacre JM. Technical aspects of bile duct evaluation and exploration. Surg Clin North Am. 2014;94(2):281–96.

10. Strasberg SM, Hertl M, Soper NJ. An analysis of the problem of biliary injury during laparoscopic cholecystectomy. J Am Coll Surg. 1995;180(1):101–25.

11. Peters JH, Ollila D, Nichols KE, Gibbons GD, Davanzo MA, Miller J, Front ME, Innes JT, Ellison EC. Diagnosis and management of bile leaks following laparoscopic cholecystectomy. Surg Laparosc Endosc. 1994;4(3):163–70.

12. Christoforidis E, Goulimaris I, Tsalis K, Kanellos I, Demetriades H, Betsis D. The endoscopic management of persistent bile leakage after laparoscopic cholecystectomy. Surg Endosc. 2002;16(5):843–6.

13. Baron TH. Endoscopic management of biliary disorders: diagnostic and therapeutic. Surg Clin North Am. 2014;94(2):395–411.

14. Thomson BNJ, Parks RW, Madhavan KK, Wigmore SJ, Garden OJ. Early specialist repair of biliary injury. Br J Surg. 2006;93(2):216–20.

15. Lillemoe KD, Martin SA, Cameron JL, Yeo CJ, Talamini MA, Kaushal S, Coleman J, Venbrux AC, Savader SJ, Osterman FA, Pitt HA. Major bile duct injuries during laparoscopic cholecystectomy. Follow-up after combined surgical and radiologic management. Ann Surg. 1997;225(5):459–68. discussion 468–71.

16. Mercado MA, Chan C, Jacinto JC, Sanchez N, Barajas A. Voluntary and involuntary ligature of the bile duct in iatrogenic injuries: a nonadvisable approach. J Gastrointest Surg. 2008;12(6):1029–32.

17. Misra S, Melton GB, Geschwind JF, Venbrux AC, Cameron JL, Lillemoe KD. Percutaneous management of bile duct strictures and injuries associated with laparoscopic cholecystectomy: a decade of experience. J Am Coll Surg. 2004;198(2):218–26.

18. Brittain RS, Marchioro TL, Hermann G, Waddell WR, Starzl TE. Accidental hepatic artery ligation in humans. Am J Surg. 1964;107:822–32.

19. Koffron A, Ferrario M, Parsons W, Nemcek A, Saker M, Abecassis M. Failed primary management of iatrogenic biliary injury: incidence and significance of concomitant hepatic arterial disruption. Surgery. 2001;130(4):722–8. discussion 728–31.

20. Girard RM, Legros G. Retained and recurrent bile duct stones. Surgical or nonsurgical removal? Ann Surg. 1981;193(2):150–4.

21. Shojaiefard A, Khorgami Z, Ghafouri A, Soroush A, Hedayat A, Kaveie E. Outcome of common bile duct exploration without intraoperative cholangiography: a case series and review of literature. Acad J Surg. 2014;1(2):30–3.

22. Gurusamy KS, Koti R, Davidson BR. T-tube drainage versus primary closure after open common bile duct exploration. Cochrane Database Syst Rev. 2013;6, CD005640.

23. Zhang W-J, Xu G-F, Wu G-Z, Li J-M, Dong Z-T, Mo X-D. Laparoscopic exploration of common bile duct with primary closure versus T-tube drainage: a randomized clinical trial. J Surg Res. 2009;157(1):e1–5.

24. ElGeidie AA. Single-session minimally invasive management of common bile duct stones. World J Gastroenterol. 2014;20(41):15144–52.

25. Hameed K, Azami R, Jaffery W, Hameed T. Retained stones in the common bile duct: results of management. J Pak Med Assoc. 1993;43(5):90–2.

26. Chiappetta Porras LT, Nápoli ED, Canullán CM, Quesada BM, Petracchi JE, Oría AS. Laparoscopic bile duct reexploration for retained duct stones. J Gastrointest Surg. 2008;12(9):1518–20.

27. Escarce JJ, Shea JA, Chen W, Qian Z, Schwartz JS. Outcomes of open cholecystectomy in the elderly: a longitudinal analysis of 21,000 cases in the prelaparoscopic era. Surgery. 1995;117(2):156–64.

28. Sheridan WG, Williams HO, Lewis MH. Morbidity and mortality of common bile duct exploration. Br J Surg. 1987;74(12):1095–9.

29. Paganini AM, Guerrieri M, Sarnari J, De Sanctis A, D'Ambrosio G, Lezoche G, Lezoche E. Long-term results after laparoscopic transverse choledochotomy for common bile duct stones. Surg Endosc. 2005;19(5):705–9.

30. Lee HM, Min SK, Lee HK. Long-term results of laparoscopic common bile duct exploration by choledo-

chotomy for choledocholithiasis: 15-year experience from a single center. Ann Surg Treat Res. 2014;86(1):1–6.

31. Deutsch AA, Nudelman I, Gutman H, Reiss R. Choledochoduodenostomy an important surgical tool in the management of common bile duct stones. A review of 126 cases. Eur J Surg. 1991;157(9): 531–3.

32. Strasberg SM, Picus DD, Drebin JA. Results of a new strategy for reconstruction of biliary injuries having an isolated right-sided component. J Gastrointest Surg. 2001;5(3):266–74.

33. Mercado MA, Orozco H, de la Garza L, López-Martínez LM, Contreras A, Guillén-Navarro E. Biliary duct injury: partial segment IV resection for intrahepatic reconstruction of biliary lesions. Arch Surg. 1999;134(9):1008–10.

34. Lillemoe KD, Pitt HA, Cameron JL. Postoperative bile duct strictures. Surg Clin North Am. 1990;70(6): 1355–80.

35. de Reuver PR, Grossmann I, Busch OR, Obertop H, van Gulik TM, Gouma DJ. Referral pattern and timing of repair are risk factors for complications after reconstructive surgery for bile duct injury. Ann Surg. 2007;245(5):763–70.

36. Khaled YS, Malde DJ, de Souza C, Kalia A, Ammori BJ. Laparoscopic bile duct exploration via choledochotomy followed by primary duct closure is feasible and safe for the treatment of choledocholithiasis. Surg Endosc. 2013;27(11):4164–70.

37. Sahajpal AK, Chow SC, Dixon E, Greig PD, Gallinger S, Wei AC. Bile duct injuries associated with laparoscopic cholecystectomy: timing of repair and long-term outcomes. Arch Surg. 2010;145(8):757–63.

38. Walsh RM, Henderson JM, Vogt DP, Brown N. Long-term outcome of biliary reconstruction for bile duct injuries from laparoscopic cholecystectomies. Surgery. 2007;142(4):450–6. discussion 456–7.

39. Monteiro da Cunha JE, Machado MC, Herman P, Bacchella T, Abdo EE, Penteado S, Jukemura J, Montagnini A, Machado MA, Pinotti HW. Surgical treatment of cicatricial biliary strictures. Hepatogastroenterology. 1998;45(23):1452–6.

40. Fujii T, Kato H, Suzaki M, Noguchi T, Isaji S. Is it possible to predict the development of an incisional surgical site infection and its severity after biliary tract surgery for benign disease? J Hepatobiliary Pancreat Sci. 2012;19(4):389–96.

41. Mohammed S, Evans C, VanBuren G, Hodges SE, Silberfein E, Artinyan A, Mo Q, Issazadeh M, McElhany AL, Fisher WE. Treatment of bacteriobilia decreases wound infection rates after pancreaticoduodenectomy. HPB (Oxford). 2014;16(6):592–8.

42. Sourrouille I, Gaujoux S, Lacave G, Bert F, Dokmak S, Belghiti J, Paugam-Burtz C, Sauvanet A. Five days of postoperative antimicrobial therapy decreases infectious complications following pancreaticoduodenectomy in patients at risk for bile contamination. HPB (Oxford). 2013;15(6):473–80.

43. Malik AA, Bari SU, Rouf KA, Wani KA. Pyogenic liver abscess: changing patterns in approach. World J Gastrointest Surg. 2010;2(12):395–401.

44. Ochsner A, DeBakey M, Murray S. Pyogenic abscess of the liver. Am J Surg. 1938;40(1):292–319.

45. Bari S, Sheikh KA, Malik AA, Wani RA, Naqash SH. Percutaneous aspiration versus open drainage of liver abscess in children. Pediatr Surg Int. 2007;23(1): 69–74.

46. Hunt DR, Blumgart LH. Iatrogenic choledochoduodenal fistula: an unsuspected cause of postcholecystectomy symptoms. Br J Surg. 1980; 67(1):10–3.

47. Cotton PB, Garrow DA, Gallagher J, Romagnuolo J. Risk factors for complications after ERCP: a multivariate analysis of 11,497 procedures over 12 years. Gastrointest Endosc. 2009;70(1):80–8.

48. Loperfido S, Angelini G, Benedetti G, Chilovi F, Costan F, De Berardinis F, De Bernardin M, Ederle A, Fina P, Fratton A. Major early complications from diagnostic and therapeutic ERCP: a prospective multicenter study. Gastrointest Endosc. 1998;48(1):1–10.

49. Masci E, Toti G, Mariani A, Curioni S, Lomazzi A, Dinelli M, Minoli G, Crosta C, Comin U, Fertitta A, Prada A, Rubis Passoni G, Testoni PA. Complications of diagnostic and therapeutic ERCP: a prospective multicenter study. Am J Gastroenterol. 2001;96(2): 417–23.

50. Jeurnink SM, Siersema PD, Steyerberg EW, Dees J, Poley JW, Haringsma J, Kuipers EJ. Predictors of complications after endoscopic retrograde cholangiopancreatography: a prognostic model for early discharge. Surg Endosc. 2011;25(9):2892–900.

51. Vandervoort J, Soetikno RM, Tham TCK, Wong RCK, Ferrari AP, Montes H, Roston AD, Slivka A, Lichtenstein DR, Ruymann FW, Van Dam J, Hughes M, Carr-Locke DL. Risk factors for complications after performance of ERCP. Gastrointest Endosc. 2002;56(5):652–6.

52. Wilcox CM, Canakis J, Mönkemüller KE, Bondora AW, Geels W. Patterns of bleeding after endoscopic sphincterotomy, the subsequent risk of bleeding, and the role of epinephrine injection. Am J Gastroenterol. 2004;99(2):244–8.

53. Ferreira LEVVC, Baron TH. Post-sphincterotomy bleeding: who, what, when, and how. Am J Gastroenterol. 2007;102(12):2850–8.

54. Shah JN, Marson F, Binmoeller KF. Temporary self-expandable metal stent placement for treatment of post-sphincterotomy bleeding. Gastrointest Endosc. 2010;72(6):1274–8.

55. Aslinia F, Hawkins L, Darwin P, Goldberg E. Temporary placement of a fully covered metal stent to tamponade bleeding from endoscopic papillary balloon dilation. Gastrointest Endosc. 2012;76(4): 911–3.

56. Mutignani M, Seerden T, Tringali A, Feisal D, Perri V, Familiari P, Costamagna G. Endoscopic hemostasis with fibrin glue for refractory postsphincterotomy and

postpapillectomy bleeding. Gastrointest Endosc. 2010;71(4):856–60.

57. Saeed M, Kadir S, Kaufman SL, Murray RR, Milligan F, Cotton PB. Bleeding following endoscopic sphincterotomy: angiographic management by transcatheter embolization. Gastrointest Endosc. 1989;35(4): 300–3.

58. Jersek M, Vracko J. Sphincterotomy of Oddi's muscle through posterior distal duodenum: a modified technique with low morbidity and mortality. Hepatogastroenterology. 1996;43(8):377–80.

59. Makary MA, Elariny HA. Laparoscopic transduodenal sphincteroplasty. J Laparoendosc Adv Surg Tech A. 2006;16(6):629–32.

60. Sulkowski U, Kautz G, Nottberg H, Förster E. [Surgical therapy of hemorrhage after endoscopic sphincterotomy. Indications and technique]. Chirurg. 1996;67(1):26–31.

61. Stapfer M, Selby RR, Stain SC, Katkhouda N, Parekh D, Jabbour N, Garry D. Management of duodenal perforation after endoscopic retrograde cholangiopancreatography and sphincterotomy. Ann Surg. 2000; 232(2):191–8.

62. Assalia A, Suissa A, Ilivitzki A, Mahajna A, Yassin K, Hashmonai M, Krausz MM. Validity of clinical criteria in the management of endoscopic retrograde cholangiopancreatography related duodenal perforations. Arch Surg. 2007;142(11):1059–64.

63. Genzlinger JL, McPhee MS, Fisher JK, Jacob KM, Helzberg JH. Significance of retroperitoneal air after endoscopic retrograde cholangiopancreatography with sphincterotomy. Am J Gastroenterol. 1999;94(5):1267–70.

64. Pannu HK, Fishman EK. Complications of endoscopic retrograde cholangiopancreatography: spectrum of abnormalities demonstrated with CT. Radiographics. 2001;21(6):1441–53.

65. Machado NO. Management of duodenal perforation post-endoscopic retrograde cholangiopancreatography. When and whom to operate and what factors determine the outcome? A review article. JOP. 2012;13(1):18–25.

66. Avgerinos DV, Llaguna OH, Lo AY, Voli J, Leitman IM. Management of endoscopic retrograde cholangiopancreatography: related duodenal perforations. Surg Endosc. 2009;23(4):833–8.

67. Preetha M, Chung Y-FA, Chan W-H, Ong H-S, Chow PKH, Wong W-K, Ooi LLPJ, Soo K-C. Surgical management of endoscopic retrograde cholangiopancreatography-related perforations. ANZ J Surg. 2003;73(12):1011–4.

68. Wu HM, Dixon E, May GR, Sutherland FR. Management of perforation after endoscopic retrograde cholangiopancreatography (ERCP): a population-based review. HPB (Oxford). 2006; 8(5):393–9.

69. Knudson K, Raeburn CD, McIntyre RC, Shah RJ, Shaw RJ, Chen YK, Brown WR, Stiegmann G. Management of duodenal and pancreaticobiliary perforations associated with periampullary endoscopic procedures. Am J Surg. 2008;196(6):975–81. discussion 981–2.

70. Warren J, Hardy D, MacFadyen Jr B. Management of endoscopic complications. In: Principles of flexible endoscopy for surgeons. New York: Springer; 2013. p. 227.

71. Fukino N, Oida T, Kawasaki A, Mimatsu K, Kuboi Y, Kano H, Amano S. Impaction of a lithotripsy basket during endoscopic lithotomy of a common bile duct stone. World J Gastroenterol. 2010;16(22):2832–4.

72. Cid JA, Lobo DN. Impacted biliary basket. Gastrointest Endosc. 2005;61(1):110–1.

73. Schutz SM, Chinea C, Friedrichs P. Successful endoscopic removal of a severed, impacted Dormia basket. Am J Gastroenterol. 1997;92(4):679–81.

74. Attila T, May GR, Kortan P. Nonsurgical management of an impacted mechanical lithotriptor with fractured traction wires: endoscopic intracorporeal electrohydraulic shock wave lithotripsy followed by extra-endoscopic mechanical lithotripsy. Can J Gastroenterol. 2008;22(8):699–702.

75. Pruitt A, Schutz SM, Baron T, McClendon D, Lang KA. Fractured hydrophilic guidewire during ERCP: a case series. Gastrointest Endosc. 1998;48(1):77–80.

76. Subramaniam N, Kudari AK, Naik BM. Complications of endoscopic retrograde cholangiopancreatography requiring surgical intervention: one-year experience in a tertiary care centre. J Surg. 2015;3(1):12–6.

77. Silviera ML, Seamon MJ, Porshinsky B, Prosciak MP, Doraiswamy VA, Wang CF, Lorenzo M, Truitt M, Biboa J, Jarvis AM, Narula VK, Steinberg SM, Stawicki SP. Complications related to endoscopic retrograde cholangiopancreatography: a comprehensive clinical review. J Gastrointestin Liver Dis. 2009;18(1):73–82.

Teresa S. Jones and Vimal K. Narula

Introduction

Morbid obesity and rapid weight loss are two well known risk factors for the development of gall-stones. Bariatric surgery and the resultant weight loss increase the frequency of gallstones from 6 to 9 % to 30–53 % [1]. The mechanism for the increase in gallstone development is multifactorial and includes altered bile composition (increased cholesterol saturation and mucin), decreased gall-bladder motility and stimulation as well as vagal nerve disruption [2]. Symptomatic gallstones are more likely to occur in female patients who lose 25 % or more of their excess body weight in the first 3 months. This risk returns to baseline as weight loss slows. Cholecystectomy is needed postoperatively in 7–15 % of these patients (com-pared to 3 % in the normal population) [3].

Choledocholithiasis is found in 15 % of all patients with cholelithiasis and can be managed via Endoscopic Retrograde Cholangiopancreatography (ERCP) following gastric banding or gastric sleeve procedures. However, the Roux-en-Y gastric bypass (RYGB) and the duodenal switch (DS) create long mal-absorptive limbs that are not easily traversed for endoscopic intervention (Fig. 15.1a, b). Biliary access can be created at the time of surgery in patients who are expected to need future proce-dures (i.e., primary hepatolithiasis, known biliary stricture, etc.). This can be done via gastropexy of the gastric remnant, gastrostomy placement in the gastric remnant or tunneling of a limb of jejunum in the sub-fascial plane for future percutaneous or endoscopic access [4, 5]. Alternative techniques for the management of choledocholithiasis after RYGB or DS include balloon enteroscopy with ERCP, transgastric ERCP, surgical (laparoscopic or open) bile duct explorations, and percutaneous transhepatic cholangiography.

Prevention

Due to high complexity of the techniques required to treat gallstones and their complications after RYGB, there has been significant interest in pre-vention. In the early days of bariatric surgery, many centers practiced routine cholecystectomy. This practice increased operative time during laparoscopic RYGB by 20 min but did not alter

T.S. Jones, M.D. (✉)
Department of Surgery, The Ohio State University
Wexner Medical Center, Columbus, OH, USA
e-mail: Teresa.Jones@OSUMC.edu

V.K. Narula, M.D.
Department of Surgery, The Ohio State University
Wexner Medical Center, N 724 Doan Hall, 410 West
10th Avenue, Columbus, OH 43210, USA
e-mail: raaja.narula@osumc.edu

© Springer International Publishing Switzerland 2016
J.W. Hazey et al. (eds.), *Multidisciplinary Management of Common Bile Duct Stones*,
DOI 10.1007/978-3-319-22765-8_15

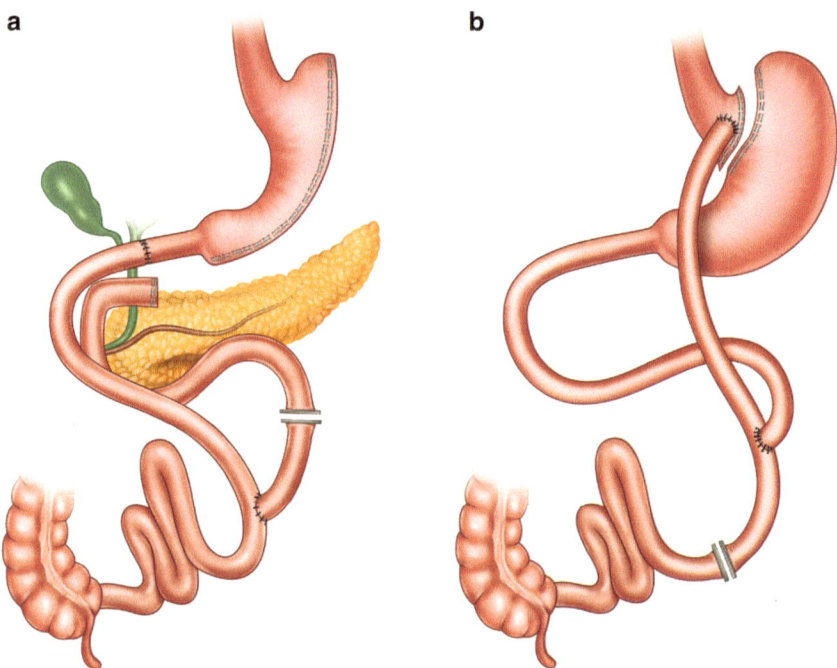

Fig. 15.1 (**a**) Dudodenal switch anatomy; (**b**) Roux-en-Y gastric bypass anatomy

morbidity or hospital length of stay [6]. Unfortunately, there remains no consensus in the bariatric literature with regard to prophylactic cholecystectomy and centers are advised to make decisions based upon their own experience [7–9].

An alternative to the surgical removal of the gallbladder is postoperative gallstone chemoprophylaxis. Ursodeoxycholic acid inhibits biliary cholesterol crystallization. Randomized control trials have shown that ursodeoxycholic acid following any type of bariatric surgery can significantly decrease the rate of gallstone formation [10, 11]. Many centers now practice routine administration of this medication for 3–6 months during the highest risk period following bariatric surgery in order to reduce the incidence of gallbladder-related complications.

In patients who develop symptomatic gallbladder disease (with or without chemoprophylaxis), laparoscopic cholecystectomy can still be done following laparoscopic RYGB. However, the management of choledocholithiasis is significantly more difficult and requires specialized techniques

and personnel. The specific techniques are discussed below and are generally performed at large referral centers.

Techniques to Treat Choledocholithiasis After Weight Reduction Surgery

ERCP via Balloon Enteroscopy

In order to access the biliary system after RYGB or DS, an endoscope must traverse the roux limb of jejunum (75–150 cm in length), cross the jejuno-jejunal anastomosis and travel retrograde through the bilio-pancreatic limb (30–40 cm) to the ampulla of Vater. Traversing this distance is not achievable with a standard side-viewing endoscope. Specialized endoscopes utilizing single- or double-balloons and overtubes have proven successful at "telescoping" the small intestine onto the endoscope and traveling up to 270 cm. This technique remains challenging; success rates of ERCP with double balloon enteroscopy in RYGB patients remain at 39–66 % [12]. Long Roux limbs (>100 cm) and sharp angulation of the intestine at the jejuno-jejunal anastomosis contribute to the difficulty of this procedure. Even after achieving access, there are few ERCP instruments long enough to be used with these enteroscopes. The double lumen enteroscope has a working length of 200 cm, compared to 103 cm in a standard ERCP duodenoscope. Additionally, the double lumen enteroscope does not have an elevator, limiting the ability to access and manipulate perpendicular to the scope.

Transgastric ERCP

An alternative to traversing both the malabsorptive segment and biliopancreatic limb of a RYGB is to access the gastric remnant via a percutaneous or laparoscopically created gastrostomy. Transgastric ERCP after RYGB was first reported in 1998 by Baron and Vickers [13]. This technique was initially performed via an open gastrostomy followed by ERCP through the gastrostomy 2 weeks later. As comfort with laparoscopy increased, laparoscopic-assisted transgastric ERCP has replaced open gastrotomy/gastrostomy [14]. The technique involves the creation of a laparoscopic gastrotomy with a 15 mm laparoscopic port through which the ERCP scope is introduced [15] (Figs. 15.2 and 15.3).

Biliary access can then be performed with a standard ERCP scope and equipment under the same general anesthetic. Once the ERCP is complete, the gastrotomy can be closed with suture or laparoscopic staples. If the patient has a high likelihood of requiring repeat ERCPs, a 24 fr gastrostomy tube can be placed in the site of the 15 mm trocar to maintain access. If access is required within 6 weeks, the gastric remnant should be secured to the abdominal wall via laparoscopic suture.

In lieu of going to the operating room for a laparoscopic-assisted procedure, a gastrostomy can be created percutaneously (with radiographic assistance) and the fistula tract matured for 4–6 weeks. This tract can then accessed with a pediatric side-viewing duodenoscope or dilated to permit a standard ERCP scope [16]. Due to the delay for tract maturation and dilation, urgent biliary decompression should not be attempted in this manner.

Both techniques of access via the remnant stomach can result in high rates of successful cannulation. The largest series of patients to undergo trans-gastric ERCP reported successful ampullary cannulation 93 % of the time regardless of the technique of gastric access (percutaneous gastrostomy or laparoscopic-assisted gastrotomy) [17]. In this series of 85 ERCPs, there was a 19 % complication rate with 88 % of those complications related to access. Most complications were minor and only two required operative intervention.

Fig. 15.2 Laparoscopic gastrotomy for transgastric ERCP. Two stay sutures (*long arrows*) are placed on either side of the planned gastrotomy site which is entered with electrocautery (*short arrow*)

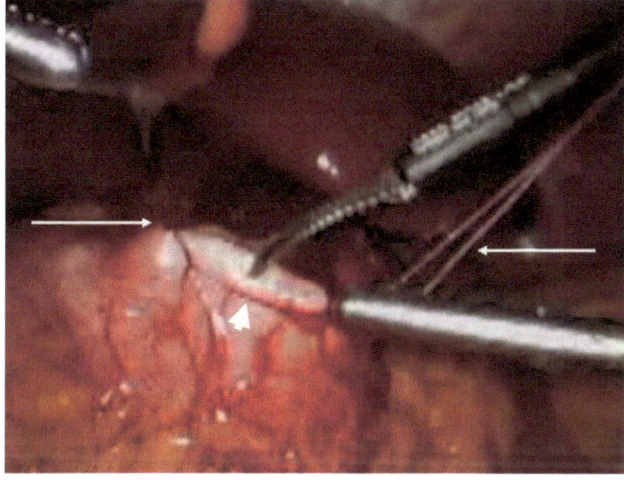

Fig. 15.3 Laparoscopic transgastric port placement. A 15 mm laparscopic port is placed through the abdominal wall and into the stomach to permit introduction of the duodenoscope

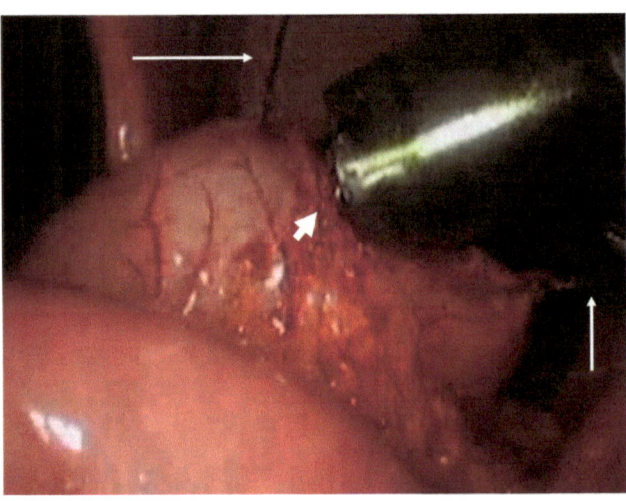

An added benefit of the laparoscopic-assisted approach is the ability to assist with difficult cannulations via a laparoscopic rendezvous technique. This is done by laparoscopic insertion of a guidewire into the common bile duct (or via the cystic duct stump) that is passed antegrade through the ampulla of Vater and into the duodenum (Fig. 15.4). This wire can then be grasped by the endoscopist to facilitate cannulation.

Laparoscopic Biliary Access

Despite concerns about the reoperative field, laparoscopic cholecystectomy can be performed without added morbidity after laparoscopic RYGB. Similarly, there are no anatomic alterations that prohibit laparoscopic common bile duct exploration. First reported in 1991, laparoscopic common bile duct exploration can be performed through the cystic duct stump or a choledochotomy [18]. Concomitant fluoroscopy and/or choledochoscopy is then used to remove stones via saline flush, Fogarty balloon catheterization, basket extraction, extracorporeal shockwave lithotripsy (ESWL), electrohydraulic lithotripsy (EHL), or holmium:YAG laser [19]. Success rates of stone clearance with laparoscopic common bile duct exploration are comparable to ERCP and have the benefit of avoiding the risks and cost of a second anesthetic [20].

In patients with a stone impacted at the ampulla or who have numerous (>15) stones, open common bile duct exploration can be the most successful at duct clearance. A minimally invasive alternative, laparoscopic choledochoduodenostomy, has recently been reported in a series of 11 patients after RYGB [21]. The technique includes a longitudinal choledochotomy followed by stone removal via methods discussed above. Once complete, a duodenotomy is created in the first portion of the duodenum and, using intracorporeal sutures, a side-to-side choledochoduodenostomy is created. No cases of stone recurrence were reported and only one patient suffered a postoperative bile leak.

Percutaneous Radiographic Biliary Access

Percutaneous transhepatic biliary access has been highly successful in cases of RYGB and other anatomic variations when ERCP cannot be accomplished [22]. Transhepatic access does require biliary dilation in order to initially access the bile ducts but, once accessed, a complete range of instruments are available for duct clearance, including standard Fogarty balloons, baskets, EHL and ESWL. A 7 French choledochoscope can also be inserted via the transhepatic sheath for direct visualization and treatment of biliary

Fig. 15.4 Laparoscopic transcystic rendezvous ERCP. A guidewire is placed place laparoscopically through the cystic or common bile duct and travels antegrade through the ampulla of Vater to assist in biliary cannulation via the duodenoscope

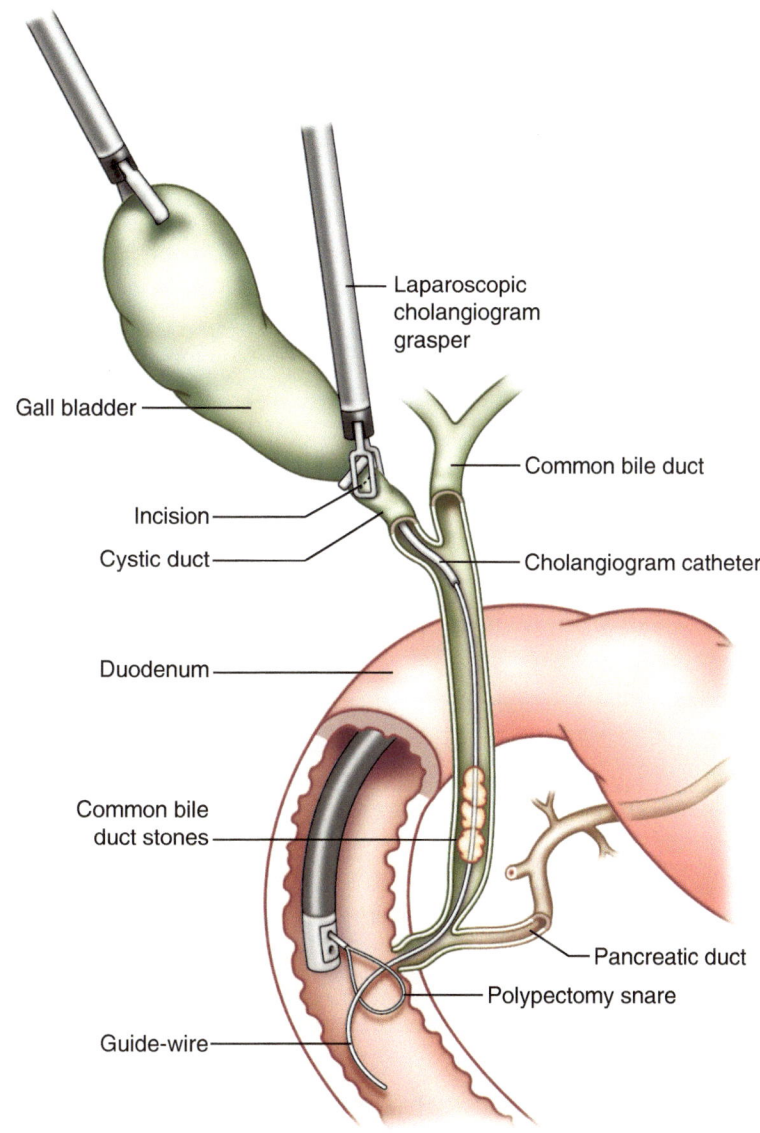

Laparoscopic cholangiogram grasper

Gall bladder

Common bile duct

Incision

Cystic duct

Cholangiogram catheter

Duodenum

Common bile duct stones

Pancreatic duct

Polypectomy snare

Guide-wire

obstruction. This requires dilation of the tract to at least 12 French but allows for the use of standard instruments as well as the holmium:YAG laser and EHL to clear stones even in the proximal hepatic ducts [23].

Percutaenous jejunal access for ERCP has also been described. This technique most frequently occurs in patients with a "Hutson loop": intentional tunneling of jejunum in the subfascial plane of the abdominal wall during their bariatric procedure to provide biliary access [24]. This type of access can provide long-term biliary access in patients who are expected to require frequent biliary intervention (hepatolithiasis, biliary stricture, primary lithiasis).

Conclusions

Following bariatric surgery, patients are at an increased risk of gallstone formation and subsequent common bile duct stones. Patients who have undergone sleeve gastrectomy or placement of a restrictive gastric band can be managed in the standard fashion with ERCP. Patients who have undergone a Roux-en-Y gastric bypass or a duodenal switch require specialized techniques to treat their common bile duct stones. These complex techniques require specialized equipment and training and are typically performed at large referral centers. The selection of the preferred technique is dependent upon the available expertise and urgency of biliary intervention.

References

1. Tsirline VB, Keilani ZM, El Djouzi S, Phillips RC, Kuwada TS, Gersin K, Simms C, Stefanidis D. How frequently and when do patients undergo cholecystectomy after bariatric surgery? Surg Obes Relat Dis. 2014;10(2):313–21. doi:10.1016/j.soard.2013.10.011.

2. Li VK, Pulido N, Fajnwaks P, Szomstein S, Rosenthal R, Martinez-Duartez P. Predictors of gallstone formation after bariatric surgery: a multivariate analysis of risk factors comparing gastric bypass, gastric banding, and sleeve gastrectomy. Surg Endosc. 2009;23(7):1640–4. doi:10.1007/s00464-008-0204-6.

3. Everhart JE, Khare M, Hill M, Maurer KR. Prevalence and ethnic differences in gallbladder disease in the United States. Gastroenterology. 1999;117(3):632–9.

4. Hutson DG, Russell E, Schiff E, Levi JJ, Jeffers L, Zeppa R. Balloon dilatation of biliary strictures through a choledochojejuno-cutaneous fistula. Ann Surg. 1984;199(6):637–47.

5. Amitha Vikrama KS, Keshava SN, Surendrababu NR, Moses V, Joseph P, Vyas F, Sitaram VJ. Jejunal access loop cholangiogram and intervention using image guided access. Med Imaging Radiat Oncol. 2010;54(1):5–8. doi:10.1111/j.1754-9485.2010.02130.x.

6. Kim J, Schirmer B. Safety and efficacy of simultaneous cholecystectomy at Roux-en-Y gastric bypass. Surg Obes Relat Dis. 2009;5:48–53.

7. Mason EE, Renquist KE. Gallbladder management in obesity surgery. Obes Surg. 2002;12(2):222–9.

8. Swartz DE, Feliz EK. Elective cholecystectomy after Roux-en-Y gastric bypass: why should asymptomatic gallstones be treated differently in morbidly obese patients? Surg Obes Relat Dis. 2005;1:555–60.

9. Patel KR, White SC, Tejirian T, et al. Gallbladder management during laparoscopic Roux-en-Y gastric bypass surgery: routine preoperative screening for gallstones and postoperative prophylactic medical treatment are not necessary. Am Surg. 2006;72:857–61.

10. Sugarman HJ, Brewer WH, Shiffman ML, et al. A multicenter, placebo-controlled, randomized, double-blind, prospective trial of prophylactic ursodiol for the prevention of gallstone formation following gastric bypass induced rapid weight loss. Am J Surg. 1995;169:91–6.

11. Miller K, Hell E, Lang B, et al. Gallstone formation prophylaxis after gastric restrictive procedures for weight loss. Ann Surg. 2003;238:697–702.

12. Grover BT, Kothari SN. Biliary issues in the bariatric population. Surg Clin North Am. 2014;94(2):413–25. doi:10.1016/j.suc.2014.01.003.

13. Baron TH, Vickers SM. Surgical gastrostomy placement as access for diagnostic and therapeutic ERCP. Gastrointest Endosc. 1998;22:640–1.

14. Peters M, Papsavas PK, Caushak PF, et al. Laparoscopic transgastric endoscopic retrograde cholangiopancreatography for benign common bile duct stricture after Roux-en-Y gastric bypass. Surg Endosc. 2002;16:1106.

15. Facchiano E, Quartararo G, Pavoni V, et al. Laparoscopic-assisted transgastric endoscopic retrograde cholangiopancreatography (ERCP) after Roux-en-Y gastric bypass: technical features. Obes Surg. 2014;25:373.

16. Richardson JF, Lee JG, Smith BR, Nguyen B, Pham KP, Nguyen NT. Laparoscopic transgastric endoscopy after Roux-en-Y gastric bypass: case series and review of the literature. Am Surg. 2012;78(10):1182–6.

17. Grimes KL, Maciel VH, Mata W, et al. Complications of laparoscopic transgastric ERCP in patients with Roux-en-Y gastric bypass. Surg Endosc. 2015;29:1753.

18. Koc B, Karahan S, Adas G, et al. Comparison of laparoscopic common bile duct exploration and endoscopic retrograde cholangiopancreatography plus laparoscopic cholecystectomy for choledocholithiasis: a prospective randomized study. Am J Surg. 2013;206:457–63.

19. Buxbaum J. Modern management of common bile duct stones. Gastrointest Endosc Clin N Am. 2013;23(2):251–75. doi:10.1016/j.giec.2012.12.003.

20. Dasari BV, Tan CJ, Gurusamy KS, Martin DJ, Kirk G, McKie L, Diamond T, Taylor MA. Surgical versus endoscopic treatment of bile duct stones. Cochrane Database Syst Rev 2013; 9: CD003327. doi:10.1002/14651858.CD003327.pub3

21. Ducoin C, Moon RC, Teixeira AF, et al. Laparoscopic choledochoduodenostomy as an alternate treatment for common bile duct stones after Roux-en-Y gastric bypass. Surg Obes Relat Dis. 2014;10:647–53.

22. Ozcan N, Kahriman G, Mavili E. Percutaneous transhepatic removal of bile duct stones: results in 261 patients. Cardiovasc Intervent Radiol. 2012;35:621–7.

23. Hazey JW, McCreary M, Guy G, Melvin WS. Efficacy of percutaneous treatment of biliary tract calculi using the holmium: YAG laser. Surg Endosc. 2007; 21(7):1180–3.

24. Fonetin DB, Gibson RN, Collier NA. Two decades of percutaneous transjejunal biliary intervention for benign biliary disease: a review of the intervention nature and complication. Insights Imaging. 2011;5:557–65.

Management of Choledocholithiasis in the Cirrhotic Patient

16

Eliza W. Beal and Sylvester M. Black

Introduction

Common bile duct stones (choledocholithiasis) are one of the most common manifestations of cholelithiasis. The consequences of common bile duct stones can be significant and include gallstone pancreatitis, septic cholangitis, and secondary biliary cirrhosis [1].

The presence of gallstones in patients with cirrhosis is higher than in the general population with rates reported to be between 23.3 and 38 % [2, 3]. The calculated annual incidence is 3.4 % [2]. The total prevalence of cirrhosis between 1999 and 2010 in the USA is 0.27 % with peak prevalence between 45 and 54 years old and increasing incidence with increasing age [4]. This corresponds to greater than 600,000 adults in the USA living with cirrhosis [4].

The Child–Turcotte–Pugh (CTP) score (Table 16.1) is one of the most common scoring systems used to predict operative risk and prognosis in patients with chronic liver disease. The CTP score was initially designed to predict outcomes in patients with cirrhosis undergoing por-

tacaval shunts and esophageal transection for bleeding related to portal hypertension. The CTP score uses five clinical measures of liver disease: total bilirubin, prothrombin time (PT) or international normalized ratio (INR), ascites, and hepatic encephalopathy [5]. In one of the early studies, which looked at 38 patients undergoing ligation of bleeding esophageal varices, class A patients had 71 % 6-month survival, class B had 36 % 6-month survival and there were no survivors at 6-months in the class C group. The authors concluded that, "in grade C the results were so poor that operation on such patients does not seem justified unless there is a clear additional and reversible factor which may partially account for the poor liver function." [6].

Garrison et al., in a study of cirrhotic patients undergoing laparotomy for nonshunt abdominal procedures, reported 10 % mortality for CTP class A patients, 31 % for CTP class B patients and 76 % for CTP class C patients [7]. In a review of mortality rates after a variety of abdominal procedures, Mansour et al. report 10 % mortality for CTP class A patients, 30 % for CTP class B patients and 82 % for CTP class C patients [8].

Clinical factors that have been shown to be associated with increased mortality rate in cirrhotic patients with choledocholithiasis include: total bilirubin >5, serum glutamic oxalacetic transaminase level greater than 100 units, PT <40 %, platelet count <100,000, CTP class C classification, nonsuppurative cholangitis or

E.W. Beal, M.D. • S.M. Black, M.D., Ph.D. (✉)
Department of General Surgery, The Ohio State University Wexner Medical Center,
395 W. 12th Ave. Suite 150, Columbus, OH 43210, USA
e-mail: sylvester.black@osumc.edu

© Springer International Publishing Switzerland 2016
J.W. Hazey et al. (eds.), *Multidisciplinary Management of Common Bile Duct Stones*,
DOI 10.1007/978-3-319-22765-8_16

Table 16.1 Child–Turcotte–Pugh (CTP) Score [5]

	Points[a]		
	1	2	3
Encephalopathy	None	Grade 1–2 (or precipitant induced)	Grade 3–4 (or chronic)
Ascites	None	Mild/moderate (diuretic responsive)	Severe (diuretic resistance)
Bilirubin (mg/dL)	<2	2–3	>3
Albumin (g/dL)	>3.5	2.8–3.5	<2.8
PT (sec prolonged) or	<4 or <1.7	4–6 or 1.7–2.3	>6 or >2.3

[a]CTP score is obtained by adding the score for each parameter. Class A = 5–6 points, Class B = 7–9 points, Class C = 10–15 points

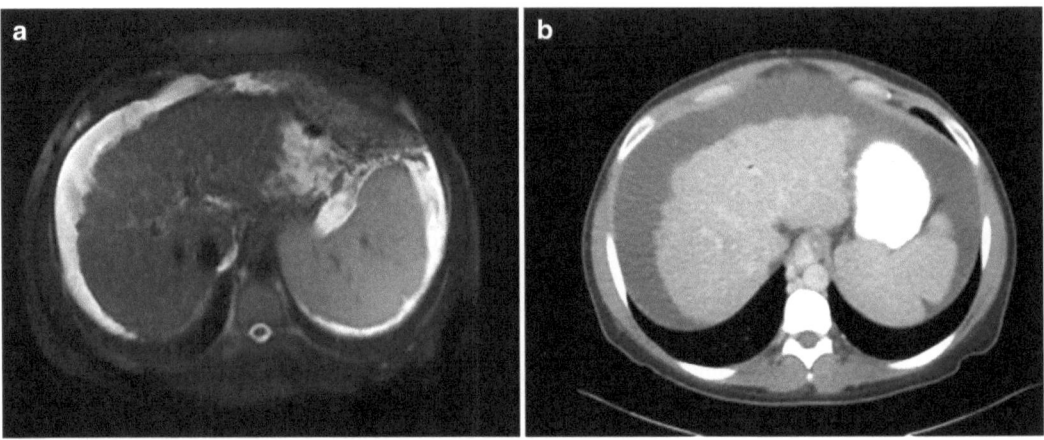

Fig. 16.1 44-year-old female patient with change in the liver consistent with cirrhosis including nodularity and ascites on magnetic resonance imaging (MRI) (**a**) and computed tomography (CT) (**b**)

acute obstructive suppurative cholangitis, and emergency surgery or emergency endoscopic retrograde cholangiopancreatography (ERCP) with endoscopic sphincterotomy (ES) [9].

The diagnosis and management of choledocholithiasis in patients with cirrhosis presents a unique challenge. Liver dysfunction requires expert perioperative management. It may result in prolonged duration of action of anesthetic agents and requires avoidance of anesthetic agents that may precipitate hepatic encephalopathy [10]. Cirrhotic patients undergoing surgery are at risk for hepatic decompensation with worsening or new ascites, upper GI bleeding, worsening or new acute renal failure, hepatorenal syndrome, liver failure, coagulopathy, increased prothrombin time, increased partial thromboplastin time [10]. Cirrhotic patients are also at risk for surgical wound complications including infection, dehiscence, eventration, fistula, abscess, bleeding, and more general complications including pneumonia, Acute Respiratory Distress Syndrome (ARDS),

ventilation dependence, chronic obstructive pulmonary disease (COPD), chronic heart failure, arrhythmia, myocardial infarction, urinary tract infections, paralytic ileus, phlebitis/PE, and death [10]. Additionally, ERCP with ES, which is the most commonly performed intervention for choledocholithiasis, has special risks in cirrhotic patients. It has been demonstrated that cirrhosis is a known risk factor for overall complications of ERCP, may be associated with hemorrhage after ES, but is not thought to be associated with post-ERCP pancreatitis [11].

Diagnosis

Clinical exam, laboratory studies, imaging studies including ultrasound, computed tomography (CT), and magnetic resonance cholangiopancreatography (MRCP) are used in the diagnosis of choledocholithiasis in patients with cirrhosis (Fig. 16.1). In addition, endoscopic retrograde cholangiopancreatography (ERCP) can be both diagnostic and therapeutic for patients with common bile duct stones.

Patients are diagnosed with cirrhosis based on clinical exam, nodular macroscopic appearance of the liver (noted for example during abdominal surgery), previous liver biopsy interpretation, a radiological exam revealing a liver with an irregular contour or clinical findings characteristic of decompensated liver disease in a patient with risk factors for cirrhosis [11].

Due to the potential complications of ERCP it is important to use appropriate imaging to assess high-risk patients prior to undertaking an invasive procedure. Imaging studies that have been shown to be useful to diagnose common bile duct stones include magnetic resonance MRCP and endoscopic ultrasound (EUS). In the general population it has been demonstrated that MRCP and EUS have sensitivities and specificities for identifying common bile duct stones comparable to ERCP and intraoperative cholangiogram in the general patient population [12, 13]. In a single center study in patients with suspected choledocholithiasis, Prat et al. demonstrated that EUS had a sensitivity of 93 %, specificity of 97 %, positive predictive value of 98 %, and negative predictive value of 88 % [12]. However, EUS is an invasive procedure with its' own complications and this study did not specifically focus on patients with cirrhosis. In another small, single center study, Laokpessi et al. demonstrated that the sensitivity of magnetic resonance cholangiopancreatography was 93 % and specificity was 100 % [13].

Treatment

Prior to invasive intervention cirrhotic patients should be medically optimized, which may include hyperalimentation, fresh frozen plasma, vitamin K, diuretics, antibiotics for malnutrition, coagulopathy, ascites, and cholangitis. Management may be continued after treatment of common bile duct stones as needed [9]. Bleeding with endoscopic sphincterotomy (ES) can be avoided with correction of coagulopathy (INR < 1.5) with FFP and/or vitamin K and appropriate platelet count (>50,000) [14].

There are both endoscopic and surgical treatment options for choledocholithiasis in cirrhotic patients. Endoscopic treatment options include endoscopic retrograde cholangiopancreatography (ERCP) with ES, which is the gold standard for removing common bile duct stones in the general population, mechanical lithotripsy and stent placement, laser and electrohydraulic stone fragmentation, and endoscopic papillary dilation [1, 15, 16].

Although endoscopic management is more commonly undertaken, there is still a role for surgical management in the case of complicated choledocholithiasis, altered intestinal anatomy and failure of endoscopic management. Surgical options include: cholecystectomy with choledochotomy and T-tube placement or choleodochotomy with T-tube placement, and open common bile duct exploration [9, 16, 17].

Surgical Treatment Options

Reported mortality rates for patients with cirrhosis undergoing surgery are between 8.3 and 25 % depending on source, in comparison to 1.1 % for non-cirrhotic patients. The range of mortality rate reported depends on several factors including severity of liver disease, type of surgery, demographics of patient population in included in the study, expertise of healthcare team and bias [10].

Surgical options for treatment of choledocholithiasis in general include laparoscopic or open cholecystectomy with choledochotomy and T-tube placement or choledochotomy with T-tube placement and open common bile duct exploration [9, 17].

Laparoscopic Common Bile Duct Exploration

Laparoscopic common bile duct exploration has become the gold standard in patients in whom endoscopic retrograde cholangiopancreatography (ERCP) is unsuccessful. Qiu et al. assessed the feasibility and safety of laparoscopic common bile duct exploration in choledocholithiasis patients with well-compensated cirrhosis (CTP class A and B). In comparing cirrhotic patients to non-cirrhotic patients undergoing laparoscopic common bile duct exploration at their institution, there was no significant difference in mean operation time (2.1 h vs. 1.9 h, $p=0.07$), complication rates (10.6 vs 8.8, $p=0.6$), mean hospital stay (4.2 vs. 4.0, $p=0.6$), conversion rate (5.3 vs. 6.1 $p=0.77$), and retained choledocholithiasis rate (8.3 vs. 7.1, $p=0.65$). They did not encounter mortality in either group. There was a significant difference in blood loss ($p<0.01$). The authors concluded that laparoscopic common bile duct exploration is a feasible, effective and safe surgical procedure for choledocholithiasis in patients with compensated cirrhosis. There was also no difference in analgesic requirements or visual analog scale pain score. Transcystic stone extraction can be performed, without requiring external biliary drainage, or by choledochotomy with T-tube placement [17].

Endoscopic Treatment Options

The gold standard for removing common bile duct stones in the general population is endoscopic retrograde cholangiopancreatography (ERCP) with endoscopic sphincterotomy (ES) [1, 15]. Other endoscopic treatment options include mechanical lithotripsy, stent placement, laser and electrohydraulic stone fragmentation and endoscopic papillary balloon dilation (EPBD) [1, 16].

In an analysis of the use of ERCP for common bile duct stones in liver cirrhosis, Li et al. noted that there was not a statistically significant difference in success rate of selective biliary cannulation, bile duct clearance rate or post-ERCP pancreatitis between cirrhotic and non-cirrhotic patients. They included patients who underwent ES, EPBD and mechanical lithotripsy. They noted that CTP class C patients had a statistically significant higher rate of hemorrhage than non-cirrhotic patients [18].

Endoscopic Retrograde Cholangiopancreatography (ERCP) with Endoscopic Sphincterotomy (ES)

The gold standard for removing common bile duct stones in the general population is endoscopic retrograde cholangiopancreatography (ERCP) with endoscopic sphincterotomy (ES) [1, 15]. The use of this procedure in patients with cirrhosis has been studied (Fig. 16.2). Initial concerns with its use in patients with cirrhosis related to its potential to cause sepsis or hemorrhage [14]. Risk factors for increased bleeding with ES in patients with cirrhosis include advanced Child stage and coagulopathy [14]. Cirrhosis is a well-known risk factor for overall complications of ERCP [14]. Overall morbidity and mortality of cirrhotic patients undergoing ERCP was 12.5–50 and 0–22 % and the most common associated complication is bleeding [14]. Factors associated with bleeding in cirrhotic patients include: coagulopathy, thrombocytopenia, portal hypertension, advanced Child stage [14]. Bleeding associated with ES can be treated with heat probe coagulation or epinephrine injection [14].

Prat et al. completed a large retrospective study of 52 patients who underwent endoscopic sphincterotomy between 1988 and 1993. Prat et al. report that there was no difference in morbidity and mortality in cirrhotic patients undergoing ES and age-sex and disease-matched controls [19]. Prat et al. report that portal hypertension, coagulopathy and Child–Pugh status do not influence the incidence of post-ES complications [19]. Prat et al. report that the four early deaths in their study occurred in patients with class C cirrhosis [19]. Prat et al. conclude that, "ES is a potential alternative to biliary surgery in Child Class A and B patients, and the preferred choice for Child C patients with life-threatening biliary obstruction." [19].

Cirrhosis does not increase risk of postprocedure pancreatitis [9, 11, 16, 19, 20]. Prophylactic antibiotics are recommended in all studies [9, 11, 16, 19, 20].

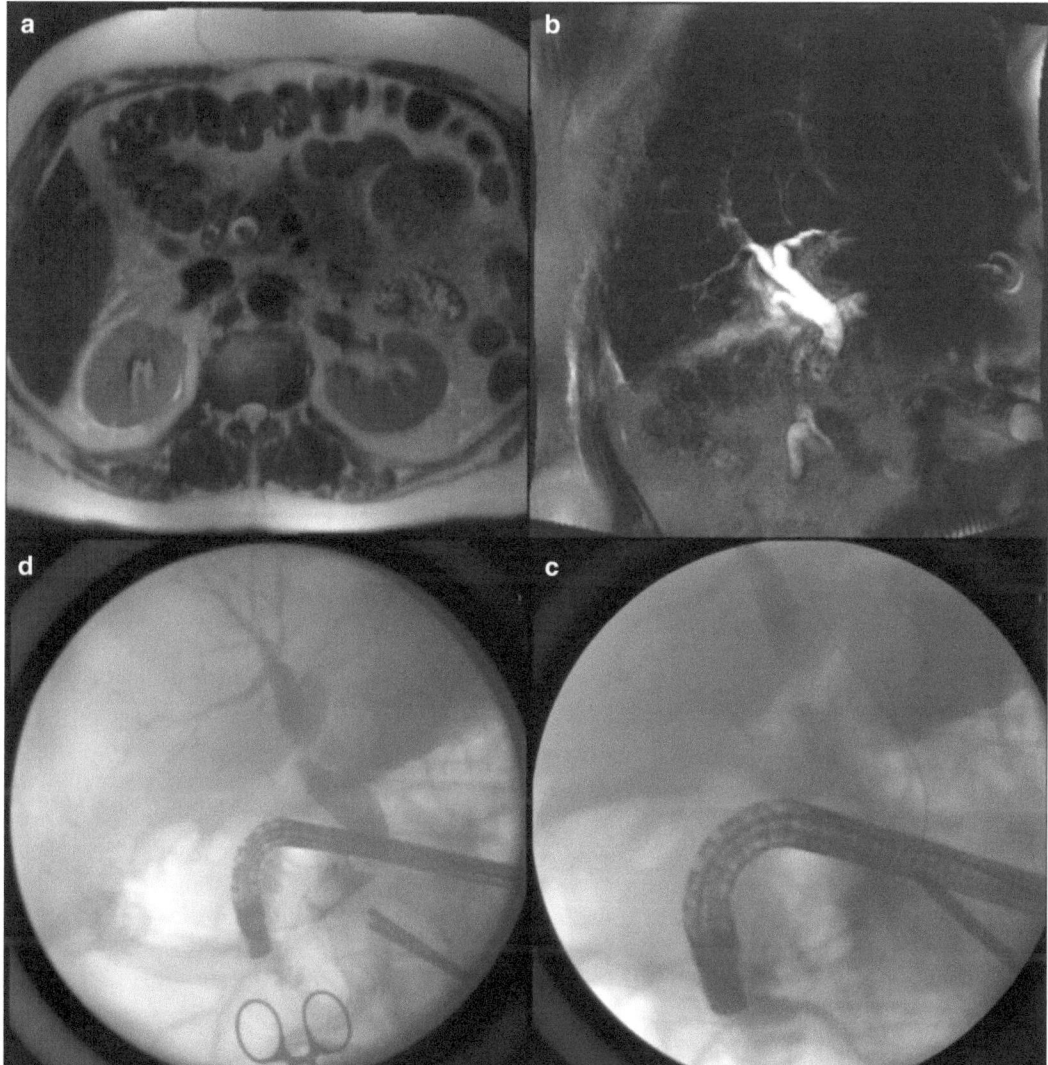

Fig. 16.2 57 year old male patient with history of roux-en-y gastric bypass and early alcoholic cirrhosis presented with pancreatitis and MRCP consistent with choledocholithiasis (**a, b**). The patient underwent cholecystectomy with intraoperative cholangiogram and then transgastric endoscopic retrograde cholangiopancreatography with removal of a common duct stone (**c, d**)

ES is performed with high-frequency alternating current passing through papillary tissue producing coagulation and/or cutting, using one or more of three types of current: pure cut, coagulation, and mixed current. Alternating current provides alternating cutting and coagulation phases and in a database study completed in Turkey,

Parlak et al. report that patients with cirrhosis who underwent endoscopic sphincterotomy with alternating mixed current in pulse-cut mode had bleeding associated with their ES less often than those who underwent ES with blended current [13]. Pulse cut and blended current are forms of mixed current. In blended, both cutting and coagulation wave-forms are delivered together in one waveform. In pulse cut they are alternated in short bursts with an intermittent pause [13].

Suprapapillary puncture (SPP) might be safer than standard cannulation techniques for ES in cirrhotic patients or other patients with coagulopathy [21]. Suprapapillary puncture is an alternative technique for accessing and treating conditions of the biliary tree. In suprapapillary puncture a transmural puncture of the distal common bile duct through the roof of the major ampulla using a modified needle catheter ("Artifon Catheter") is performed [21]. The same group has reported low rates of bleeding and post-ERCP pancreatitis with this technique. Artifon et al. compared 42 patients who underwent suprapapillary puncture (SPP) to a control group of 63 patients undergoing standard cannulation (SC). There was no significant difference in complications between the two groups. SPP was also shown to be a cost effective alternative. The authors concluded that, "SPP is a safe and effective technique for the management of common bile duct stones in decompensated cirrhotic patients. Conditional to the willingness-to-pay and to the local ERCP-related costs, SPP is also a cost-effective alternative to the SC methods. SPP is associated with a lower rate of complications but larger studies to validate these findings are necessary." [21] In previously reported studies the authors noted that complications were lower in the SPP group, including post-ERCP pancreatitis and bleeding [22–24]. In cirrhotic patients undergoing procedures for choledocholithiasis there was a lower overall rate of complications with SPP than with ES, but this did not reach statistical significance [21]. The authors also report that SPP is slightly more expensive than ES, but that this cost may be overcome by a reduction in post-procedural complications [21].

Endoscopic Papillary Balloon Dilation (EPBD)

Endoscopic papillary balloon dilation (EPBD) has been advocated in place of endoscopic sphincterotomy (ES) secondary to its ability to preserve the sphincter of Oddi function and to reduce complications including hemorrhage and pancreatitis (Fig. 16.3) [13, 16].

Park et al. compared a group of cirrhotic patients with coagulopathy undergoing EPBD (21 patients) to a historic control group (20 patients) that had undergone ES in order to explore the relationships between these procedures and the rates of post-procedural hemorrhage and procedure-related pancreatitis. They concluded that there was a significantly lower risk of hemorrhage in the group undergoing EPBD (30 % vs. 0 %, $p < 0.009$). They concluded that there was no difference in procedure related pancreatitis between the two groups (10 % vs. 4.7 %, $p > 0.05$). They concluded that in patients with coagulopathy and cirrhosis EPBD should be the procedure of choice for the treatment of choledocholithiasis [16].

Park et al. specifically report results for patients with CTP class C cirrhosis. Five of fourteen patients in the ES group developed hemorrhage (35.7 %). Hemorrhage did not occur in any of the patients in the EPBD group (0/16, 0 %, $p = 0.014$). There was no significant difference for patients with CTP class B cirrhosis [16]. There was no significant difference in post-procedure pancreatitis or cholangitis between the two groups [16]. Deaths secondary to hemorrhage occurred exclusively in the ES group in patients with Child–Pugh C cirrhosis [16]. EPBD is more commonly performed in Japan and less commonly in the USA, likely secondary to concern for post-procedure pancreatitis. Park et al. demonstrated no significant difference in post-procedure pancreatitis between the ES and EPBD groups [16]. Kawabe et al. demonstrate that EPBD is a safe and effective technique for the removal of common bile duct stones with liver cirrhosis [25].

Comparing Endoscopic Sphincterotomy and Endoscopic Balloon Dilation in the General Population

Baron et al. performed a meta-analysis of randomized controlled trials reported that there were eight prospective, randomized trials published in English involving 1106 patients (552 EPBD, 554 ES) which were referenced for their study. These studies did not specifically involve patients with

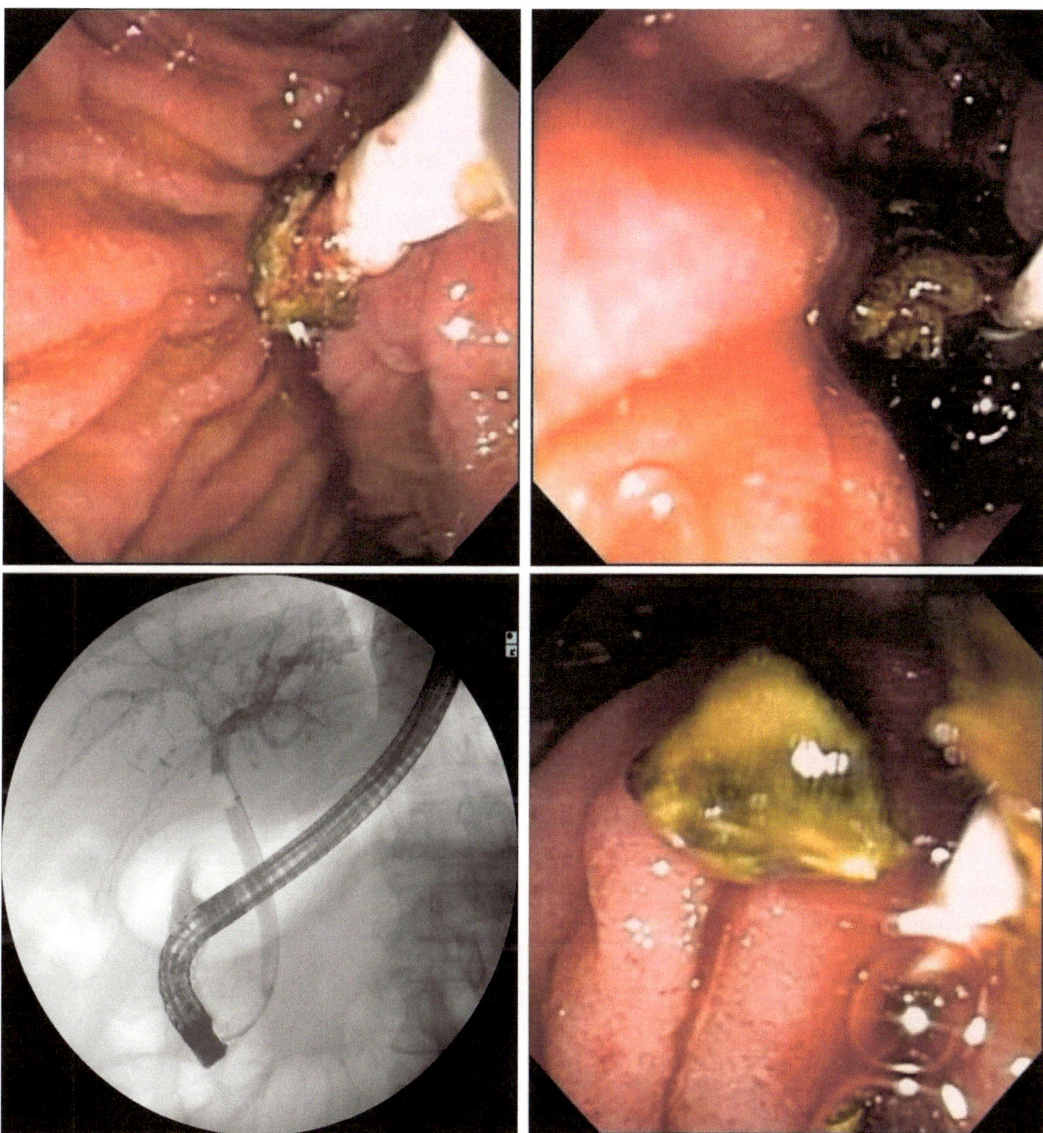

Fig. 16.3 Endoscopic papillary balloon dilation (EPBD) with cannulation of the bile duct, balloon dilation of the sphincter, and stone extraction

cirrhosis or coagulopathy. They reported similar success in removal of CBD stones (94.3 % vs. 96.5 %) and similar rates of complications overall (10.5 % vs. 10.3 %). Bleeding was less commonly a complication of endoscopic balloon dilation (EPBD) (0 % vs. 2 %, $p=0.001$). Post-ERCP pancreatitis was more common in the EPBD group (7.4 % vs. 4.3 %, $p=0.05$). There was no significant difference in the rates of perforation or infection.

Patients undergoing EPBD were more likely to undergo mechanical lithotripsy for stone extraction (20.9 % vs. 14.8 %, $p=0.014$). The authors of this study recommended that secondary to reduced bleeding EPBD should be the procedure of choice for patients with coagulopathy for removal of common bile duct stones, but that in general EPBD cannot be recommended secondary to increased rates of post-ERCP pancreatitis [15].

Although these authors note that the studies included in their meta-analysis excluded patients with preexisting coagulopathy EPBD is the appropriate technique to use in coagulopathic patients or those patients who require full anticoagulation within 72 h of stone removal. The authors do suggest that EPBD may prevent the long-term consequences of permanent loss of the biliary sphincter [15].

Park et al. reports reduced risk of bleeding and no difference in post-procedure pancreatitis between ES and balloon dilation [16]. Baron et al. report two times higher risk of pancreatitis after endoscopic large-diameter balloon dilation [15].

Other Endoscopic Options

The use of expandable stents has also been advocated, especially in patients with obvious stricture or when patients could not tolerate stone removal [1, 26]. Mechanical lithotripsy can be used for large stones which could not be removed with maximum sphincterotomy or when the stone is greater than 1 cm in diameter [26]. Methods for lithotripsy include mechanical, electrohydraulic, laser and extracorporeal shock-wave lithotripsy [26]. PTC is also a treatment option, but may have higher complication and lower success rates in patients with cirrhosis [14].

Surgery Versus Endoscopy

In a study of 16 patients with cirrhosis and choledocholithiasis Suigyiama et al. compared surgical intervention and endoscopic sphincterotomy. They noted that there was excessive intraoperative hemorrhage (mean 1576 ml) in the surgical group, an overall mortality rate of 44.4 % and a morbidity rate of 66.7 %. Causes of early postoperative death included hemorrhage, liver failure and sepsis. The authors noted that the mortality rate in patients with CTP class A and B cirrhosis was 0 % and that it was 80 % in patients with CTP class C cirrhosis [9].

Sugiyama et al. also compared ES in cirrhotic patients to ES in patients without cirrhosis and noted that there was a significant difference in mortality (14.3 % versus 6.5 %, no *p*-value given).

There was no significant difference in morbidity (14.3 % versus 6.5 %). Complications that they reported associated with ES included hepatic dysfunction, coagulopathy, cholangitis and that these were predictive of an increased mortality rate [9].

Summary

Endoscopic Retrograde Cholangiopancreatography (ERCP) with Endoscopic Sphincterotomy (ES) or Endoscopic Papillary Balloon Dilation (EPBD) is the most commonly used approaches for choledocholithiasis in cirrhotic patients. When these procedures fail or patients have altered anatomy other options include transgastric ERCP with ES or EPBD, expandable stents and/or lithotripsy. Although cirrhotic patients have some increased risk of bleeding, there does not appear to be an increased risk of post-ERCP pancreatitis and patients generally do well with ERCP with ES or EPBD. There is some risk associated with these procedures and it is important to confirm the presence of choledocholithiasis if suspicion is not high, with imaging studies including magnetic resonance cholangiography (MRCP). Surgery is an option in the case of failed endoscopic management. Surgical options include laparoscopic cholecystectomy with choledochotomy, laparoscopic common bile duct exploration and T-tube placement. CTP class A and B patients tolerate these procedures with moderate mortality risk, while CTP class C patients have high associated mortality.

References

1. Buxbaum J. Modern management of common bile duct stones. Gastrointest Endosc Clin N Am. 2013;23(2):251–75. doi:10.1016/j.giec.2012.12.003.
2. Del Olmo JA, García F, Serra MA, Maldonado L, Rodrigo JM. Prevalence and incidence of gallstones in liver cirrhosis. Scand J Gastroenterol. 1997;32(10): 1061–5.
3. Maggi A, Solenghi D, Panzeri A, Borroni G, Cazzaniga M, Sangiovanni A, De Fazio C, Salerno F. Prevalence and incidence of cholelithiasis in patients with liver cirrhosis. Ital J Gastroenterol Hepatol. 1997;29(4):330–5.

4. Scaglione S, Kliethermes S, Cao G, Shoham D, Durazo R, Luke A, Volk ML. The epidemiology of cirrhosis in the United States: a population-based study. J Clin Gastroenterol 2015 Sep;49(8):690–6.

5. Ziser A, Plevak DJ, Wiesner RH, Rakela J, Offord KP, Brown DL. Morbidity and mortality in cirrhotic patients undergoing anesthesia and surgery. Anesthesiology. 1999;90(1):42–53.

6. Pugh RN, Murray-Lyon IM, Dawson JL, Pietroni MC, Williams R. Transection of the oesophagus for bleeding oesophageal varices. Br J Surg. 1973;60(8):646–9. doi:10.1002/bjs.1800600817.

7. Garrison RN, Cryer HM, Howard DA, et al. Clarification of risk factors for abdominal operations in patients with hepatic cirrhosis. Ann Surg. 1984;199:648–55.

8. Mansour A, Watson W, Shayani V, et al. Abdominal operations in patients with cirrhosis: still a major surgical challenge. Surgery. 1997;122:730–5.

9. Sugiyama M, Atomi Y, Kuroda A, Muto T. Treatment of choledocholithiasis in patients with liver cirrhosis. Surgical treatment or endoscopic sphincterotomy? Ann Surg. 1993;218(1):68–73.

10. Millwala F, Nguyen GC, Thuluvath PJ. Outcomes of patients with cirrhosis undergoing non-hepatic surgery: risk assessment and management. World J Gastroenterol. 2007;13(30):4056–63.

11. Freeman ML. Complications of endoscopic retrograde cholangiopancreatography: avoidance and management. Gastrointest Endosc Clin N Am. 2012;22(3):567–86. doi:10.1016/j.giec.2012.05.001.

12. Prat F, Amouyal G, Amouyal P, Pelletier G, Fritsch J, Choury AD, Buffet C, Etienne JP. Prospective controlled study of endoscopic ultrasonography and endoscopic retrograde cholangiography in patients with suspected common-bile duct lithiasis. Lancet. 1996;347(8994):75–9.

13. Laokpessi A, Bouillet P, Sautereau D, Cessot F, Desport JC, Le Sidaner A, Pillegand B. Value of magnetic resonance cholangiography in the preoperative diagnosis of common bile duct stones. Am J Gastroenterol. 2001;96(8):2354–9.

14. Parlak E, Köksal AŞ, Öztaş E, Dişibeyaz S, Ödemiş B, Yüksel M, Yıldız H, Şaşmaz N, Şahin B. Is there a safer electrosurgical current for endoscopic sphincterotomy in patients with liver cirrhosis? Wien Klin Wochenschr 2015 Jan 10.

15. Baron TH, Harewood GC. Endoscopic balloon dilation of the biliary sphincter compared to endoscopic biliary sphincterotomy for removal of common bile duct stones during ERCP: a metaanalysis of randomized, controlled trials. Am J Gastroenterol. 2004; 99(8):1455–60.

16. Park DH, Kim MH, Lee SK, Lee SS, Choi JS, Song MH, Seo DW, Min Y. Endoscopic sphincterotomy vs. endoscopic papillary balloon dilation for choledocholithiasis in patients with liver cirrhosis and coagulopathy. Gastrointest Endosc. 2004;60(2):180–5.

17. Qiu J, Yuan H, Chen S, Wu H. Laparoscopic common bile duct exploration in cirrhotic patients with choledocholithiasis. J Clin Gastroenterol. 2015;49(2):132–6. doi:10.1097/MCG.0000000000000068.

18. Li DM, Zhao J, Zhao Q, Qin H, Wang B, Li RX, Zhang M, Hu JF, Yang M. Safety and efficacy of endoscopic retrograde cholangiopancreatography for common bile duct stones in liver cirrhotic patients. J Huazhong Univ Sci Technolog Med Sci. 2014;34(4):612–5. doi:10.1007/s11596-014-1325-x.

19. Prat F, Tennenbaum R, Ponsot P, Altman C, Pelletier G, Fritsch J, Choury AD, Bernades P, Etienne JP. Endoscopic sphincterotomy in patients with liver cirrhosis. Gastrointest Endosc. 1996;43(2 Pt 1):127–31.

20. Chijiiwa K, Kozaki N, Naito T, Kameoka N, Tanaka M. Treatment of choice for choledocholithiasis in patients with acute obstructive suppurative cholangitis and liver cirrhosis. Am J Surg. 1995;170(4):356–60.

21. Artifon EL, da Silveira EB, Aparicio D, Takada J, Baracat R, Sakai CM, Garcia RT, Teich V, Couto DS. Management of common bile duct stones in cirrhotic patients with coagulopathy: a comparison of supra-papillary puncture and standard cannulation technique. Dig Dis Sci. 2011;56(6):1904–11. doi:10.1007/s10620-011-1593-2.

22. Artifon EL, Kumar A, Eloubeidi MA, Chu A, Halwan B, Sakai P, Bhutani MS. Prospective randomized trial of EUS versus ERCP-guided common bile duct stone removal: an interim report (with video). Gastrointest Endosc. 2009;69(2):238–43. doi:10.1016/j.gie.2008.05.020.

23. Artifon EL, Paulo S, Cardillo GZ, Ishioka S. Suprapapillary needle puncture for common bile duct access: laboratory profile. Arq Gastroenterol. 2006;43(4):299–304.

24. Artifon EL, Hondo FY, Sakai P, Ishioka S. A new approach to the bile duct via needle puncture of the papillary roof. Endoscopy. 2005;37(11):1158.

25. Kawabe T, Komatsu Y, Tada M, Toda N, Ohashi M, Shiratori Y, Omata M. Endoscopic papillary balloon dilation in cirrhotic patients: removal of common bile duct stones without sphincterotomy. Endoscopy. 1996;28(8):694–8.

26. Garg PK, Tandon RK, Ahuja V, Makharia GK, Batra Y. Predictors of unsuccessful mechanical lithotripsy and endoscopic clearance of large bile duct stones. Gastrointest Endosc. 2004;59(6):601–5.

Reshi C. Kanuru and Edward Levine

Introduction

Common bile duct stones are currently managed via endoscopic retrograde cholangiopancreatography (ERCP) or surgery. Despite the relatively recent trend for endoscopic management, efforts into pharmacological management of gallstones have been in development for the past century. The advantage of medical management of common bile duct stones is highlighted in patients with multiple comorbidities who are high risk for procedural complications. Though nonprocedural management is possible it is not the standard of care and further investigation is needed to examine the efficacy of non-procedural management of biliary stones. To understand the mechanism of non-procedural management of stones it is important to understand bile salt physiology and the formation of biliary stones.

R.C. Kanuru, M.D.
Division of Gastroenterology, Hepatology, and Nutrition, Department of Internal Medicine,
The Ohio State University Wexner Medical Center,
Columbus, OH, USA
e-mail: Reshi.Kanuru@osumc.edu

E. Levine, M.D. (✉)
Department of Internal Medicine, The Ohio State University Wexner Medical Center,
395 W. 12th Avenue, Columbus,
OH 43210-1228, USA
e-mail: Edward.Levine@osumc.edu

Pathophysiology

Bile salts are produced by hepatocytes through the metabolism of cholesterol. The bile salt pool consists of primary and secondary bile salts. Primary bile salts are directly synthesized from cholesterol within the liver. Primary bile salts consist of chenodeoxycholic acid and cholic acid. Secondary bile salts are created by bacteria that conjugate primary bile salts, within the small bowel and colon, into secondary bile salts. These secondary bile salts are reabsorbed to enter the bile salt pool. Secondary bile salts include lithocholic acid, ursodeoxycholic acid, and deoxycholic acid [1]. Both primary and secondary bile acids need to undergo conjugation with taurine or glycine to be water soluble and assist in cholesterol absorption [2]. Once bile salts are conjugated they are released into the small bowel to assist in gastrointestinal absorption of cholesterol.

Bile salts are able to assist in cholesterol absorption as they contain hydrophobic and hydrophilic components. The bile salt polarity allows them to form micelles, which are spherical structures with a hydrophilic outer layer and a hydrophobic inner component [3]. Micelles allow absorption of cholesterols and fat soluble vitamins within the enterocytes of the gastrointestinal system. Cholesterol absorption is feasible if the balance between the concentration of bile salts and

© Springer International Publishing Switzerland 2016
J.W. Hazey et al. (eds.), *Multidisciplinary Management of Common Bile Duct Stones*,
DOI 10.1007/978-3-319-22765-8_17

the concentration of cholesterol is maintained. Without bile salts, the absorption of cholesterol and fat soluble vitamins is significantly impaired. Biliary stones form when the concentration of excreted cholesterol exceeds that of bile salts leading to cholesterol precipitation [4].

Cholesterol gallstones compose a majority of all stones with the minority being pigmented stones [5]. Cholesterol stones form due to a higher cholesterol concentration in excreted bile as compared to bile salt concentration [6]. If bile cholesterol levels are high, cholesterol can become supersaturated and crystallize into cholesterol stones. Cholesterol excretion can be increased in comparison to bile salts as a result of a high cholesterol diet, familial hypercholesterolemia syndromes, or loss of bile salts through inadequate reabsorption. An imbalance between cholesterol and bile salts explains why obese patients with rapid weight loss have a higher risk of developing cholesterol gallstones. As more cholesterol is mobilized from the adipose tissue through diet and exercise, more cholesterol is excreted in bile. With a higher concentration of cholesterol in bile in relation to bile salts, cholesterol becomes supersaturated and forms cholesterol gallstones. Biliary stones are generally managed endoscopically but in patients with a high risk of peri-procedural complications medical management can be considered.

Chenodeoxycholic Acid

Since bile cholesterol concentrations plays such a significant role in cholesterol stone formation, bile cholesterol concentration acts as a natural target for stone dissolution therapy. One of the first attempts at biliary stone dissolution therapy was the use of chenodeoxycholic acid (CDCA). Chenodeoxycholic acid is part of the natural composition of bile salts and composes up to one third of the normal bile salt pool [6]. CDCA has been extensively studied to determine the effect of CDCA on cholesterol secretion by the liver. It is believed that CDCA suppresses the hepatic synthesis of cholesterol and cholic acid [1]. With decreased hepatic cholesterol secretion there is a

decrease in biliary cholesterol. As a result of its effects on bile acid composition, cholesterol saturation is kept low in comparison to bile salts leading to a lower likelihood of forming and dissolution of cholesterol stones [7].

The hallmark paper evaluating CDCA for gallstone dissolution therapy was Danzinger et al. [8]. Previous studies have shown that CDCA decreased the saturation of cholesterol in bile but few prior studies had examined CDCA's role in the dissolution of gallstones [8]. In this case-series by Danzinger et al., seven female patients with asymptomatic radiolucent calculi underwent cholecystograms to evaluate the presence and size of gallstones. Each patient in the case series was given CDCA with a range in dosages from 0.75 to 4.5 g per day. In addition, each patient underwent cholecystokinin stimulated bile collection both prior to CDCA exposure and after administration of CDCA to evaluate any changes in bile acid composition.

Four of the seven subjects within the case-series had a decrease in the size of their gallstones. Through analysis of bile acid composition there was a notable increase in the bile salt concentration compared to cholesterol in the excreted bile salt pool. The change in composition was believed to account for the dissolution and prevention of gallstones in four of the subjects studied [8].

Ursodeoxycholic Acid

Despite the decrease in gallstone size in a majority of patients, CDCA even on initial evaluation was shown to cause significant diarrhea at therapeutic levels and can lead to a notable transaminitis. The adverse effects of CDCA are associated with the large increase in lithocholic acid levels within the bile salt pool that results from CDCA therapy [9].

Despite the effects of gallstone dissolution, CDCA therapy led to significant diarrhea and transaminitis prohibiting the use of CDCA. Alternative bile salts were examined to identify those that could promote gallstone dissolution without the side effects seen with CDCA. One agent that was identified was ursodeoxycholic acid (UDCA). Unlike CDCA, UDCA does not increase the levels of lithocholic acid and therefore does not cause similar side effects as CDCA [9]. UDCA is a naturally occurring secondary bile acid that normally composes about 5 % of the circulating bile salt pool. UDCA administration alters the chemical composition of the bile salt pool to where UDCA composes 30–50 % of the entire pool, as opposed to only 5 % [9].

One of the preliminary studies that evaluated UDCA as a dissolution agent was Tint et al. [9]. In this study 53 patients with cholesterol gallstones less than 30 mm in diameter, identified on cholecystography, were placed on UDCA with varying dosages. All subjects completed therapy for at least 6 months with the maximum extent being 38 months. Subjects were randomly assigned to one of three treatment arms. The arms included low dose UDCA of 250–300 mg per day, medium dose 500–600 mg per day, and high dose 900–1000 mg per day in divided doses. There was no placebo group used. Of the 53 subjects, 42 of them had at least partial dissolution of their stones with 27 patients having complete dissolution [9]. In four patients calcium rims developed during treatment (three patients in the low dose arm and one in the medium dose arm). Several factors were highlighted as possible contributors to gallstone dissolution. Gallstone size was noted to play a role as the mean gallstone size in those who had complete dissolution was 8.9 mm while those without dissolution had a mean of 13.6 mm [9]. In addition the number of stones seemed to be a contributing factor. Those subjects with five or fewer gallstones had significantly higher dissolution rates than those with greater than five gallstones. Lastly the dosage of UDCA influenced the gallstone dissolution rate. Patients with gallstones less than 10 mm who were in the high dosage group had completed dissolution on average in 5 months while those with stones less than 10 mm in the medium dosage arm had a dissolution time of 10.3 months [9]. A complicating factor was rim calcification that occurred in the low dose and high dose arms. Rim calcification has been associated with poor response to dissolution therapy [9]. From this study it is unclear if rim calcification is a product of the lower UDCA dosages of if calcification

provided increased resistance to dissolution in low and medium dose arms. No subjects developed diarrhea during the study and liver enzymes did not significantly vary from normal.

This study highlights several key points. First there are several factors that influence the dissolution of gallstones with size and number of stones being significant factors to achieving successful dissolution. Second, UDCA has clearly been identified as an effective method for gallstone dissolution with greater response with a higher dosage. Lastly, UDCA is not associated with the significant side effects that CDCA has been associated with making UDCA a safe effective alternative.

Pro-motility Agents

The formation of gallstones is affected by multiple processes. Cholesterol saturation appears to play a large role in stone formation but also gallbladder function is believed to be a contributing factor. Stasis of bile within the gallbladder has been suggested to influence the formation of gallstones [10]. Given these influences on gallstone formation, studies have examined optimizing dissolution therapy by evaluating pro-motility agents in conjunction with UDCA in gallstone dissolution. One study compared combination therapy of UDCA and domperidone against UDCA alone in the dissolution of gallbladder stones [10]. Seventy five patients were randomized to two separate test groups with one group receiving monotherapy with UDCA and the other group receiving UDCA, as well as, domperidone. There was no statistical significance between the two groups in terms of gallstone formation or dissolution. This study highlights that pro-motility agents do not seem to play a significant role in gallstone dissolution therapy.

Combination Therapy: CDCA and UDCA

Another method in optimizing dissolution therapy includes dual therapy with CDCA and UDCA. A meta-analysis was performed that compared

CDCA to UDCA to combination therapy with CDCA and UDCA [11]. The meta-analysis only utilized randomized controlled trials and noted that UDCA was superior to CDCA therapy as mono-therapies. In addition combination therapy with CDCA and UDCA was superior to UDCA therapy alone; however, the effectiveness of combination therapy was based on only two randomized trials possibly skewing the true effectiveness of combination therapy [11]. The true effectiveness of UDCA over CDCA is not clear but tolerability remains the main advantage of UDCA. Compliance can be an issue with long term therapy with CDCA since significant side effects like diarrhea are more prevalent in patients who use CDCA than those that are treated with UDCA.

UDCA has shown some promise in gallstone dissolution, but keep in mind that several studies have demonstrated the recurrence rate to be as high as 61 % within 11 years [12]. UDCA is not definitive therapy but may be considered a tool to use in a select group of patients with cholesterol stones where there risk of procedural intervention outweighs the potential benefit of more definitive therapy. Unfortunately there are no significant studies that help characterize in which populations dissolution therapy should be used.

Statins

UDCA and CDCA are not the only definitive therapies available for gallstone dissolution. Statins have become a popular and effective tool in the management of dyslipidemia. Statins work by inhibiting HMG-CoA reductase, the rate limiting enzyme in cholesterol synthesis. As a result, statins lead to a decrease in LDL, triglycerides, and VLDL within the body. Given the effect of statins on regulating cholesterol synthesis, a natural application was to see how this class of medications affected biliary tract stones.

The cholesterol content in bile, otherwise known as the cholesterol saturation index (CSI), has shown to play a role in the formation of cholesterol gallstones [13]. In fact statins have been shown to decrease the CSI in non-insulin dependent diabetics who were treated with statins for

12 weeks [14]. Given statins decrease the CSI the next step was to evaluate whether statins could truly affect biliary stone dissolution. Chapman et al. explored this question evaluating 27 patients who had gallstones and who were placed on simvastatin therapy [13]. Twenty-seven subjects were given simvastatin 20 mg once a day for 12 months. They underwent a cholecystogram, cholecystokinin stimulated bile collection via a polyvinyl tube, and evaluation of serum lipids. With simvastatin therapy there was a significant drop in CSI in 11 subjects but there was no decrease in the size of the gallstones. Even five subjects with non-calcified gallstones and a well-functioning gallbladder showed no significant improvement in gallstone diameter at 12 months. Of these 27 subjects only six had a significant decrease in gallstone diameter. When these six responders were continued on therapy for another 12 months there was no further decrease in gallstone size. Chapman et al. raised two concerns. The first concern is that statin therapy for the treatment of gallstones may not be an effective therapy as some studies have led us to believe and secondly there may be an alternative mechanism that is playing a role besides just decreasing the cholesterol saturation index.

Combination Therapy: UDCA and Statins

As we previously discussed UDCA has been shown to have some effect in a select group of patients in dissolving cholesterol biliary stones. With investigation of statins and their role in stone dissolution, the question that arises is whether combination therapy with UDCA and statins provides a more profound effect on stone dissolution. A randomized controlled trial conducted by Tazuma et al. identified 50 patients with radiolucent gallbladder stones [15]. These patients were split into two separate groups. One group received simvastatin 10 mg per day with 600 mg per day of UDCA, while the other received UDCA 600 g per day only. Cholecystography and RUQ US, along with LFTs, were drawn every 3 months for the span of 12 months. Partial dissolution was defined as a 50 % reduction in stone volume, stone number, or both. The study demonstrated dissolution in 58 % of patients on combination therapy with 4 of 26 patients having complete dissolution. The dissolution rates were significantly higher in the combination therapy group than the monotherapy group. On the other hand 33 % of patients with monotherapy with UDCA achieved dissolution. Interestingly the rates of dissolution in patients with monotherapy and combination therapy were not different for those with solitary gallstones. Surprisingly the cholesterol saturation index of bile was decreased in both groups but they were not statistically different [15]. This study was the first trial comparing the combination therapy of statins with UDCA versus UDCA alone. The comparison highlighted some interesting results including that despite combination therapy and greater dissolution rates in the combination group, as compared to monotherapy, the cholesterol saturation index was not statistically significant. This observation begs the question whether statins have an alternate pathway that leads to cholesterol dissolution.

Besides utilizing statins for dissolution therapy, statins have also been investigated for the role in decreasing symptomatic cholelithiasis and complications rates with gallbladder disease. Pulkkinen et al. investigated 1140 patients who presented with symptomatic gallstones [16]. These patients were placed into two cohorts. One cohort consisted of those on statin therapy and the second cohort were those who were not on statin therapy. The hypothesis was that with the use of stain therapy there should be less gallbladder inflammation, fewer stones in the common bile duct, and fewer overall complications. There were no notable differences in CRP and LDL between the two cohorts. There was also no difference in need for laparoscopic versus open cholecystectomy, complications such as CBD stones, and mortality between the statin and statin free group. Statins seem to not play a role as a preventive measure for symptomatic cholelithiasis or the prevention of CBD stones.

Ezetimibe

An evolving tool in the medical management of cholelithiasis and choledocholithiasis is ezetimibe. Ezetimibe is commonly used as an adjunct therapy in cholesterol management. Ezetimibe decreases the jejunal absorption of cholesterol by inhibiting the Niemann–Pick C1-Like 1 protein (NPCIL1) [17]. NPCIL1 is a cholesterol transport protein that assists in the movement of cholesterol across jejunal enterocytes. Ezetimibe undergoes glucuronidation by enterocytes and is recirculated through the liver. It is excreted in the bile in a conjugated form eventually entering the small bowel allowing repetitive inhibition of NPCIL1.

Bile cholesterol concentration plays a significant role in the creation of cholesterol biliary stones. The concept behind the use of ezetimibe is similar to that of statins, to decrease the cholesterol content of bile. One of the first studies looking at ezetimibe as an agent for gallstone dissolution therapy was Wang et al. where C57L mice on a lipogenic diet were given ezetimibe to assess its role in cholesterol stone dissolution [18]. C57L mice are a strain of mice that are prone to gallstone formation when on a high fat content diet. Four groups of 20 mice were formed with each being exposed to a different dosage of ezetimibe. The dosages used include 0, 0.8, 4, and 8 mg/kg/day. These mice were then transitioned to a normal chow diet to see if this change led to dissolution but the size of the gallstones was not significantly smaller [18]. The mice were then fed a normal chow diet with their respective doses of ezetimibe. After completion of 8 weeks of therapy the 0.8 mg/kg/day group had stones with a mean size of 0.27 mm in 5 % of the mice while no stones were noted in the 4 and 8 mg/kg/day groups [18]. Though only demonstrated in mice, Wang et al. demonstrate a potentially new therapeutic tool in gallstone dissolution therapy. Human efficacy trials still need to be completed to see if ezetimibe can truly be used as dissolution therapy.

Summary

Cholesterol stone dissolution therapy has been shown to be effective in certain situations, but dissolution can take years and recurrence is fairly common. As a result there are many factors to consider when choosing medical dissolution therapy over procedural therapies. UDCA appears to be the most effective and tolerable therapy currently available. Statins and Ezetimibe are currently being evaluated to assess their efficacy but are not considered definitive therapy. In the end, endoscopic or surgical removal of stones is the standard of care with medical dissolution being a last resort for patients who may be too high risk for procedural intervention.

References

1. Barrett KE. Chapter 11: Bile formation and secretion. In: Gastrointestinal physiology. New York, NY: Lange Medical/McGraw-Hill, Medical Pub. Division; 2006.
2. Reshetnyak VI. Physiological and molecular biochemical mechanisms of bile formation. World J Gastroenterol. 2013;19(42):7341–60.
3. Barrett KE. Chapter 16: Lipid assimilation. In: Gastrointestinal physiology. New York, NY: Lange Medical/McGraw-Hill, Medical Pub. Division; 2006.
4. Wang DQH, Cohen DE, Carey MC. Biliary lipids and cholesterol gallstone disease. J Lipid Res. 2009; 50(Suppl):S406–11.
5. Trotman BW, Soloway RD. Pigment vs cholesterol cholelithiasis: clinical and epidemiological aspects. Am J Dig Dis. 1975;20(8):735–40.
6. Carey MC, Small DM. The physical chemistry of cholesterol solubility in bile. Relationship to gallstone formation and dissolution in man. J Clin Invest. 1978;61(4):998–1026.
7. Einarsson C, Hillebrant CG, Axelson M. Effects of treatment with deoxycholic acid and chenodeoxycholic acid on the hepatic synthesis of cholesterol and bile acids in healthy subjects. Hepatology. 2001;33(5): 1189–93.
8. Danzinger RG, Hofmann AF, Schoenfield LJ, Thistle JL. Dissolution of cholesterol gallstones by chenodeoxycholic acid. N Engl J Med. 1972;286:1–8.
9. Tint GS, Salen G, Colalillo A, et al. Ursodeoxycholic acid: a safe and effective agent for dissolving cholesterol gallstones. Ann Intern Med. 1982;97(3):351–6.
10. Tuncer I, Harman M, Colak Y, Arslan I, Turkdogan MK. Effect of ursodeoxycholic acid alone and ursodeoxycholic acid plus domperidone on radiolucent gallstones and gallbladder contractility in humans. Gastroenterol Res Pract. 2012;2012:1–6.
11. Petroni ML, Jazrawi RP, Pazzi P, et al. Ursodeoxycholic acid alone or with chenodeoxycholic acid for dissolution of cholesterol gallstones: a randomized multicentre trial. The British-Italian Gallstone Study group. Aliment Pharmacol Ther. 2001;15(1):123–8.
12. Villanova N, Bazzoli F, Taroni F, et al. Gallstone recurrence after successful oral bile acid treatment. A 12-year follow-up study and evaluation of long-term postdissolution treatment. Gastroenterology. 1989;97(3):726–31.
13. Chapman BA, Burt MJ, Chisholm RJ, Allan RB, Yeo KH, Ross AG. Dissolution of gallstones with simvastatin, an HMG CoA reductase inhibitor. Dig Dis Sci. 1998;43(2):349–53.
14. Wilson IR, Hurrell MA, Pattinson NR, Chapman BA. The effect of simvastatin and bezafibrate on bile composition and gall-bladder emptying in female non-insulin-dependent diabetics. J Gastroenterol Hepatol. 1994;9(5):447–51.
15. Tazuma S, Kajiyama G, Mizuno T, et al. A combination therapy with simvastatin and ursodeoxycholic acid is more effective for cholesterol gallstone dissolution than is ursodeoxycholic acid monotherapy. J Clin Gastroenterol. 1998;26(4):287–91.
16. Pulkkinen J, Eskelinen M, Kiviniemi V, et al. Effect of statin use on outcome of symptomatic cholelithiasis: a case-control study. BMC Gastroenterol. 2014;14:119.
17. Ahmed MH. Ezetimbe as potential treatment for cholesterol gallstones: the need for clinical trials. World J Gastroenterol. 2010;16(13):1555–7.
18. Wang HH, Portincasa P, Mendez-sanchez N, Uribe M, Wang DQ. Effect of ezetimibe on the prevention and dissolution of cholesterol gallstones. Gastroenterology. 2008;134(7):2101–10.

Index

© Springer International Publishing Switzerland 2016
J.W. Hazey et al. (eds.), *Multidisciplinary Management of Common Bile Duct Stones*,
DOI 10.1007/978-3-319-22765-8